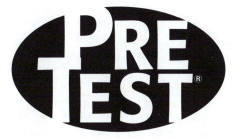

Biochemistry and Genetics

PreTest® Self-Assessment and Review

Notice

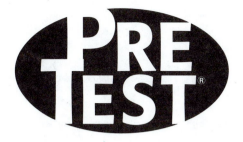

Biochemistry and Genetics
PreTest® Self-Assessment and Review

Golder N. Wilson, M.D., Ph.D.
Mary McDermott Cook Distinguished Professor of Pediatric Genetics
University of Texas Southwestern Medical School
Dallas, Texas

Student Reviewers
Rakhi Chaudhuri
Ohio State University College of Medicine
Columbus, Ohio
Class of 2002

Brian T. Schroeder
University of Iowa College of Medicine
Iowa City, Iowa
Class of 2002

Junda C. Woo
State University of New York at Buffalo
School of Medicine
Class of 2002

McGraw-Hill
Medical Publishing Division
New York   Chicago   San Francisco   Lisbon   London   Madrid   Mexico City
Milan   New Delhi   San Juan   Seoul   Singapore   Sydney   Toronto

McGraw-Hill

A Division of The **McGraw·Hill** Companies

Biochemistry and Genetics: PreTest® Self-Assessment and Review

2 3 4 5 6 7 8 9 0   DOC/DOC   0 9 8 7 6 5 4 3 2

ISBN 0-07-137578-3

This book was set in Berkeley by North Market Street Graphics.
The editor was Catherine A. Johnson.
The production supervisor was Phil Galea.
Project management was provided by North Market Street Graphics.
The cover designer was Li Chen Chang / Pinpoint.
R.R. Donnelley & Sons was printer and binder.

This book is printed on acid-free paper.

Library of Congress Cataloging-in-Publication Data

PreTest biochemistry and genetics: PreTest self-assessment and review / edited by Golder N. Wilson.—1st ed.
    p.; cm.
   New edition partially based on titles formerly issued separately.
   Includes bibliographical references and index.
   ISBN 0-07-137578-3 (alk. paper)
    1. Biochemistry—Examinations, questions, etc. 2. Genetics—Examinations, questions, etc. I. Title: Biochemistry and genetics. II. Wilson, Golder. III. Biochemistry. IV. Genetics.
    [DNLM: 1. Biochemistry—Examination Questions. 2. Genetics, Medical—Examination Questions. QU 18.2 T942 2001]
   QP518.5 .P74 2001
   572'.076—dc21   2001034274

Contents

INTERMEDIARY METABOLISM
Carbohydrate Metabolism

Bioenergetics and Energy Metabolism

Amino Acid, Lipid, and Nucleotide Metabolism

NUTRITION
Vitamins and Minerals

Hormones and Integrated Metabolism

INHERITANCE MECHANISMS
AND BIOCHEMICAL GENETICS
Inheritance Mechanisms/Risk Calculations

Genetic and Biochemical Diagnosis

Preface

This new edition of *Biochemistry and Genetics PreTest®: Self-Assessment and Review* is based in part on the earlier biochemistry editions prepared by Francis J. Chlapowski, Ph.D., Department of Biochemistry and Molecular Biology, University of Massachusetts Medical School. All questions are now in single-best-answer format and a large number are analogous to those of the United States Medical Licensing Examination (USMLE), Part I. Questions are updated to the most current editions of leading textbooks in medical biochemistry and medical genetics.

Introduction

Each *PreTest® Self-Assessment and Review* allows medical students to comprehensively and conveniently assess and review their knowledge of a particular basic science, in this instance biochemistry. The 500 questions parallel the format and degree of difficulty of the questions found in the United States Medical Licensing Examination (USMLE), Step 1. Appendix 1 lists the major subject areas of the biochemistry, genetics, and nutrition portions of the USMLE Step 1 content outline together with questions in this book that cover those areas. Practicing physicians who want to hone their skills before USMLE Step 3 or recertification may find this to be a good beginning in their review process.

Each question is accompanied by an answer, a paragraph explanation, and a specific page reference to an appropriate textbook. Over 20 reference figures have been added to help with review, and there are an additional 40 figures geared to specific questions. A bibliography listing sources can be found following the second appendix of this text, and a list of abbreviations used in the text follows this introduction. As listed in Appendix 2, over 100 clinical disorders or processes are discussed and related to biochemical and/or genetic mechanisms. For genetic disorders, a McKusick number is included that allows the reader to immediately access information about the disorder using the Online Mendelian Inheritance in Man Internet site (see the bibliography).

An effective way to use this PreTest® is to allow yourself one minute to answer each question in a given chapter. As you proceed, indicate your answer beside each question. By following this suggestion, you approximate the time limits imposed by the USMLE Step 1 examination. After you finish going through the questions in the section, spend as much time as you need verifying your answers and carefully reading the explanations provided. Pay special attention to the explanations for the questions you answered incorrectly—but read every explanation. The authors of this material have designed the explanations to reinforce and supplement the information tested by the questions. If you feel you need further information about the material covered, consult and study the text or online references indicated.

The High-Yield Facts in this book are provided to facilitate rapid review of biochemistry and genetics. It is anticipated that the reader will use the High-Yield Facts as a "memory jog" before proceeding through the questions.

Abbreviations

ACAT	acyl CoA–cholesterol acyl transferase
ACTH	adrenocorticotropic hormone
ADP	adenosine diphosphate
AMP	adenosine monophosphate
ATP	adenosine triphosphate
ATPase	adenosine triphosphatase
CAP	catabolite activator protein
CDP	cytidine diphosphate
CMP	cytidine monophosphate (cytidylic acid)
CoA	coenzyme A
cyclic AMP	adenosine 3',5'-cyclic monophosphate (3',5'-cyclic adenylic acid)
DHAP	dihydroxyacetone phosphate
DNA	deoxyribonucleic acid
DNP	2,4-dinitrophenol
DPG	diphosphoglycerate
dTMP	deoxythymidine monophosphate
dUMP	deoxyuridine monophosphate
EF	elongation factor
FAD (FADH)	flavin adenine dinucleotide (reduced form)
FMN	flavin mononucleotide
FSH	follicle-stimulating hormone
GDP	guanosine diphosphate
GMP	guanosine 5'-monophosphate (guanylic acid)
GTP	guanosine triphosphate
hCG	human chorionic gonadotropin
HDL	high-density lipoprotein
HGPRT	hypoxanthine-guanine phosphoribosyltransferase
HMG CoA	3-hydroxy-3-methylglutaryl coenzyme A
hnRNA	heterogeneous RNA of the nucleus
IDL	intermediate-density lipoprotein
IMP	inosine 5'-monophosphate (inosinic acid)
IP_3	inositol 1,4,5-triphosphate
LDH	lactate dehydrogenase
LDL	low-density lipoprotein
LH	luteinizing hormone

mRNA	messenger RNA
MSH	melanocyte-stimulating hormone
NAD (NADH)	nicotinamide adenine dinucleotide (reduced form)
NADP (NADPH)	nicotinamide adenine dinucleotide phosphate (reduced form)
PGH	pituitary growth hormone
P_i	inorganic orthophosphate
PP_i	inorganic pyrophosphate
PRPP	5-phosphoribosylpyrophosphate
RNA	ribonucleic acid
RQ	respiratory quotient
rRNA	ribosomal RNA
TMP	thymidine monophosphate
TPP	thymidine pyrophosphate
tRNA	transfer RNA
TSH	thyroid-stimulating hormone
TTP	thymidine triphosphate
UDP	uridine diphosphate
UMP	uridine monophosphate
UTP	uridine triphosphate
VLDL	very-low-density lipoprotein

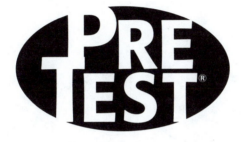

Biochemistry and Genetics

PreTest® Self-Assessment and Review

High-Yield Facts in Biochemistry and Genetics

HORMONAL CONTROL OF METABOLISM

Metabolism is precisely regulated by hormones controlling the level of blood fuels and their delivery to tissues. The primary control hormones of metabolism are insulin and glucagon. Epinephrine has effects similar to those of glucagon, except that glucagon has a greater effect on the liver while epinephrine has a greater effect on muscle. Blood levels of glucose, amino acids, fatty acids, and ketone bodies are maintained by variations in the [insulin]/[glucagon] ratio. When blood sugar is high, the ratio increases and insulin signals the fed state, promoting anabolic activities. The ratio decreases as glucagon is released to direct catabolic activities when blood glucose falls between meals, during fasting, and during starvation. Epinephrine or norepinephrine is released during exercise to promote catabolism of glucose and fat that supports muscular activity. Under normal conditions, the very precise interplay between insulin and glucagon maintains homeostatic blood fuel levels at about: glucose, 4.5 mM; fatty acids, 0.5 mM; amino acids, 4.5 mM; ketone bodies, 0.02 mM. Blood levels of ketone bodies and fatty acids rise during fasting or during starvation, with blood glucose levels being maintained. However, during uncontrolled juvenile diabetes, blood glucose levels rise greatly. The lack of insulin in this disease otherwise mimics starvation. The activity of various pathways during different metabolic states is summarized in the following table.

ACTIVITY OF METABOLIC PATHWAYS

Pathway	Fed	Fasted	Diabetes
Glycogen synthesis	+	−	−
Glycolysis (liver)	+	−	−
Triacylglyceride synthesis	+	−	−
Fatty acid synthesis	+	−	−
Protein synthesis	+	−	−
Cholesterol synthesis	+	−	−
Glycogenolysis	−	+	+
Gluconeogenesis (liver)	−	+	+
Lipolysis	−	+	+
Fatty acid oxidation	−	+	+
Protein breakdown	−	+/−	+/−
Ketogenesis (liver)	−	+	+
Ketone body utilization (non-hepatic tissues)	−	+	+

KEY FACTS ABOUT INHERITANCE

- Human gametes have 23 chromosomes (haploid chromosome number $n = 23$), while most somatic cells have 46 chromosomes (diploid chromosome number $2n = 46$).

- Genes occupy sites on chromosomes (loci) and occur in alternative forms (alleles).

- Mendelian diseases exhibit autosomal dominant, autosomal recessive, or X-linked inheritance, while multifactorial diseases (e.g., cleft palate, diabetes mellitus, schizophrenia, hypertension) are determined by multiple genes plus the environment.

- Characteristics of autosomal dominant diseases include a vertical pedigree pattern, affliction of both males and females, variable expressivity (variable severity among affected individuals), frequent new mutations, and a 50% recurrence risk for offspring of affected individuals (see pedigree A on chart). *Corollary:* germ-line mosaicism may produce affected siblings with autosomal dominant disease when neither parent is affected.

- Characteristics of autosomal recessive diseases include a horizontal pedigree pattern, affliction of males and females, frequent consanguinity (inbreeding), frequent carriers (heterozygotes without manifestations of disease), and a 25% recurrence risk for carrier parents (see pedigree B on chart). *Corollary:* normal siblings of individuals with autosomal recessive disease have a 2/3 chance of being carriers.

- Characteristics of X-linked recessive diseases include an oblique pedigree pattern, affliction of males only, frequent female carriers, and a 25% recurrence risk for carrier females (see pedigree C on chart). *Corollary:* Haldane's law predicts a 2/3 chance that the mother of an affected male with X-linked recessive disease is a carrier (and a 1/3 chance the affected male represents a new mutation).

- Ethnic correlations with Mendelian disorders include higher frequencies of cystic fibrosis in whites, sickle cell anemia in blacks, β-thalassemia in Italians and Greeks, α-thalassemia in Asians, and Tay-Sachs disease in Jews.

- Advanced maternal age is associated with higher risks for chromosomal disorders (e.g., Down's syndrome, trisomy 13), while advanced paternal age is associated with higher risks for new mutations (e.g., those producing achondroplasia or Marfan's syndrome).

- The Hardy-Weinberg law predicts allele frequencies in an idealized population according to the formula $p^2 + 2pq + q^2 = 1$. Applied to cystic fibrosis, the law predicts that homozygotes (q^2) have a frequency of 1 in 1600, predicting that carriers ($2pq$) have a frequency of 1 in 20.

- A karyotype is an ordered arrangement of chromosomes that is described by cytogenetic notation. A karyotype can be obtained from dividing cells (blood leukocytes, bone marrow, fibroblasts, amniocytes), but not from frozen or formalin-fixed cells.

- Cytogenetic notation includes the chromosome number (usually 46), description of the sex chromosomes (usually XX or XY), and indication of missing, extra, or rearranged chromosomes. Examples include 47,XY,+21 (male with Down's syndrome); 47,XX,+13 (female with trisomy 13); 45,X (female with monosomy X or Turner's syndrome); 46,XX,del(5p) (female with deletion of the chromosome 5 short arm).

- DNA diagnosis examines specific regions of genes for altered nucleotide sequences or deletions that affect gene expression and function; techniques include Southern blotting, gene amplification with the polymerase chain reaction (PCR), and mutant allele detection by

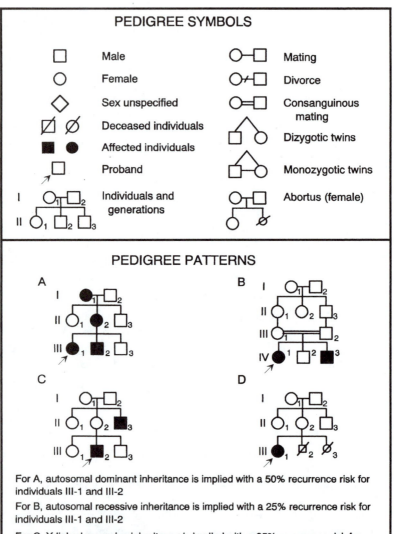

For A, autosomal dominant inheritance is implied with a 50% recurrence risk for individuals III-1 and III-2

For B, autosomal recessive inheritance is implied with a 25% recurrence risk for individuals III-1 and III-2

For C, X-linked recessive inheritance is implied with a 25% recurrence risk for individuals I-1 and II-2

For D, chromosomal inheritance is implied with individual II-2 being a translocation carrier

Pedigree symbols and pedigree patterns.

hybridization with allele-specific oligonucleotides (ASOs). Chromosome microdeletions encompass several genes and are detected by fluorescent in situ hybridization (FISH).

- Non-Mendelian inheritance mechanisms include mitochondrial inheritance (exhibiting maternal transmission), expansion of triplet repeats (exhibiting anticipation in pedigrees as in the fragile X syndrome), and genomic imprinting (exhibiting different phenotypes according to maternal or paternal origin of the aberrant genes).

- Prenatal diagnosis can include fetal ultrasound, maternal serum studies, or sampling of cells from the fetoplacental unit by chorionic villus sampling [CVS at 8 to 10 weeks, amniocentesis at 12 to 18 weeks, or percutaneous umbilical sampling (PUBS) from 16 weeks to term].

GENETICALLY BASED BIOCHEMICAL DISEASES

Disease and Incidence*	Defect	Symptoms
Glycolysis-based hemolytic anemias	Deficient glycolytic enzymes	Hemolytic anemia
Glucose-6-P dehydrogenase deficiency (up to 1 in 3)	Deficient enzyme of pentose phosphate shunt	Hemolytic anemia with antimalarial drugs
Glycogen storage diseases (one type XLR)	Deficient glycogen catabolism	Glycogen accumulation
Type 1a von Gierke's disease (1 in 100,000)	Glucose-6-phosphatase deficiency	Large liver, hypoglycemia
Type II Pompe's disease (1 in 100,000)	Lysomal α-glucosidase deficiency	Short PR interval on ECG, fatal
Type III Cori's disease	Debranching enzyme deficiency	Large liver, mild myopathy
Type V McArdle's disease (1 in 100,000)		
Lipid storage diseases	Deficiencies of sphingolipid metabolism	Sphingolipid storage neurodegeneration
Tay-Sachs disease [1 in 4,000 (Jews); 1 in 100,000]	Hexosaminidase A deficiency	Cherry red spot, neurodegeneration
Krabbe's disease (1 in 100,000)	Galactosylceramide β-galactosidase deficiency	Neurodegeneration, demyelination
Niemann-Pick disease type A (1 in 50,000)	Sphingomyelinase deficiency	Organomegaly, neurodegeneration
Gaucher's disease type I [1 in 1,000 (Jews); 1 in 100,000]	Glucosylceramide β-glucosidase deficiency	Organomegaly, fractures
Fabry's disease (XLR) (1 in 40,000)	β-galactosidase deficiency	Angiokeratoma, nerve pains
Lipid transport diseases (most AD)	Abnormality in plasma lipoprotein receptors or enzymes	Fatty serum, atherosclerosis

GENETICALLY BASED BIOCHEMICAL DISEASES (CONT.)

Disease and Incidence*	Defect	Symptoms
Familial hypercholesterolemia type IIa [1 in 500 (AD)]	Defective apo-B100 LDL receptors	Xanthomas, hypercholesterolemia
Familial hypertriglyceridemia type IV [1 in 50,000 (AD)]	Increased synthesis or decreased catabolism of VLDLs	Hypertriglyceridemia, atherosclerosis
Ion channel diseases (cystic fibrosis)	Sodium transport deficiency	High sweat chloride, lung disease
Nucleotide catabolism diseases (some XLR)	PRPP synthetase abnormalities	Gouty arthritis
Lesch-Nyhan syndrome [(XLR) 1 in 100,000]	Deficient HGPRT	Self-mutilation
DNA repair diseases (xeroderma pigmentosum)	Exonuclease deficiency	Skin cancer
Hereditary nonpolyposis colorectal cancer [(AD) 1 in 50,000]	DNA mismatch repair defects	Colon cancer
RNA-processing diseases [thalassemias (1 in 50,000; higher in Mediterraneans (β) or Asians (α)]	Imbalance of α- or β- hemoglobin chains	Anemia
Porphyrias [(one form AD) 1 in 1 million]	Heme biosynthesis enzyme defects	Abdominal pain, psychosis, skin rash
Amino acid metabolism diseases [Phenylketonuria (1 in 12,000)	Phenylalanine hydroxylase deficiency	Mousy odor, pale skin, blond hair
Maple syrup urine disease (1 in 100,000)]	Branched-chain amino acid dehydrogenase deficiency	Seizures, acidosis

*All diseases are autosomal recessive unless otherwise indicated. AD, autosomal dominant; XLR, X-linked recessive; PRPP, 5-phosphoribosyl-1-pyrophosphate; HGPRT, hypoxanthine-guanine phosphoribosyl-transferase.

Storage and Expression of Genetic Information

DNA Structure, Replication, and Repair

Questions

DIRECTIONS: Each item below contains a question or incomplete statement followed by suggested responses. Select the **one best** response to each question.

1. Patients with Hurler's syndrome (252800) are known to have mutations at the L-iduronidase locus. The diagnosis of Hurler's syndrome is most efficiently made by analyzing a patient's DNA for

a. A region of DNA that does not encode RNA
b. Alternative forms of the L-iduronidase gene
c. The entire set of genes in one leukocyte
d. A nucleotide substitution in the L-iduronidase gene
e. The position of the L-iduronidase gene on a chromosome

2. Which of the following statements regarding a double-helical molecule of DNA is true?

a. All hydroxyl groups of pentoses are involved in linkages
b. Bases are perpendicular to the axis
c. Each strand is identical
d. Each strand has parallel, 5′ to 3′ direction
e. Each strand replicates itself

3. A sample of human DNA is subjected to increasing temperature until the major fraction exhibits optical density changes due to disruption of its helix (melting or denaturation). A smaller fraction is atypical in that it requires a much higher temperature for melting. This smaller, atypical fraction of DNA must contain a higher content of

a. Adenine plus cytosine
b. Cytosine plus guanine
c. Adenine plus thymine
d. Cytosine plus thymine
e. Adenine plus guanine

4. A newborn baby has a sibling with sickle cell anemia (141900) and is at risk for the disease. The appropriate diagnostic test for sickle cell anemia in this baby will include

a. DNA amplification
b. Hemoglobin antibodies
c. DNA restriction
d. Red cell counting
e. DNA fingerprinting

5. A polymorphism is best defined as

a. Cosegregation of alleles
b. One phenotype, multiple genotypes
c. Nonrandom allele association
d. One locus, multiple abnormal alleles
e. One locus, multiple normal alleles

6. The process that occurs at the 5 position of cytidine and often correlates with gene inactivation is

a. Gene conversion
b. Sister chromatid exchange
c. Pseudogene
d. Gene rearrangement
e. DNA methylation

7. The average size of a human gene is

a. 1,000 bp
b. 40,000 bp
c. 2×10^6 bp
d. 1.5×10^8 bp
e. 3×10^9 bp

8. Restriction fragment length polymorphism (RFLP) analysis can only be used to follow the inheritance of a genetic disease if

a. mRNA probes are used in combination with antibodies
b. The disease-causing mutation is at or closely linked to an altered restriction site
c. Proteins of mutated and normal genes migrate differently upon gel electrophoresis
d. Mutations are outside of restriction sites so that cleaving still occurs
e. Restriction fragments remain the same size but their charge changes

9. It is well known that DNA polymerases synthesize DNA only in the 5' to 3' direction. Yet, at the replication fork, both strands of parental DNA are being replicated with the synthesis of new DNA. How is it possible that while one strand is being synthesized in the 5' to 3' direction, the other strand appears to be synthesized in the 3' to 5' direction? This apparent paradox is explained by

a. 3' to 5' DNA repair enzymes
b. 3' to 5' DNA polymerase
c. Okazaki fragments
d. Replication and immediate crossover of the leading strand
e. Lack of RNA primer on one of the strands

10. Given that the chromosomes of mammalian cells may be 20 times as large as those of *Escherichia coli,* how can replication of mammalian chromosomes be carried out in just a few minutes?

a. Eukaryotic DNA polymerases are extraordinarily fast compared with prokaryotic polymerases
b. The higher temperature of mammalian cells allows for an exponentially higher replication rate
c. Hundreds of replication forks work simultaneously on each piece of chromosomal DNA
d. A great many different RNA polymerases carry out replication simultaneously on chromosomal DNA
e. The presence of histones speeds up the rate of chromosomal DNA replication

11. A farming couple in Northern Michigan consult their physician about severe skin rashes and ulcers noted over the past year. They also have lost many cattle over the past year, and claim that their cattle feed changed in consistency and smell about 1 year ago. Chemical analysis of the feed shows high concentrations of polychlorinated biphenyls, a fertilizer related to known carcinogens. The physician sends the chemical to a laboratory for carcinogen testing, which is performed initially and rapidly by

a. Inoculation of the chemical into nude mice
b. Incubation of mutant bacteria with the chemical to measure the rate of reverse or "back" mutations
c. Incubation with stimulated white blood cells to measure the impact on DNA replication
d. Computer modeling based on the structures of related carcinogens
e. Incubation with mammalian cell cultures to measure the rates of malignant transformation

12. A child presents with severe growth failure, accelerated aging that causes adult complications such as diabetes and coronary artery disease, and microcephaly (small head) due to increased nerve cell death. In vitro assay of labeled thymidine incorporation reveals decreased levels of DNA synthesis compared to controls, but normal-sized labeled DNA fragments. The addition of protein extract from normal cells, gently heated to inactivate DNA polymerase, restores DNA synthesis in the child's cell extracts to normal. Which of the enzymes used in DNA replication is likely to be defective in this child?

a. DNA-directed DNA polymerase
b. Unwinding proteins
c. DNA polymerase I
d. DNA-directed RNA polymerase
e. DNA ligase

13. Patients with hereditary nonpolyposis colon cancer [HNPCC (114500)] have genes with microsatellite instability, that is, many regions containing abnormal, small loops of unpaired DNA. This is a result of a mutation affecting

a. Mismatch repair
b. Chain break repair
c. Base excision repair
d. Depurination repair
e. Nucleotide excision repair

14. If a completely radioactive double-stranded DNA molecule undergoes two rounds of replication in a solution free of radioactive label, what is the radioactivity status of the resulting four double-stranded DNA molecules?

a. Half should contain no radioactivity
b. All should contain radioactivity
c. Half should contain radioactivity in both strands
d. One should contain radioactivity in both strands
e. None should contain radioactivity

15. Sickle cell anemia (141900) is the clinical manifestation of homozygous genes for an abnormal hemoglobin molecule. The mutation in the β chain is known to produce a single amino acid change. The most likely mechanism for this mutation is

a. Crossing over
b. Two-base insertion
c. Three-base deletion
d. Nondisjunction
e. Single-base substitution (point mutation)

16. Parents bring their newborn daughter to you for consultation about diagnosis and management. Their first two children, a boy and a girl, have a complete form of albinism (203100) with pink irides, blond hair, and pale skin. Which of the following represents your correct advice concerning the newborn child?

a. A 1/8 risk for albinism and skin cancer from DNA deletions
b. A 1/8 risk for albinism and skin cancer from DNA cross-linkage
c. A 1/4 risk for albinism and skin cancer from DNA point mutations
d. A 1/4 risk for albinism and skin cancer from DNA deletions
e. A 1/4 risk for albinism and skin cancer from DNA cross-linkage

17. A culture of bacteria not resistant to tetracycline develops an infection from a virus that is derived from the lysis of tetracycline-resistant bacteria. Most of the bacterial progeny of the original culture is found to have become resistant to tetracycline. What phenomenon has occurred?

a. Conjugation
b. Colinearity
c. Recombination
d. Transformation
e. Transduction

18. Following ultraviolet damage of DNA in skin

a. A specific excinuclease detects damaged areas
b. Purine dimers are formed
c. Both strands are cleaved
d. Endonuclease removes the strand
e. DNA hydrolysis does not occur

19. Which of the following statements correctly describes eukaryotic nuclear chromosomal DNA?

a. Each discontinuous piece making up the chromosomes of eukaryotes is about the same size as each prokaryotic chromosome
b. Unlike bacterial DNA, no histones are associated with it
c. It is not replicated semiconservatively
d. It is a linear and unbranched molecule
e. It is not associated with a specific membranous organelle

20. Xeroderma pigmentosum (278700) is an inherited human skin disease that causes a variety of phenotypic changes in skin cells exposed to sunlight. The molecular basis of the disease appears to be

a. Rapid water loss caused by defects in the cell membrane permeability
b. The inactivation of temperature-sensitive transport enzymes in sunlight
c. The induction of a virulent provirus on ultraviolet exposure
d. The inability of the cells to synthesize carotenoid-type compounds
e. A defect in an excision-repair system that removes thymine dimers from DNA

21. Which of the following statements describes both the spiral structure of double-stranded DNA and the spiral structure found in certain segments of protein?

a. They are repeating spiral structures with intervals of pleated sheets
b. They have four alternative units arranged in polymeric chains
c. They are held together by hydrogen bonding
d. They are α-helical
e. They have covalently linked backbones

22. Which of the following descriptions of DNA replication is not common to the synthesis of both leading and lagging strands?

a. RNA primer is synthesized
b. DNA polymerase III synthesizes DNA
c. Helicase (rep protein) continuously unwinds duplex DNA at the replication fork during synthesis
d. Nucleoside monophosphates are added in a 5′ to 3′ direction along the growing DNA chain
e. DNA ligase repeatedly joins the ends of DNA along the growing strand

23. Which of the following statements describing restriction endonucleases is true?

a. They always yield overhanging single-stranded ends
b. They recognize methylated DNA sequences
c. They recognize triplet repeats
d. They cleave both strands in duplex DNA
e. They always yield blunt ends

24. DNA fingerprinting is used for paternity testing and forensic identification of suspects. Which of the following is the most accurate description of DNA fingerprinting?

a. DNA can be isolated from blood, skin, or sperm and analyzed for variable patterns of restriction fragments arising from tandemly repeated sequences (microsatellites)
b. DNA is copied from blood, skin, or sperm RNA using reverse transcriptase and analyzed for the pattern of complementary DNAs
c. DNA is isolated from blood, skin, or sperm and its fragment size distribution is analyzed by gel electrophoresis
d. DNA is isolated from blood, skin, or sperm and hybridized with probes from the HLA locus to visualize HLA gene patterns
e. DNA is isolated from blood, skin, or sperm, centrifuged to separate satellite DNA fractions, and analyzed by gel electrophoresis

25. The first drug to be effective against AIDS, including the reduction of maternal-to-child AIDS transmission by 30%, was AIDS drug azidothymidine (AZT). Which of the following describes its mechanism of action?

a. It inhibits viral protein synthesis
b. It inhibits RNA synthesis
c. It inhibits viral DNA polymerase
d. It stimulates DNA provirus production
e. It inhibits viral reverse transcriptase

26. Which of the following enzymes can polymerize deoxyribonucleotides into DNA?

a. Primase
b. DNA ligase
c. DNA gyrase
d. RNA polymerase III
e. Reverse transcriptase

27. Which of the following statements correctly describes the recombinant DNA tool known as plasmids?

a. They are found more commonly in viruses than in bacteria
b. They are single-stranded circles
c. They sometimes enhance bacterial susceptibility to antibiotics
d. They sometimes enhance bacterial resistance to antibiotics
e. They are too small to be useful as vectors for the cloning of mammalian DNA segments

28. Which of the following molecules is found in a nucleoside?

a. A pyrophosphate group
b. A 1' base linked to a pentose sugar
c. A 5'-phosphate group linked to a pentose sugar
d. A 3'-phosphate group linked to a pentose sugar
e. A terminal triphosphate

29. Which is the most correct sequence of events in gene repair mechanisms in patients without a mutated repair process?

a. Nicking, excision, replacement, sealing, recognition
b. Sealing, recognition, nicking, excision, replacement
c. Recognition, nicking, excision, replacement, sealing
d. Nicking, sealing, recognition, excision, replacement
e. Nicking, recognition, excision, sealing, replacement

30. Which of the following enzymes can be described as a DNA-dependent RNA polymerase?

a. DNA ligase
b. Primase
c. DNA polymerase III
d. DNA polymerase I
e. Reverse transcriptase

31. Radiation therapy is employed for many cancers, including irradiation of the central nervous system to destroy lymphoblasts in leukemia. Which of the following accounts for the destruction of rapidly growing cells?

a. Cross-linking of DNA
b. Demethylation of DNA
c. Cleavage of DNA double strands
d. Disruption of DNA-RNA transcription complexes
e. Disruption of purine rings in DNA

32. Mammalian chromosomes have specialized structures with highly repetitive DNA at their ends (telomeres). Which aspect of telomeric DNA replication is different from that of other chromosomal regions?

a. The DNA polymerase uses an RNA primer but does not degrade it
b. The DNA polymerase contains an RNA molecule that serves as template for DNA synthesis
c. The DNA polymerase must cross-link the 5′ and 3′ termini
d. The DNA polymerase has a σ subunit that facilitates binding to repetitive DNA
e. The DNA polymerase does not use an RNA template or primer

DNA Structure, Replication, and Repair

Answers

1. **The answer is b.** *(Murray, pp 412–434. Scriver, pp 3–45. Sack, pp 3–29. Wilson, pp 99–121.)* The most efficient DNA diagnosis would involve analysis of the two L-iduronidase genes in an individual, looking for any change in DNA sequence (nucleotide substitutions, deletions, duplications) that would alter function of the L-iduronidase protein. Alternative forms of a gene are called alleles, and an allele that has changed during transmission from parent to child may be called a mutant allele. Many human characteristics are encoded by genes, each occupying a particular address or locus on a chromosome. Genes consist of DNA segments that encode RNA along with flanking DNA sequences that regulate gene expression (see the figures below). Within the coding regions are DNA segments that are transcribed and then translated into protein (exons), and those that are transcribed but removed by RNA splicing (introns). If a DNA mutation produces a disease through its altered protein, as with L-iduronidase gene mutations in Hurler's syndrome, the mutant gene (strictly, the mutant allele) may be called abnormal. Human autosomes (chromosomes 1 through 22) and X chromosomes in females have two homologous loci in each individual, harboring two identical (homozygous) or different (heterozygous) alleles. Males have only one X chromosome and often only one allele per sex chromosome locus because the Y has minimal coding material. The complete set of genetic material (all the genes and loci) in each biological species is called the genome.

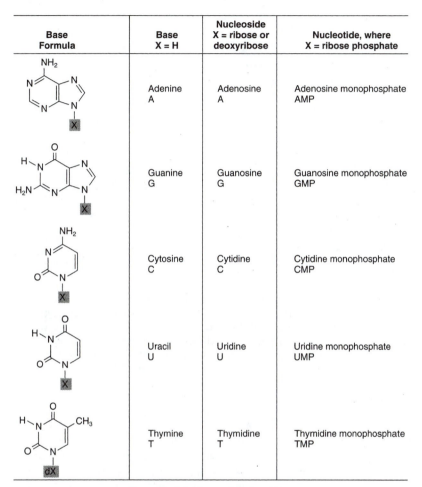

Base Formula	Base X = H	Nucleoside X = ribose or deoxyribose	Nucleotide, where X = ribose phosphate
	Adenine A	Adenosine A	Adenosine monophosphate AMP
	Guanine G	Guanosine G	Guanosine monophosphate GMP
	Cytosine C	Cytidine C	Cytidine monophosphate CMP
	Uracil U	Uridine U	Uridine monophosphate UMP
	Thymine T	Thymidine T	Thymidine monophosphate TMP

Bases, nucleotides, and nucleosides.
(Reproduced, with permission, from Murray RK, Granner DK, Mayes PA, Rodwell VW: Harper's Biochemistry, 25/e. New York, McGraw-Hill, 2000: 376.)

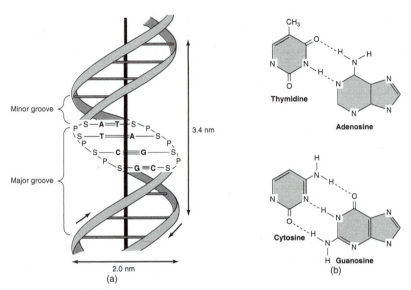

(a) Structure of DNA (B form) showing the double helix with antiparallel strands (arrows). One complete turn (3.4 nm) includes 10 base pairs (bp). A, adenine; C, cytosine; G, guanine; T, thymine; P, phosphate; S, deoxyribose sugar. (b) Base pairing showing two hydrogen bonds (broken lines) between A and T, and three bonds between C and G.
(Reproduced, with permission, from Murray RK, Granner DK, Mayes PA, Rodwell VW: Harper's Biochemistry, 25/e. New York, McGraw-Hill, 2000: 404.)

2. The answer is b. *(Murray, pp 412–434. Scriver, pp 3–45. Sack, pp 3–29. Wilson, pp 99–121.)* In the classic double-helical model of DNA proposed by Watson and Crick, the purine (adenosine and guanine) and pyrimidine (cytosine and thymine) bases (see the figure above) attached to the sugar backbone are perpendicular to the axis and parallel to each other. They are paired (A to G or T to C) and held together by hydrogen bonds. The DNA strands (nucleotide polymers) are joined by linkages between the 3′-hydroxyl of each pentose (deoxyribose) and the 5′-phosphate of its deoxyribose neighbor. Each strand composing the double helix is different and antiparallel. The 3′ end of one strand is opposite the 5′ end of its complement and vice versa (see the figure above). It is this complementary nature of DNA that allows the strands to be templates for one another during DNA replication.

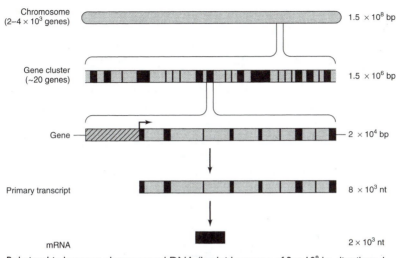

Relationship between chromosomal DNA (haploid genome of 3×10^9 bp distributed among 23 chromosomes) and mRNA [average gene length 20,000 bp, yielding a mature RNA of 2,000 nucleotides (nt) after introns (gray areas) are removed by splicing].
(Reproduced, with permission, from Murray RK, Granner DK, Mayes PA, Rodwell VW:
Harper's Biochemistry, 25/e. New York, McGraw-Hill, 2000: 418.)

3. The answer is b. *(Murray, pp 412–434. Scriver, pp 3–45. Sack, pp 3–29.*
Wilson, pp 99–121.) The melting temperature T_m of duplex DNA is the temperature at which half the base pairs are denatured. Adenine-thymine (A-T) base pairs have two hydrogen bonds, in contrast to cytosine-guanine (C-G) base pairs, which have three hydrogen bonds. Duplex DNA molecules rich in A-T base pairs have a much lower T_m than those rich in C-G base pairs. As DNA is heated, fractions with a higher A-T content melt or denature before those with a higher C-G content. Most mammals, including humans, have satellite DNA fractions that are highly repetitive and clustered in particular chromosome regions. Satellite DNAs are named for their altered density (satellite band) on centrifugation, caused by higher G-C content. Their function is unknown.

4. The answer is a. *(Murray, pp 412–434. Scriver, pp 3–45. Sack, pp 3–29.*
Wilson, pp 99–121.) Sufficient DNA for analysis can be obtained by amplification of leukocyte DNA using the polymerase chain reaction (PCR).

Short segments of DNA (oligonucleotide primers) are designed to be complementary to areas flanking the DNA region of interest—in this case, the portion of the β-globin gene that may harbor the sickle cell anemia (141900) mutation. Some 20 to 30 cycles of cooling (to anneal the primers), synthesis (with heat-stable DNA polymerase), and heating (to melt the DNA and allow the next cycle) can amplify the targeted DNA segment over 1 million-fold. Hybridization in duplicate to allele-specific oligonucleotides (ASOs; one ASO for the hemoglobin A mutation, one ASO for the S mutation) can establish the diagnosis of normal (AA alleles), sickle trait (AS alleles), or sickle cell anemia (SS alleles). Newborns have fetal hemoglobin (α- and γ-globin) with little expression of hemoglobin A (α- and β-globin genes) until 3 to 6 months of life, so testing for anemia or for abnormal hemoglobin with antibodies would not be helpful.

DNA polymorphisms (nucleotide sequence variations) occur approximately once per 200 to 500 base pairs (bp) of human DNA. If the sequence variation affects the recognition site for a restriction endonuclease, the altered segment sizes produced by endonuclease digestion allow detection of the sequence change [restriction fragment length polymorphism (RFLP)]. If the nucleotide change causing the RFLP is adjacent to (linked with) or coincident with a disease mutation, then one size variant of the RFLP may be diagnostic. However, mutations of known sequence (such as that for sickle cell anemia) are better detected by PCR and ASOs. The use of several highly variable RFLPs produces a pattern of restriction fragments that is highly distinctive for each individual (DNA fingerprinting) but not diagnostic for a particular disease.

5. The answer is e. *(Murray, pp 412–434. Scriver, pp 3–45. Sack, pp 3–29. Wilson, pp 99–121.)* Polymorphic loci have multiple alleles because of DNA sequence variation, including one or more with frequencies greater than 1%. This higher frequency and benign connotation differentiate polymorphic loci from those that harbor multiple disease-causing alleles. The DNA sequence changes may alter restriction sites [producing restriction fragment length polymorphisms (RFLPs)], change the numbers of repeated segments [producing variable numbers of tandem repeats (VNTRs)], or alter the genetic code (producing variant proteins, or protein polymorphisms). Polymorphisms may cosegregate (be inherited together) with disease alleles, allowing diagnosis by linkage analysis or estimates of risk through allele association (a.k.a. linkage disequilibrium, as with certain HLA alleles and diabetes mellitus). Different mutant alleles may cause indistinguishable phenotypes (allelic heterogeneity), as may mutations at different loci (genetic heterogeneity).

6. The answer is e. *(Murray, pp 412–434. Scriver, pp 3–45. Sack, pp 3–29. Wilson, pp 99–121.)* DNA methylation occurs mainly at CpG dinucleotides that often cluster in at the upstream promoter regions of genes (CpG islands). While these are generally correlated with gene inactivation, there are many exceptions. Double crossovers at meiosis can substitute a normal allele for a mutant allele (conversion), and reverse transcriptases can copy intronless mRNA into complementary DNAs (cDNAs) that integrate into the genome as pseudogenes. Immunoglobulin genes undergo gene rearrangement to unite variable, joining, and constant regions for expression of a unique antibody. Unequal crossing over between sister chromatids is thought to be an important mechanism for variation in copy number within gene clusters.

7. The answer is b. *(Murray, pp 412–434. Scriver, pp 3–45. Sack, pp 3–29. Wilson, pp 99–121.)* The 6×10^9 bp of DNA in each human diploid cell are apportioned among 46 chromosomes. Even with the highest-resolution karyotype, the average chromosome band equals about 2×10^6 bp. These measurements emphasize the vastly greater precision of molecular analysis in detecting gene deletions (each gene averages 40,000 bp in size) or codon (3 bp) deletions, as in the ΔF_{508} mutation [the deletion of a phenylalanine codon that is common in cystic fibrosis (219700)].

8. The answer is b. *(Murray, pp 488–504. Scriver, pp 3–45. Sack, pp 41–45. Wilson, pp 151–186.)* A variety of genetic diseases, such as sickle cell anemia (141900), Huntington's chorea (143100), and cystic fibrosis (219700), can be detected by restriction fragment length polymorphism (RFLP) analysis. In order for RFLP to be able to detect and follow the inheritance of these genes, the detected mutation must be at or closely linked to an altered restriction site. Mutations within the restriction sites change the size of restriction fragments. The different-sized fragments migrate in different positions during electrophoresis of bands visualized by Southern blot analysis, which utilizes fluorescent or radiolabeled DNA probes.

9. The answer is c. *(Murray, pp 412–434. Scriver, pp 3–45. Sack, pp 3–29. Wilson, pp 99–121.)* Since both strands of parental DNA serve as templates for the synthesis of new DNA, it appears that DNA synthesis must be 5′ to 3′ for one daughter strand and 3′ to 5′ for the other daughter strand at the replication fork. Despite the apparent need for 3′ to 5′ synthesis, all DNA polymerases and repair enzymes can only synthesize DNA in the 5′ to 3′ direction. The apparent contradiction is solved by understanding that one strand of DNA is synthesized continuously in the 5′ to 3′ direction while the other strand is made up of small fragments known as Okazaki fragments. The small Okazaki fragments are, in fact, synthesized in a 5′ to 3′ direction and then joined together by DNA ligase. Each Okazaki fragment is about 1000 nucleotides long. Thus, while the overall direction of growth of the lagging strand that is made up of small fragments is in fact in the 3′ to 5′ direction, the actual polymerization of individual nucleotides is in the 5′ to 3′ direction. Crossing over of the DNA strands does not occur during replication.

10. The answer is c. *(Murray, pp 412–434. Scriver, pp 3–45. Sack, pp 3–29. Wilson, pp 99–121.)* Despite the great length of the chromosomes of eukaryotic DNA, the actual replication time is only minutes. This is because eukaryotic DNA is replicated bidirectionally from many points of origin. The hundreds of initiation sites for DNA replication on chromosomes share a consensus sequence called an autonomous replication sequence (ARS). Thus, while the process of DNA replication in mammals is similar to that in bacteria, with DNA polymerases of similar optimal temperatures and speed, the many replication forks allow for a rapid synthesis of chromosomal DNA. Proteins such as histones, which are bound to mammalian chromosomes, inhibit DNA replication or transcription. Dissociation of the protein-DNA complex (chromatin) and unwinding of DNA supercoils (followed by chromatin reassembly) is part of the replication process.

11. The answer is b. *(Murray, pp 412–434. Scriver, pp 3–45. Sack, pp 3–29. Wilson, pp 99–121.)* The Ames test is a rapid and relatively inexpensive bacterial assay for determining mutagenicity of potential toxic chemicals. Since many chemical carcinogens are mutagenic, it seems obvious that damage to DNA is a central event in carcinogenesis as well as mutagenesis. Dr. Bruce Ames developed a tester strain of *Salmonella* that has been modified not to grow in the absence of histidine because of a mutation in one of the genes for the biosynthesis of histidine. Toxic chemicals that are mutagens are placed in the center of the plate and result in reversions of the original mutations, so that histidine is synthesized and the mutated revertants multiply in histidine-free media. Since many carcinogens are converted to active forms by metabolism in the liver, preliminary incubation with liver homogenates may precede the bacterial assay. Essentially all chemicals known as carcinogens in humans cause mutagenesis in the Ames test. The other options—carcinogenicity screening in immunosuppressed (nude) mice, computer modeling, or incubation with mammalian cell cultures—may provide some information, but are less efficient and validated than the Ames test. Contamination of Michigan cattle feed with polychlorinated biphenyls (PCBs) did occur through an industrial mistake.

12. The answer is b. (*Murray, pp 412–434. Scriver, pp 3–45. Sack, pp 3–29. Wilson, pp 99–121.*) Before DNA replication can actually begin, unwinding protein must open segments along the DNA double helix. A defective unwinding protein slows the overall rate of DNA synthesis, but does not alter the size of replicated DNA fragments. Defects in DNA synthesis or transcription may produce a phenotype of accelerated aging, as in Cockayne's syndrome [216400 (usually defective in a transcription factor)]. After unwinding, DNA-directed RNA polymerase (primase) catalyzes the synthesis of a complementary RNA primer of approximately 50 to 100 bases on each DNA strand. Then DNA-directed DNA polymerase III adds deoxyribonucleotides to the 3′ end of the primer RNA, which replicates a segment of DNA, the Okazaki fragment. DNA polymerase I then removes the primer RNA and adds deoxyribonucleotides to fill the gaps between adjacent Okazaki fragments. The fragments are finally joined together by DNA ligase to create a continuous DNA chain.

13. The answer is a. (*Murray, pp 412–434. Scriver, pp 769–784. Sack, pp 3–29. Wilson, pp 99–121.*) One of the most common types of inherited cancers is nonpolyposis colon cancer [HNPCC (114500)]. Most cases are associated with mutations of either of two genes that encode proteins critical in the surveillance of mismatches. Mismatches are due to copying errors leading to one- to five-base unmatched pieces of DNA. Two- to five-base-long unmatched bases form miniloops. Normally, specific proteins survey newly formed DNA between adenine methylated bases within a GATC sequence.

Mismatches are removed and replaced. First, a GATC endonuclease nicks the faulty strand at a site complementary to GATC, then an exonuclease digests the strand from the GATC site beyond the mutation. Finally, the excised faulty DNA is replaced. In HNPCC, the unrecognized mismatches accumulate, leading to malignant growth of colon epithelium. The other forms of DNA repair are important for rectifying damage from ultraviolet light.

14. The answer is a. (*Murray, pp 412–434. Scriver, pp 3–45. Sack, pp 3–29. Wilson, pp 99–121.*) The replication of double-stranded DNA is semiconservative, meaning that each strand separates and serves as a template for synthesis of a new complementary strand. The first round of replication of a labeled DNA helix in a cold (unlabeled) solution will yield two daughter double-stranded molecules, each with one labeled and one unlabeled strand. The second round of replication will yield four double-stranded DNA molecules. Two of these will have one original labeled strand and one unlabeled strand; the other two will have two unlabeled strands and contain no radioactivity.

15. The answer is e. (*Murray, pp 412–434. Scriver, pp 3–45. Sack, pp 3–29. Wilson, pp 99–121.*) In the β-globin chain of hemoglobin S (141900), a valine residue replaces a glutamic acid at the sixth amino acid position from the N-terminus. The amino acid substitution is the result of a single-base change (point mutation) from thymine to adenine at the second position of the sixth codon. Crossing over among homologous β-globin genes might exchange alleles, if equal, or generate mutant alleles with duplicated/deficient nucleotides, if unequal. Two-base insertions would change the reading frame of the genetic code (frame-shift mutation) and produce a nonsense peptide after the point of insertion. Three-base deletions could also cause frame shifts or, if one codon were removed, delete one amino acid. Nondisjunction involves abnormal segregation of chromosomes at meiosis or mitosis, and would produce nonviable individuals or somatic cells with additional or missing copies of chromosome 11 and its β-globin locus.

16. The answer is e. (*Murray, pp 412–434. Scriver, pp 5587–5628. Sack, pp 3–29. Wilson, pp 99–121.*) Normal parents having two affected children, male and female, is suggestive of autosomal recessive inheritance. This interpretation fits with the usual inheritance of oculocutaneous albinism (203100), implying a 1/4 risk for a newborn in whom signs and symptoms of albinism are not yet evident. The defect in melanin synthesis in albinism decreases the amount of this protective pigment in skin and increases the exposure of DNA in skin cells to sunlight. Ultraviolet rays from sunlight cause DNA cross-linkage between at least two bases in the same or opposite strands of DNA. Cross-linking occurs through the formation of thymine-thymine dimers. The DNA cross-links cause higher rates of mutation and skin cancer in albinism, mandating the wearing of protective clothing, sunglasses, and sunscreens by affected individuals. DNA deletions and point mutations are less common than DNA cross-links after sunlight exposure.

17. The answer is e. *(Murray, pp 412–434. Scriver, pp 3–45. Sack, pp 3–29. Wilson, pp 99–121.)* The process of transduction involves the transfer of a portion of DNA from one bacterium to the chromosome of another bacterium by means of a viral infection. Conjugation is the transfer of a so-called male chromosomal DNA to the DNA of an acceptor, or female, bacterial cell. Colinearity defines the relationship between genes and proteins in that the sequence of amino acids in proteins is a result of the sequence of base triplets in template genes. Recombination is simply the exchange of sequences between two molecules of DNA. Transformation results when exogenous DNA fragments are incorporated into the chromosome of another organism, as in the transformation of pneumococcal bacteria that led Avery and McLeod to recognize the genetic significance of DNA.

18. The answer is a. *(Murray, pp 412–434. Scriver, pp 3–45. Sack, pp 3–29. Wilson, pp 99–121.)* Ultraviolet irradiation causes thymine dimers to form in DNA. Replication is inhibited in cells until the pyrimidine dimers are removed. Removal of the damaged areas occurs in two ways. The process can be simply reversed by a photoreactivating enzyme that cleaves the dimers and yields the original bases. Blue light is required for this. Alternatively, the dimer is removed. A UV-specific excinuclease nicks the dimer on its 5′ side. DNA polymerase I replicates the damaged sequence, while the damaged sequence swings out. Finally, the damaged piece is hydrolyzed by the 5′ to 3′ exonuclease activity of the DNA polymerase I. DNA ligase then joins the new piece to the original DNA at the cleavage site.

19. The answer is d. *(Murray, pp 412–434. Scriver, pp 3–45. Sack, pp 3–29. Wilson, pp 99–121.)* Like bacterial DNA, eukaryotic DNA is replicated in a semiconservative manner. However, in contrast to most bacterial DNA, which is circular in structure, nuclear chromosomal DNA is a single, uninterrupted molecule that is linear and unbranched. A eukaryotic chromosome contains a strand of DNA at least 100 times as large as the DNA molecules found in prokaryotes. Eukaryotic, but not prokaryotic, DNA molecules are bound to small basic proteins called histones. The histone-DNA complex formed is referred to as chromatin.

20. The answer is e. *(Murray, pp 412–434. Scriver, pp 677–704. Sack, pp 3–29. Wilson, pp 99–121.)* Xeroderma pigmentosum (278700) appears to be due to the inability of an excision-repair system to remove thymine dimers, which are formed on exposure of DNA to ultraviolet radiation. This results in a deficiency in the ability to repair the damaged DNA. Mutagenesis by this mechanism is presumably the basis for the multiple neoplasms that occur in patients who have this disease.

21. The answer is e. *(Murray, pp 412–434. Scriver, pp 3–45. Sack, pp 3–29. Wilson, pp 99–121.)* Double-stranded DNA is arranged in a double helix as originally deduced by Watson and Crick. The double-helical structure of duplex DNA is different than the α-helical structure of portions of proteins. The α-helical structure of proteins is formed of one chain of proteins stabilized by individual hydrogen bonds between components of the amide bonds, that is, between the carbonyl oxygens and the amide nitrogens. In contrast, the hydrogen bonding in double-stranded DNA is important to allow each strand to act as a template for the other complementary strand, with adenine bonding to thiamine and cytosine bonding to guanine. Hydrophobic stacking between bases in the hydrophobic interior of the double strand actually makes a greater contribution to the stability of the DNA double helix than does hydrogen bonding. DNA and protein helices are both composed of polymers of subunits (amino acids and nucleotides) held together by a covalently linked backbone. As pointed out above, hydrogen bonding is important to both the double helix of DNA and the α-helix of proteins. Finally, both are, in fact, spiral structures, although only the helix of proteins is an α helix.

22. The answer is e. *(Murray, pp 412–434. Scriver, pp 3–45. Sack, pp 3–29. Wilson, pp 99–121.)* In the leading strand, DNA is synthesized continuously in the 5′ to 3′ direction by DNA polymerase. In contrast, in the lagging strand, which is in the 3′ to 5′ direction, DNA polymerase III synthesizes small (approximately 1000 nucleotides) Okazaki fragments. For the synthesis of these small fragments, all the same roles and steps apply except that additional enzymes are needed to fill the gap between the fragments and join the fragments. Consequently, DNA ligase is repeatedly needed to join the ends of the DNA fragments along the growing lagging strand. DNA ligase catalyzes the formation of a phosphodiester bond between the 3′ hydroxyl group at the end of one DNA chain and the 5′ DNA phosphate group at the end of the other. DNA ligase is only functional when double-helical DNA molecules are the substrate. It does not work on single-stranded DNA. DNA ligase effects the joining of strands of DNA not only during the normal synthesis of DNA, but during the splicing of DNA chains in genetic recombination as well as the repair of damaged DNA.

23. The answer is d. *(Murray, pp 488–504. Scriver, pp 3–45. Sack, pp 41–45. Wilson, pp 151–186.)* Restriction endonucleases are produced by prokaryotes for cleaving both strands of foreign DNA. The host cell's DNA is not degraded because the recognition sites are specifically methylated. The endonucleases recognize specific short symmetrical sequences known as palindromes. These cleavage sites contain twofold rotational symmetry in that the sequence is identical but antiparallel in the complementary strands. In some cases, single-stranded cohesive ends on each of the complementary strands are produced, while in other cases double-stranded blunt ends are formed. Modern analysis of DNA structure is highly dependent upon the use of different restriction endonucleases that permit the specific hydrolysis of DNA into large polynucleotides.

24. The answer is a. *(Murray, pp 488–504. Scriver, pp 3–45. Sack, pp 41–45. Wilson, pp 151–186.)* Restriction fragment length polymorphisms (RFLPs) arising from variable numbers of tandem repeats (VNTRs) are the basis of the DNA fingerprinting technique. The process is: (1) isolation of DNA from parent/child or forensic specimens using blood, skin, or semen; (2) PCR amplification and radioactive labeling of DNA from variable regions in each sample; (3) separation of the variable DNA fragments by gel electrophoresis; and (4) comparison of the DNA fragment patterns among samples. Since numbers of arrays of repeats of two, three, or four base pairs (microsatellites) may vary from 5 to 100 at a particular chromosome locus, particular alleles may occur in less than 1% of the population. As a result, analysis of three loci, each with two alleles, can produce odds as high as $(100)^6$ that the pattern matches a putative father or suspect as compared to a random person from the general population. Reverse transcription based upon RNA-directed DNA synthesis is not utilized in DNA fingerprinting, and the size distribution of undigested DNA reflects its integrity during isolation rather than individual identify. HLA typing uses antibodies to define the constellation of alleles from various loci in the HLA region on chromosome 6. The tendency for certain HLA alleles to occur together (associate) on the same chromosome as haplotypes greatly reduces their odds of identity when compared to DNA fingerprinting.

25. The answer is e. *(Murray, pp 412–434. Scriver, pp 3–45. Sack, pp 3–29. Wilson, pp 99–121.)* The AIDS treatment drug azidothymidine (AZT) exerts its effect by inhibiting viral reverse transcriptase. Thus, it prevents replication of the human immunodeficiency virus. Reverse transcriptase is an RNA-directed DNA polymerase. The RNA of retroviruses utilizes reverse transcriptase to synthesize DNA provirus, which in turn synthesizes new viral RNA. AZT inhibits DNA provirus production, but does not directly inhibit synthesis of new viral RNA.

26. The answer is e. *(Murray, pp 412–434. Scriver, pp 3–45. Sack, pp 3–29. Wilson, pp 99–121.)* Reverse transcriptase is an RNA-dependent DNA polymerase that can synthesize first a single strand and then a double-stranded DNA from a single-strand RNA template. It was originally found in animal retroviruses. Primase is a DNA-dependent RNA polymerase enzyme that synthesizes an RNA molecule 10 to 200 nucleotides in length that initiates or "primes" DNA synthesis. DNA ligase joins DNA fragments and DNA gyrase winds or unwinds DNA. Transfer RNA, 5SRNA, and other small RNAs are synthesized by RNA polymerase III (RNA polymerase I synthesizes ribosomal RNA and RNA polymerase II synthesizes messenger RNA).

27. The answer is d. (*Murray, pp 488–504. Scriver, pp 3–45. Sack, pp 41–45. Wilson, pp 151–186.*) Plasmids are duplex DNA circles that may carry genes determining antibiotic resistance (R factors), sex (F factors), or toxin production (colicinogenic factors) in their bacterial hosts. They can replicate independently of the host chromosome or insert into the host chromosome. Plasmids are one class of mobile genetic elements (transposons) that are normally found in bacteria. Restriction of plasmid vector DNA and mammalian DNA with the same endonuclease produces cohesive ends that may be joined together with DNA ligase. The ligated molecules, which consist of one or more mammalian DNA segments inserted between plasmid DNA ends, are recombinant DNA molecules that can be replicated in the host bacteria. Isolation of the recombinant plasmid DNA by centrifugation and excision of the inserted mammalian DNA segment(s) then provides a pure and abundant sample of the mammalian gene segment that is separated from all other DNA segments in the mammalian genome. Plasmid vectors are useful for gene segments under about 10 kilobases (kb) in size, but bacteriophage and recently yeast artifical chromosomes (YACs) can incorporate DNA segments up to 1000 kb or 1 megabase (Mb) in size. These larger vectors allow genomes like those of humans or mice (3000 Mb in size) to be entirely represented in a collection (library) of about 3000 recombinant molecules.

28. The answer is b. (*Murray, pp 412–434. Scriver, pp 3–45. Sack, pp 3–29. Wilson, pp 99–121.*) A nucleoside consists of a purine or pyrimidine base linked to a pentose sugar. The 1′ carbon of the pentose is linked to the nitrogen of the base. In DNA, 2′-deoxyribose sugars are used; in RNA, ribose sugars are used. Nucleotides are phosphate esters of nucleosides with one to three phosphate groups, such as adenosine monophosphate (AMP), adenosine diphosphate (ADP), or adenosine triphosphate (ATP). The nitrogenous bases are adenine, thymine, guanine, and cytosine in DNA, with thymine replaced by uridine in RNA. Nucleotide polymers are chains of nucleotides with single phosphate groups, joined by bonds between the 3′-hydroxyl of the preceding pentose and the 5′-phosphate of the next pentose. Polymerization requires high-energy nucleotide triphosphate precursors that liberate pyrophosphate (broken down to phosphate) during joining. The polymerization reaction is given specificity by complementary RNA or DNA templates and rapidity by enzyme catalysts called polymerases.

29. The answer is c. (*Murray, pp 412–434. Scriver, pp 3–45. Sack, pp 3–29. Wilson, pp 99–121.*) In all of the forms of DNA repair in normal cells, a common sequence of events occurs.

1. The single or multiple base abnormality is surveyed and detected by a specific protein or proteins.
2. The DNA is nicked on one side of the damaged DNA.
3. A specific enzyme excises the damaged portion (steps 2 and 3 can be combined if an excinuclease cuts on both sides of the damaged DNA).
4. The damaged portion of the strand is replaced by resynthesis catalyzed by DNA polymerase I.
5. A ligase seals the final gap.

With some variability, these general principles apply in nucleotide excision repair (segments of about 30 nucleotides), base excision repair of single bases, and mismatch repair of copying errors (one to five bases).

30. The answer is b. (*Murray, pp 435–451. Scriver, pp 3–45. Sack, pp 3–29. Wilson, pp 99–121.*) Primase is a DNA-dependent RNA polymerase located in the primosome at the replication fork of DNA. Primase initiates DNA synthesis by synthesizing a 10-base RNA primer. The DNA-RNA helix formed binds DNA polymerase III, which synthesizes a DNA fragment (the Okazaki fragment) in a 5′ to 3′ direction. When the RNA primer of the previous Okazaki fragment is met, DNA polymerase I replaces III and digests the RNA primer, replacing it with appropriate DNA bases. When the RNA primer is completely removed, DNA ligase synthesizes the last phosphodiester bond, thereby sealing the space. What is left is a new lagging strand extended by the new Okazaki fragment with the 10-base RNA primer at its 5′ end. Reverse transcriptase is a DNA polymerase that uses RNA as a template found in retroviruses as well as normal eukaryotic cells. Unlike DNA polymerase I and III, which proofread for errors during normal synthesis, reverse transcriptase has no proofreading capabilities. Hence, it has an exceedingly high error rate that contributes to the high rate of mutation in retroviruses like HIV.

31. The answer is e. (*Murray, pp 412–434. Scriver, pp 3–45. Sack, pp 3–29. Wilson, pp 99–121.*) The major effects of radiation are to damage cellular DNA by opening purine rings and rupturing phosphodiester bonds. Chemical agents such as formaldehyde can cross-link DNA, and inhibitors of DNA methylation, such as methotrexate (an inhibitor of folic acid), were the first anticancer drugs. Experimental gene therapies for cancer include the inhibition of oncogene expression and the enhancement of tumor suppressor gene activity. These therapies target particular DNA-RNA transcription complexes or signal transduction cascades that are active in cancer cells.

32. The answer is b. (*Murray, pp 412–434. Scriver, pp 3–45. Sack, pp 3–29. Wilson, pp 99–121.*) A special DNA polymerase called telomerase is responsible for replication of the telomeric DNA. Telomerase contains an RNA molecule that guides the synthesis of complementary DNA. Telomerase is therefore an RNA-dependent DNA polymerase in a category with reverse transcriptase. Telomerase does not require an RNA primer, initiating synthesis of the leading strands at 3′ ends within the telomeric DNA. Synthesis of the lagging strands uses primase, DNA polymerase III, and DNA polymerase I, as with the replication of other chromosomal regions.

Gene Expression

Questions

DIRECTIONS: Each item below contains a question or incomplete statement followed by suggested responses. Select the **one best** response to each question.

33. Which statement about the "genetic code" is most accurate?

a. Information is stored as sets of dinucleotide repeats called codons
b. The code is degenerate (i.e., more than one codon may exist for a single amino acid)
c. Information is stored as sets of trinucleotide repeats called codons
d. There are 64 codons, all of which code for amino acids
e. The sequence of codons that make up a gene exhibits an exact linear correspondence to the sequence of amino acids in the translated protein

34. Sickle cell anemia (141900) is caused by a point mutation in the hemoglobin gene, resulting in the substitution of a single amino acid in the β-globin peptides of hemoglobin. This mutation is best detected by which of the following?

a. Isolation of DNA from red blood cells followed by polymerase chain reaction (PCR) amplification and restriction enzyme digestion
b. Isolation of DNA from blood leukocytes followed by Southern blot analysis to detect globin gene exon sizes
c. Isolation of DNA from blood leukocytes followed by DNA sequencing of globin gene introns
d. Isolation of DNA from blood leukocytes followed by polymerase chain reaction (PCR) amplification and allele-specific oligonucleotide (ASO) hybridization
e. Western blot analysis of red blood cell extracts

35. The DNA sequence M, shown below, is the sense strand from a coding region known to be a mutational "hot spot" for a gene. It encodes amino acids 21 to 25. Given the genetic and amino acid codes CCC = proline (P), GCC = alanine (A), TTC = phenylalanine (F), and TAG = stop codon, which of the following sequences is a frame-shift mutation that causes termination of the encoded protein?

M 5′-CCC-CCT-AGG-TTC-AGG-3′

a. -CCA-CCT-AGG-TTC-AGG-
b. -GCC-CCT-AGG-TTC-AGG-
c. -CCA-CCC-TAG-GTT-CAG-
d. -CCC-CTA-GGT-TCA-GG—
e. -CCC-CCT-AGG-AGG——

36. Which of the following results is provided by northern blot analysis?

a. Detects specific base pairs
b. Detects DNA molecules
c. Detects RNA molecules
d. Detects proteins
e. Determines chromosome structure

37. The hypothetical "stimulin" gene contains two exons that encode a protein of 100 amino acids. They are separated by an intron of 100 bp beginning after the codon for amino acid 10. Stimulin messenger RNA (mRNA) has 5′ and 3′ untranslated regions of 70 and 30 nucleotides, respectively. A complementary DNA (cDNA) made from mature stimulin RNA would have which of the following sizes?

a. 500 bp
b. 400 bp
c. 300 bp
d. 100 bp
e. 70 bp

38. The hypothetical "stimulin" gene with two exons encoding a protein of 100 amino acids is found to have abnormal expression in cell culture. Which of the following mutations would produce a 500-bp stimulin mRNA and a 133–amino acid peptide that reacts with antibodies to stimulin protein?

a. Splice junction mutation preventing RNA splicing
b. Frame-shift mutation in codon #2
c. Silent point mutation in the third nucleotide of codon #50
d. Nonsense mutation at codon #2
e. Deletion of exon 1

39. In contrast to DNA polymerase, RNA polymerase

a. Fills in the gap between Okazaki fragments
b. Works only in a 5′ to 3′ direction
c. Edits as it synthesizes
d. Synthesizes RNA primer to initiate DNA synthesis
e. Adds nucleoside monophosphates to the growing polynucleotides

40. The removal of introns and subsequent self-splicing of adjacent exons occurs in some portions of primary ribosomal RNA transcripts. The splicing of introns in messenger RNA precursors is

a. RNA-catalyzed in the absence of protein
b. Self-splicing
c. Carried out by spliceosomes
d. Controlled by RNA polymerase
e. Regulated by RNA helicase

41. A promoter site on DNA

a. Transcribes repressor
b. Initiates transcription
c. Codes for RNA polymerase
d. Regulates termination
e. Translates specific proteins

42. The σ factor found in many bacteria is best described as a

a. Subunit of RNA polymerase responsible for the specificity of the initiation of transcription of RNA from DNA
b. Subunit of DNA polymerase that allows for synthesis in both 5' to 3' and 3' to 5' directions
c. Subunit of the 50S ribosome that catalyzes peptide bond synthesis
d. Subunit of the 30S ribosome to which mRNA binds
e. Factor that forms the bridge between the 30S and 50S particles constituting the 70S ribosome

43. An immigrant from eastern Europe is rushed into the emergency room with nausea, vomiting, diarrhea, and abdominal pain. His family indicates he has eaten wild mushrooms. They have brought a bag of fresh, uncooked mushrooms from a batch he had not yet prepared. You note the presence of *Amanita phalloides,* the death-cap mushroom. A liver biopsy indicates massive hepatic necrosis. Care is supportive. A major toxin of the death-cap mushroom is the hepatotoxic octapeptide α-amanitin, which inhibits

a. DNA primase
b. RNA nuclease
c. DNA ligase
d. RNA polymerase
e. RNA/DNA endonuclease

44. The consensus sequence 5' TATAAAA 3' found in eukaryotic genes is quite similar to a consensus sequence observed in prokaryotes. It is important as the

a. Only site of binding of RNA polymerase III
b. Promoter for all RNA polymerases
c. Termination site for RNA polymerase II
d. Major binding site of RNA polymerase I
e. First site of binding of a transcription factor for RNA polymerase II

45. The so-called caps of RNA molecules

a. Allow tRNA to be processed
b. Occur at the 3' end of tRNA
c. Are composed of poly A
d. Are unique to eukaryotic mRNA
e. Allow correct translation of prokaryotic mRNA

46. In bacterial RNA synthesis, the function of factor ρ is to

a. Bind catabolite repressor to the promoter region
b. Increase the rate of RNA synthesis
c. Eliminate the binding of RNA polymerase to the promoter
d. Participate in the proper termination of transcription
e. Allow proper initiation of transcription

47. Which of the following statements correctly describes the nucleolus of a mammalian cell?

a. It differs from that found in bacterial cells in that histones are present
b. It may contain hundreds of copies of genes for different types of ribosomal RNAs
c. It synthesizes 5S ribosomal RNA
d. It synthesizes 60S and 40S ribosomal subunits
e. It synthesizes all ribosomal RNA primary transcripts

48. Which one of the following statements correctly describes the synthesis of mammalian messenger RNA (mRNA)?

a. Each mRNA often encodes several different proteins
b. Several different genes may produce identical mRNA molecules
c. There is colinearity of the RNA sequence transcribed from a gene and the amino acid sequence of its encoded protein
d. The RNA sequence transcribed from a gene is virtually identical to the mRNA that exits from nucleus to cytoplasm
e. Mammalian mRNA undergoes minimal modification during its maturation

49. Studies of the genetic code in bacteria have revealed that

a. Messenger RNA (mRNA) molecules specify only one polypeptide chain
b. Many triplets can be "nonsense" triplets
c. No signal exists to indicate the end of one codon and the beginning of another
d. The nucleotide on the 5′ end of a triplet has the least specificity for an amino acid
e. Gene sequence and encoded proteins are not colinear

50. Which one of the following binds to specific nucleotide sequences that are upstream of the start site of transcription?

a. RNA polymerase
b. Primase
c. Helicase
d. Histone protein
e. Restriction endonuclease

51. Template-directed RNA synthesis occurs in which of the following?

a. Point mutation
b. Triplet repeat expansion
c. Initiation of the polymerase chain reaction
d. Expression of oncogenes
e. Repair of thymine dimers

52. Which of the following most correctly describes mammalian messenger RNAs?

a. They are usually transcribed from both DNA strands
b. They are normally double-stranded
c. Their content of uridine equals their content of adenine
d. They have an overall negative charge at neutral pH
e. Their ratio of ribose to purine bases equals 1

53. The western blot use what type of probe?

a. Antibody
b. mRNA
c. Products of polymerase chain reaction (PCR)
d. tRNA
e. Mutant and normal oligonucleotides
f. rRNA
g. cDNA clone

54. What is the correct order of the following steps in protein synthesis?

1. A peptide bond is formed.
2. The small ribosomal subunit is loaded with initiation factors, messenger RNA, and initiation aminoacyl–transfer RNA.
3. The intact ribosome slides forward three bases to read a new codon.
4. The primed small ribosomal subunit binds with the large ribosomal subunit.
5. Elongation factors deliver aminoacyl-tRNA to bind to the A site.

a. 1, 2, 5, 4, 3
b. 2, 3, 4, 5, 1
c. 4, 5, 1, 2, 3
d. 3, 2, 4, 5, 1
e. 2, 4, 5, 1, 3

55. New proteins destined for secretion are synthesized in the

a. Golgi apparatus
b. Smooth endoplasmic reticulum
c. Free polysomes
d. Nucleus
e. Rough endoplasmic reticulum

56. Which of the following statements regarding eukaryotic cells is true?

a. Formylated methionyl-tRNA is important for initiation of translation
b. Single mRNAs specify more than one gene product
c. Cycloheximide blocks elongation during translation
d. Cytosolic ribosomes are smaller than those found in prokaryotes
e. Erythromycin inhibits elongation during translation

57. Modification of mRNA so that a signal sequence is added to the amino terminus of the cytosolic protein, α-globin, results in

a. No change in physiology of the protein
b. Proteolytic cleavage within the cytosol
c. Translocation across the endoplasmic reticulum
d. Cytosolic localization of the protein
e. Signal recognition particle synthesis

58. How many high-energy phosphate-bond equivalents are utilized in the process of activation of amino acids for protein synthesis?

a. Zero
b. One
c. Two
d. Three
e. Four

59. The hydrolytic step leading to the release of a polypeptide chain from a ribosome is catalyzed by

a. Stop codons
b. Peptidyl transferase
c. Release factors
d. Dissociation of ribosomes
e. UAA

60. The function of signal recognition particles is to

a. Cleave signal sequences
b. Detect cytosolic proteins
c. Direct the signal sequences to ribosomes
d. Bind ribosomes to endoplasmic reticulum
e. Bind mRNA to ribosomes

61. Which of the following statements about ribosomes is true?

a. They are an integral part of transcription
b. They are found both free in the cytoplasm and bound to membranes
c. They are bound together so tightly they cannot dissociate under physiologic conditions
d. They are composed of RNA, DNA, and protein
e. They are composed of three subunits of unequal size

62. Guanosine triphosphate (GTP) is required by which of the following steps in protein synthesis?

a. Aminoacyl-tRNA synthetase activation of amino acids
b. Attachment of ribosomes to endoplasmic reticulum
c. Translocation of tRNA–nascent protein complex from A to P sites
d. Attachment of mRNA to ribosomes
e. Attachment of signal recognition protein to ribosomes

63. Erythromycin is the antibiotic of choice when treating respiratory tract infections in legionnaire's disease, whooping cough, and *Mycoplasma*-based pneumonia because of its ability to inhibit protein synthesis in certain bacteria by

a. Inhibiting translocation by binding to 50S ribosomal subunits
b. Acting as an analogue of mRNA
c. Causing premature chain termination
d. Inhibiting initiation
e. Mimicking mRNA binding

64. An immigrant family from rural Mexico brings their 3-month-old child to the emergency room because of whistling inspiration (stridor) and high fever. The child's physician is perplexed because the throat examination shows a gray membrane almost occluding the larynx. A senior physician recognizes diphtheria, now rare in immunized populations. The child is intubated, antitoxin is administered, and antibiotic therapy is initiated. Diphtheria toxin is often lethal in unimmunized persons because it

a. Inhibits initiation of protein synthesis by preventing the binding of GTP to the 40S ribosomal subunit
b. Binds to the signal recognition particle receptor on the cytoplasmic face of the endoplasmic reticulum receptor
c. Shuts off signal peptidase
d. Blocks elongation of proteins by inactivating elongation factor 2 (EF-2, or translocase)
e. Causes deletions of amino acid by speeding up the movement of peptidyl-tRNA from the A site to the P site

65. A potent inhibitor of protein synthesis that acts as an analogue of aminoacyl-tRNA is

a. Mitomycin C
b. Streptomycin
c. Nalidixic acid
d. Rifampicin
e. Puromycin

66. Ribosomes similar to those of bacteria are found in

a. Plant nuclei
b. Cardiac muscle cytoplasm
c. Pancreatic mitochondria
d. Liver endoplasmic reticulum
e. Neuronal cytoplasm

67. Which of the following statements is true of all transfer (t) RNAs?

a. The 3′ end is phosphorylated
b. They are duplex chains
c. No methylated bases are found
d. The anticodon loop is identical
e. The 3′ end base sequence is CCA

68. Methionyl–transfer (t) RNA is used for initiation of protein synthesis by which of the following?

a. Chloroplast ribosomes
b. Eukaryotic mitochondrial ribosomes
c. Eukaryotic cytoplasmic ribosomes
d. Bacterial ribosomes
e. Bacterial cytoplasm

69. Which of the following is required for certain types of eukaryotic protein synthesis but not for prokaryotic protein synthesis?

a. Ribosomal RNA
b. Messenger RNA
c. Signal recognition particle
d. Peptidyl transferase
e. GTP

70. An older man with severe emphysema is found to have decreased amounts and abnormal mobility of α_1 antitrypsin (AAT) protein in his serum when analyzed by serum protein electrophoresis. Liver biopsy discloses mild scarring (cirrhosis) and demonstrates microscopic inclusions due to an engorged endoplasmic reticulum (ER). The most likely explanation for these findings is

a. Defective transport from hepatic ER to the serum
b. A mutation affecting the N-terminal methionine and blocking initiation of protein synthesis
c. A mutation affecting the signal sequence
d. Defective structure of the signal recognition particles
e. Defective energy metabolism causing deficiency of GTP

Gene Expression

Answers

33. The answer is b. (*Murray, pp 452–467. Scriver, pp 3–45. Sack, pp 1–40. Wilson, pp 101–120.*) The "genetic code" uses three-nucleotide "words," or codons, to specify the 20 different amino acids (see the chart below). There are 64 different three–base pair codons (three positions with four possible nucleotides at each). It follows that the genetic code must be degenerate, i.e., different codons can specify the same amino acid. Three codons are reserved as "stop" signals that result in peptide chain termination. The linear correspondence of codons in DNA and of amino acids in protein domains is interrupted by the presence of introns in DNA. Codons differ from the dinucleotide tandem repeats that provide useful DNA polymorphisms, or the trinucleotide repeats that can be responsible for disease. The genetic code is universal in the sense that codon–amino acid relationships are the same in all organisms.

First Nucleotide	Second Nucleotide				Third Nucleotide
	U	C	A	G	
U	Phe	Ser	Tyr	Cys	U
	Phe	Ser	Tyr	Cys	C
	Leu	Ser	Term	Term	A
	Leu	Ser	Term	Trp	G
C	Leu	Pro	His	Arg	U
	Leu	Pro	His	Arg	C
	Leu	Pro	Gln	Arg	A
	Leu	Pro	Gln	Arg	G
A	Ile	Thr	Asn	Ser	U
	Ile	Thr	Asn	Ser	C
	Ile	Thr	Lys	Arg	A
	Met	Thr	Lys	Arg	G
G	Val	Ala	Asp	Gly	U
	Val	Ala	Asp	Gly	C
	Val	Ala	Glu	Gly	A
	Val	Ala	Glu	Gly	G

The genetic code (codon assignments in messenger RNA.
(*Reproduced, with permission, from Murray RK, Granner DK, Mayes PA, Rodwell VW: Harper's Biochemistry, 25/e. New York, McGraw-Hill, 2000: 453.*)

34. The answer is d. (*Murray, pp 452–467. Scriver, pp 3–45. Sack, pp 1–40. Wilson, pp 101–120.*) Sickle cell anemia (141900) is an autosomal recessive hemoglobinopathy with an incidence of 1 in 500 African American births. It is caused by a single-nucleotide substitution in codon 6 of the β-globin gene. This mutation abolishes an enzyme site so that a larger DNA fragment is obtained after Southern blot analysis with the appropriate enzyme. Single-nucleotide substitutions do not change the length of coding regions (exons). The amplification of DNA segments using the polymerase chain reaction (PCR) allows more sensitive detection of restriction enzyme differences, and can be followed by allele-specific oligonucleotide (ASO) hybridization to determine the presence of normal versus sickle alleles. The equivalence of DNA in most tissues (with the exception of red blood cells that extrude their nucleus) makes DNA diagnosis a powerful technique that is independent of gene or protein expression. Western blotting is a technique that uses antibodies to highlight the size and amount of mutant protein in cell extracts. Since single-nucleotide changes in the gene may not affect protein size or conformation, western blotting is generally less sensitive and specific than DNA diagnosis.

35. The answer is c. (*Murray, pp 452–467. Scriver, pp 3–45. Sack, pp 1–40. Wilson, pp 101–120.*) Insertion (choice c) or deletion (choice d) of nucleotides shifts the reading frame unless the change is a multiple of 3 (choice e). Frame shifts may create unintended stop codons as in choice c. Point mutations resulting in nucleotide or amino acid substitutions are conveniently named by their position in the protein, i.e., $P_{21}A$ (choice b). The protein change $P_{21}A$ could also be denoted by the corresponding change in the DNA reading frame, i.e., $C_{63}A$. Deletions may be prefixed by the letter delta, as with ΔF_{25} (choice e).

36. The answer is c. (*Murray, pp 435–451. Scriver, pp 3–45. Sack, pp 1–40. Wilson, pp 151–180.*) Northern blotting is analogous to Southern blotting, a technique that was first described by Edward Southern. DNA fragments are separated on agarose gels by electrophoresis and then transferred to nitrocellulose filters. The filters are then exposed to labeled probes, which hybridize to the DNA fragments. Northern blotting is an analogous procedure that uses more powerful denaturing substances to extend the RNA molecules and ensure that their electrophoretic migration is inversely proportional to their length. Labeled RNA or DNA segments (probes) are used to identify particular RNA species within the size-separated array. Western blotting is a technique for detecting proteins. It uses a different type of denaturing gel and labeled antibodies as probes to detect specific proteins.

37. The answer is b. *(Murray, pp 452–467. Scriver, pp 3–45. Sack, pp 1–40. Wilson, pp 101–120.)* Exons are the coding portions of genes and consist of trinucleotide codons that guide the placement of specific amino acids into protein. Introns are the noncoding portions of genes that may function in evolution to provide "shuffling" of exons to produce new proteins. The primary RNA transcript contains both exons and introns, but the latter are removed by RNA splicing. The 5′ (upstream) and 3′ (downstream) untranslated RNA regions remain in the mature RNA and are thought to regulate RNA transport or translation. A poly(A) tail is added to the primary transcript after transcription, which facilitates transport and processing from the nucleus. The discovery of introns complicated Mendel's idea of the gene as the smallest hereditary unit; a modern definition might be the colinear sequence of exons, introns, and adjacent regulatory sequences that accomplish protein expression. Using these principles, one can determine the size of the stimulin gene. It contains a coding region of 300 bp (100 amino acids × 3 bp per amino acid), plus 100 bp in the intron, plus 70 + 30 = 100 bp in the untranslated regions (total = 500 bp). The mature RNA contains the same number of bp except for the 100 bp in the intron (500 − 100 = 400 bp). Transcription begins at the start of the 5′ untranslated region (70 bp) and the splice site occurs 30 bp (10 × 3) into the coding region at the beginning of the intron.

38. The answer is a. *(Murray, pp 452–467. Scriver, pp 3–45. Sack, pp 1–40. Wilson, pp 101–120.)* Splice junction mutations will theoretically produce a larger mRNA unless the mRNA is unstable; the larger protein may have abnormal function but retain peptide regions that react with antibody to the authentic protein. Nucleotide insertions or deletions other than multiples of 3 alter the reading frame of the code and scramble the amino acid sequence distal to the frame-shift mutation. Such altered mRNAs may be of increased or smaller size, depending on their stability, as may the translated protein, depending on the presence of stop codons within the shifted reading frame. Only the protein upstream of the frame-shift mutation retains immune cross-reactivity and normal function. Point mutations (nucleotide substitutions) may have substantial functional impact if the altered codon results in an amino acid substitution. If no amino acid substitution occurs, they are called silent mutations.

39. The answer is d. *(Murray, pp 435–451. Scriver, pp 3–45. Sack, pp 1–40. Wilson, pp 101–120.)* DNA synthesis cannot occur until an RNA primer is made. A specific type of RNA polymerase called primase synthesizes a short stretch of RNA of about five nucleotides that is complementary to the template DNA strand in duplex DNA near the replication fork. This function cannot be carried out by DNA polymerase. In contrast, both DNA polymerase and RNA polymerase work in the 5′ to 3′ direction and add nucleoside monophosphates from nucleotide triphosphates to the growing polynucleotide chains of DNA or RNA. Only DNA polymerase edits as it synthesizes DNA and fills the gap between Okazaki fragments.

40. The answer is c. *(Murray, pp 435–451. Scriver, pp 3–45. Sack, pp 1–40. Wilson, pp 101–120.)* Self-splicing of the introns of some primary ribosomal RNA transcripts occurs because of the presence of catalytic RNAs (ribozymes) generated from the introns. This occurs in the absence of protein catalysis. In contrast, the splicing of messenger RNA is carried out by spliceosomes. Spliceosomes are large complexes of three kinds of small ribonucleoprotein particles (snRNPs) and the messenger RNA precursor. The snRNPs are involved in recognizing the 5′ splice site and the 3′ splice site and then binding to these sites. Once the spliceosome is bound, it mediates excision of the intron and splicing of the two adjacent exons.

41. The answer is b. *(Murray, pp 435–451. Scriver, pp 3–45. Sack, pp 1–40. Wilson, pp 101–120.)* Promoter sites are initiation sites for transcription. Transcription starts when RNA polymerase binds to the promoter. It then unwinds the closed promoter complex, where DNA is in the form of a double helix, to form the open promoter complex in which about 17 base pairs of template DNA are unwound. RNA synthesis then begins with either a pppA or a pppG inserted at the beginning 5′-terminus of the new RNA chain, which is synthesized in the 5′ to 3′ direction.

42. The answer is a. *(Murray, pp 435–451. Scriver, pp 3–45. Sack, pp 1–40. Wilson, pp 101–120.)* σ factor is a bacterial protein that can associate with and become a subunit of bacterial RNA polymerase. σ factor confers specificity of initiation on the core enzyme. In the presence of σ factor, RNA polymerase chooses the correct strand of duplex DNA for transcription and initiates transcription at the appropriate promoter region. In some bacteria, such as *Bacillus subtilis*, a specific σ factor is synthesized to change transcriptional selectivity and effect cellular changes like sporulation.

43. The answer is d. (*Murray, pp 452–467. Scriver, pp 3–45. Sack, pp 1–40. Wilson, pp 101–120.*) The deadly mushroom *A. phalloides* has several toxins. A major toxin is α-amanitin, an octapeptide that inhibits mRNA synthesis by very tightly binding RNA polymerase II (DNA-dependent RNA polymerase). As little as one of the mushrooms (know as the death-cap, death-cup, or avenging angel) delivers a lethal dose of about 10 mg α-amanitin. Severe, irreversible liver damage occurs quickly, leading to death. At higher concentrations, the toxin can inhibit RNA polymerase III and tRNA synthesis. Polymerase I is unaffected. Since α-amanitin is effective at concentrations of 10^{-9} to 10^{-8} M, it has been useful as a research tool for studying RNA polymerase function.

44. The answer is e. (*Murray, pp 435–451. Scriver, pp 3–45. Sack, pp 1–40. Wilson, pp 101–120.*) The first event that occurs in mRNA synthesis is the binding of transcription factor TFIID to the TATA box. This consensus sequence portion of virtually all eukaryotic genes coding for mRNA is centered at about −25 and is similar to a 10-sequence promoter box found in prokaryotes. TFIID contains a TATA box–binding protein. The following sequence occurs in the initiation of mRNA synthesis:

1. TFIID binding to the TATA box
2. TFIIA binding
3. TFIIB binding
4. RNA polymerase II binding
5. TFIIE binding

When all these elements are bound to DNA, the basal transcription apparatus complex is formed and can transcribe DNA slowly. Other factors are required for fast, efficient mRNA synthesis.

45. The answer is d. (*Murray, pp 452–467. Scriver, pp 3–45. Sack, pp 1–40. Wilson, pp 101–120.*) The primary transcripts of all eukaryotic mRNAs are capped at the 5′ end. Prokaryotic RNAs and eukaryotic tRNA and rRNA are not capped. The cap is composed of 7-methylguanylate attached by a pyrophosphate linkage to the 5' end. This is known as cap 0. One of the adjacent riboses is methylated in cap 1, and both of the adjacent riboses are methylated in cap 2. The cap protects the 5' ends of mRNAs from nucleases and phosphatases and is essential for the recognition of eukaryotic mRNAs in the protein-synthesizing system. When prokaryotic monocistronic mRNAs are artificially capped, translation occurs in a eukaryotic, in vitro translation system.

46. The answer is d. *(Murray, pp 435–451. Scriver, pp 3–45. Sack, pp 1–40. Wilson, pp 101–120.)* Bacterial DNA contains stop signals, some of which require ρ protein. This has been demonstrated by examining the synthesis of mRNA in the presence and absence of ρ protein. In the absence of ρ protein, longer RNA molecules are often synthesized. This would seem to indicate that mRNA length can be controlled by the cell. In addition, antiterminator proteins are needed to allow certain genes to be properly expressed. Mammalian mechanisms for transcription termination, and the likely presence of factors regulating termination, are not yet characterized.

47. The answer is b. *(Murray, pp 452–467. Scriver, pp 3–45. Sack, pp 1–40. Wilson, pp 101–120.)* The nucleolus is an organelle unique to eukaryotic cells. It is the site where hundreds of copies of genes repeated in tandem for three of the four ribosomal RNAs are transcribed by RNA polymerase I to give a 45S primary transcript. Enzymatic modification and cleavage remove spacer regions to yield 28S, 18S, and 5.8S ribosomal RNA. The 5S subunit is synthesized by RNA polymerase III in the nucleoplasm rather than in the nucleolus. Ribosomal proteins combine with the ribosomal subunits to assemble into a 60S subunit containing the 5S, 5.8S, and 28S RNAs and a 40S subunit containing the 18S RNA. Combined, the two subunits produce a functional eukaryotic ribosome with a sedimentation coefficient of 80S.

48. The answer is b. *(Murray, pp 452–467. Scriver, pp 3–45. Sack, pp 1–40. Wilson, pp 101–120.)* About 30% of the DNA of humans and other mammals consists of repeated sequences. Repetitive DNA includes numerous families of genes like those for histones. Some families of repeated genes make identical mRNA molecules, suggesting that their multiple gene copies are needed to make adequate amounts of protein. Although many genes in bacteria produce a polycistronic mRNA that encodes several different peptides, all mRNAs in mammals encode a single peptide and are monocistronic. In addition, RNA is initially transcribed from protein-encoding genes as larger molecules called heterogenous nuclear RNA (hnRNA). These immature hnRNA molecules must be spliced to remove introns and chemically modified with 5′ caps and 3′-polyA sequences before reaching the cytoplasm as functional mRNA. The initial HnRNA transcript is colinear with its encoded protein within exons but not within introns. Mature mRNAs also have 5′ and 3′ untranslated regions that are not colinear with the encoded peptide.

49. The answer is c. (*Murray, pp 452–467. Scriver, pp 3–45. Sack, pp 1–40. Wilson, pp 101–120.*) In the mRNAs of bacteria and the exonic mRNA regions of mammals, the triplet nucleotides comprising codons are continuous, without "spacers" to mark the end of one codon and the beginning of another. These RNA regions and their product peptides are also colinear with the gene (DNA) sequence. Bacterial mRNA molecules are polycistronic and code for more than one polypeptide chain or enzyme, allowing their coordinate regulation in response to metabolic or environmental signals. There are only three "nonsense" or chain-terminating codons and 61 "sense" codons that encode for 20 amino acids. Redundancy of the code (several codons code for the same amino acid) is compensated for by the "wobble" hypothesis of Crick. The complementary anticodons of charged transfer RNAs hybridize stringently at the first two positions of the codon but weakly ("wobbly") at the third position. One aminoacyl–transfer RNA can thus recognize several different codons, each identical at the first two positions but different at the third.

50. The answer is a. (*Murray, pp 435–451. Scriver, pp 3–45. Sack, pp 1–40. Wilson, pp 101–120.*) In mammals, RNA polymerase binds to promoter sites upstream from the start site. These include the TATA box (TATAAT), the CAAT box, and the GC box. DNA primase and helicase are involved in DNA replication and do not bind specifically to sequences upstream of genes. Restriction endonucleases recognize specific sequences in double-helical DNA and cleave both strands. Histones nonspecifically bind to chromosomal DNA and constitute about half the mass of mammalian chromosomes.

51. The answer is d. *(Murray, pp 435–451. Scriver, pp 3–45. Sack, pp 1–40. Wilson, pp 101–120.)* Oncogenes are cancer-producing genes. They are closely related to normal cellular genes and are often tyrosine kinases, growth factors, or receptors for growth factors. The expression of oncogenes leads to the translation and eventual transcription of the protein product of the oncogene. Thus, template-directed RNA synthesis but not DNA synthesis occurs during the expression of oncogenes. In contrast, template-directed DNA synthesis rather than RNA synthesis occurs during the repair of thymine dimers, the polymerase chain reaction, the functioning of the replication fork, and the growth of RNA tumor viruses. In the final stages of the repair of thymine dimers, once the dimer has been excised, DNA polymerase I enters the gap to carry out template-directed synthesis. In functioning of the replication fork, DNA polymerase III holoenzyme carries out synthesis of DNA during replication. Template-directed DNA synthesis is required for the growth of RNA tumor viruses (retroviruses). Once released into the host cytoplasm, retroviral RNA synthesizes both the positive and minus strands of DNA, using reverse transcriptase. This unique enzyme catalyzes the initial RNA-directed DNA synthesis, hydrolysis of RNA, and then DNA-directed DNA synthesis. The newly formed viral DNA duplex integrates into the host cell DNA prior to transcription. In this form, the retrovirus is inherited by daughter host cells. The polymerase chain reaction is a method of amplifying the amount of DNA in a sample or of enriching particular DNA sequences in a population of DNA molecules. In the polymerase chain reaction, oligonucleotides complementary to the ends of the desired DNA sequence are used as primer for multiple rounds of template-directed DNA synthesis.

52. The answer is d. *(Murray, pp 435–451. Scriver, pp 3–45. Sack, pp 1–40. Wilson, pp 101–120.)* At a physiologic pH of 7.4, mRNAs (like DNA) are polyanionic owing to the negatively charged phosphate hydroxyl groups. Mammalian mRNAs are synthesized from DNA as single-stranded linear molecules. Because they are not double-stranded, the concentrations of the different bases in mRNA are variable rather than exhibiting the A = T and G = C pattern of double-stranded DNA (A does not equal U in mRNA). The hybridization of RNA with its complementary template DNA is antiparallel. In both DNA and RNA, sugar units equal base units equal phosphate units. However, their bases consist of pyrimidines as well as purines.

53. The answer is a. (*Murray, pp 435–451. Scriver, pp 3–45. Sack, pp 1–40. Wilson, pp 101–120.*) In an expression library, cDNA clones are screened on the basis of their ability to direct bacterial synthesis of a foreign protein of interest. Radioactive antibodies specific to this protein can be used to identify the colonies of bacteria that contain the cDNA vector. As was the case for probing genomic libraries, bacteria grown on a master plate are blotted onto a nitrocellulose replica plate and then lysed. The released proteins may then be labeled with ^{125}I antibodies. In contrast, northern blotting can be used to identify RNA molecules separated by gel electrophoresis. In northern blotting, RNA molecules separated by gel electrophoresis can be identified by hybridization with probe DNA following transfer to nitrocellulose. Mutant and wild-type oligonucleotides can be used as probes to analyze polymerase chain reaction products. Conversely, the products of polymerase chain reaction can be used to analyze cDNA libraries.

54. The answer is e. (*Murray, pp 452–467. Scriver, pp 3–45. Sack, pp 1–40. Wilson, pp 101–120.*) Despite some differences, protein synthesis in prokaryotes and eukaryotes is quite similar. The small ribosomal subunit is 30S in prokaryotes and 40S in eukaryotes. The large ribosomal subunit is 50S in prokaryotes and 60S in eukaryotes. The intact ribosome is consequently larger in eukaryotes (80S) and smaller in prokaryotes (70S). At the start of translation, initiation factors, mRNA, and initiation aminoacyl-tRNA bind to the dissociated small ribosomal subunit. The initiation tRNA in prokaryotes is N-formyl methionine in prokaryotes and simply methionine in eukaryotes. Only after the small ribosomal subunit is primed with mRNA and initiation aminoacyl-tRNA does the large ribosomal subunit bind to it. Once this happens, elongation factors bring the first aminoacyl-tRNA of the nascent protein to the A site. Then peptidyl transferase forges a peptide bond between the initiation amino acid and the first amino acid of the forming peptide. The now uncharged initiation tRNA leaves the P site and the peptidyl-tRNA from the A site moves to the now vacant P site with the two amino acids attached. The ribosome advances three bases to read the next codon and the process repeats. When the stop signal is reached after the complete polypeptide has been synthesized, releasing factors bind to the stop signal, causing peptidyl transferase to hydrolyze the bond that joins the polypeptide at the A site to the tRNA. Factors prevent the reassociation of ribosomal subunits in the absence of new initiation complex.

55. The answer is e. (*Murray, pp 452–467. Scriver, pp 3–45. Sack, pp 1–40. Wilson, pp 101–120.*) Protein synthesis occurs in the cytoplasm, on groups of free ribosomes called polysomes, and on ribosomes associated with membranes, termed the rough endoplasmic reticulum. However, proteins destined for secretion are only synthesized on ribosomes of the endoplasmic reticulum and are synthesized in such a manner that they end up inside the lumen of the endoplasmic reticulum. From there the secretory proteins are packaged in vesicles. The Golgi apparatus is involved in the glycosylation and packaging of macromolecules into membranes for secretion.

56. The answer is c. (*Murray, pp 452–467. Scriver, pp 3–45. Sack, pp 1–40. Wilson, pp 101–120.*) In a general sense, the mechanism of protein synthesis in eukaryotic cells is similar to that found in prokaryotes; however, there are significant differences. Cycloheximide inhibits elongation of proteins in eukaryotes, while erythromycin causes the same effect in prokaryotes. Thus, one is an antibiotic beneficial to humans, while the other is a poison. Cytoplasmic ribosomes of eukaryotes are larger, sedimenting at 80S instead of 70S. While eukaryotic cells utilize a specific tRNA for initiation, it is not formylated as in bacteria. Finally, eukaryotic mRNA always specifies only one polypeptide, as opposed to prokaryotic mRNA, which may specify the synthesis of more than one gene product per mRNA.

57. The answer is c. (*Murray, pp 435–451. Scriver, pp 3–45. Sack, pp 1–40. Wilson, pp 101–120.*) By using recombinant DNA techniques, mRNAs can be produced that yield chimeric proteins. By forming mRNAs that produce otherwise cytosolic proteins, as when α-globin is engineered with a cleavable amino terminal signal sequence, this otherwise cytosolic protein becomes a secretory protein and is translocated into the lumen of endoplasmic reticulum. The signal sequence thus contains all the information needed to direct the translocation of protein across endoplasmic reticulum. These experiments were performed by adding chimeric mRNA to an in vitro system of protein synthesis composed of endoplasmic reticulum vesicles, ribosomes, tRNAs, and other factors required for protein synthesis. Without the modified amino terminal signal sequence, the α-globin is released into the experimental solution, and with the signal sequence it is synthesized into the lumen of the endoplasmic reticulum vesicles.

58. The answer is c. (*Murray, pp 452–467. Scriver, pp 3–45. Sack, pp 1–40. Wilson, pp 101–120.*) ATP is required for the esterification of amino acids to their corresponding tRNAs. This reaction is catalyzed by the class of enzymes known as aminoacyl-tRNA synthetases. Each one of these enzymes is specific for one tRNA and its corresponding amino acid.

$$\text{amino acid} + \text{tRNA} + \text{ATP} \rightarrow \text{aminoacyl-tRNA} + \text{AMP} + \text{PP}_i$$

As with most ATP hydrolysis reactions that release pyrophosphate, pyrophosphatase quickly hydrolyzes the product to P_i, which makes the reaction essentially irreversible. Since ATP is hydrolyzed to AMP and PP_i during the reaction, by convention the equivalent of two high-energy phosphate bonds is utilized.

59. The answer is b. (*Murray, pp 452–467. Scriver, pp 3–45. Sack, pp 1–40. Wilson, pp 101–120.*) During the course of protein synthesis on a ribosome, peptidyl transferase catalyzes the formation of peptide bonds. However, when a stop codon such as UAA, UGA, or UAG is reached, aminoacyl-tRNA does not bind to the A site of a ribosome. One of the proteins, known as a release factor, binds to the specific trinucleotide sequence present. This binding of the release factor activates peptidyl transferase to hydrolyze the bond between the polypeptide and the tRNA occupying the P site. Thus, instead of forming a peptide bond, peptidyl transferase catalyzes the hydrolytic step that leads to the release of newly synthesized proteins. Following release of the polypeptide, the ribosome dissociates into its major subunits.

60. The answer is d. (*Murray, pp 452–467. Scriver, pp 3–45. Sack, pp 1–40. Wilson, pp 101–120.*) The directing of nascent polypeptide chains to the endoplasmic reticulum is regulated by signal recognition particles (SRPs). The signal sequence of a nascent protein is recognized by an SRP, which complexes with the ribosome, mRNA, and the nascent protein. The complexed SRP then binds to an SRP receptor on the surface of the endoplasmic reticulum. After the ribosome is transferred to ribophorins and the translocation begins, SRP is released back into the cytosol. Ribosomes with nascent protein without a signal sequence do not participate in this process and instead synthesize proteins that are released into the cytosol.

61. The answer is b. *(Murray, pp 452–467. Scriver, pp 3–45. Sack, pp 1–40. Wilson, pp 101–120.)* The two subunits of ribosomes are composed of proteins and rRNA. Ribosomes are found in the cytoplasm, in mitochondria, and bound to the endoplasmic reticulum. Transcription refers to the synthesis of RNA complementary to a DNA template and has nothing immediately to do with ribosomes.

62. The answer is c. *(Murray, pp 452–467. Scriver, pp 3–45. Sack, pp 1–40. Wilson, pp 101–120.)* Two molecules of GTP are used in the formation of each peptide bond on the ribosome. In the elongation cycle, binding of aminoacyl-tRNA delivered by EF-Tu to the A site requires hydrolysis of one GTP. Peptide bond formation then occurs. Translocation of the nascent peptide chain on tRNA to the P site requires hydrolysis of a second GTP. The activation of amino acids with aminoacyl-tRNA synthetase requires hydrolysis of ATP to AMP plus PP_i.

63. The answer is a. *(Murray, pp 452–467. Scriver, pp 3–45. Sack, pp 1–40. Wilson, pp 101–120.)* Virulent strains of bacteria that cause severe, life-threatening respiratory tract infections can often be successfully treated with erythromycin. These include *Mycoplasma pneumoniae*, various *Legionella* species, and *Bordetella pertussis*. The mechanism of action of erythromycin is to specifically bind the 50S subunit of bacterial ribosomes. Under normal conditions, after mRNA attaches to the initiation site of the 30S subunit, the 50S subunit binds to the 30S complex and forms the 70S complex that allows protein chain elongation to go forward. Elongation is prevented in the presence of erythromycin.

64. The answer is d. *(Murray, pp 452–467. Scriver, pp 3–45. Sack, pp 1–40. Wilson, pp 101–120.)* The gene that produces the deadly toxin of *Corynebacterium diphtheriae* comes from a lysogenic phage that grows in the bacteria. Prior to immunization, diphtheria was the primary cause of death in children. The protein toxin produced by this bacterium inhibits protein synthesis by inactivating elongation factor 2 (EF-2, or translocase). Diphtheria toxin is a single protein composed of two portions (A and B). The B portion enables the A portion to translocate across a cell membrane into the cytoplasm. The A portion catalyzes the transfer of the adenosine diphosphate ribose unit of NAD_1 to a nitrogen atom of the diphthamide ring of EF-2, thereby blocking translocation. Diphthamide is an unusual amino acid residue of EF-2.

65. The answer is e. *(Murray, pp 452–467. Scriver, pp 3–45. Sack, pp 1–40. Wilson, pp 101–120.)* Puromycin is virtually identical in structure to the 3′-terminal end of tyrosinyl-tRNA. In both eukaryotic and prokaryotic cells, it is accepted as a tyrosinyl-tRNA analogue. As such, it is incorporated into the carboxy-terminal position of a peptide at the aminoacyl (A) site on ribosomes, causing premature release of the nascent polypeptide. Thus, puromycin inhibits protein synthesis in both human and bacterial cells. Streptomycin, like tetracycline and chloramphenicol, inhibits ribosomal activity. Mitomycin covalently cross-links DNA, which prevents cell replication. Rifampicin is an inhibitor of bacterial DNA-dependent RNA polymerase.

66. The answer is c. *(Murray, pp 452–467. Scriver, pp 3–45. Sack, pp 1–40. Wilson, pp 101–120.)* Prokaryotic ribosomes have a sedimentation coefficient of 70S and are composed of 50S and 30S subunits. Eukaryotic cytoplasmic ribosomes, either free or bound to the endoplasmic reticulum, are larger—60S and 40S subunits that associate to an 80S ribosome. Nuclear ribosomes are attached to the endoplasmic reticulum of the nuclear membrane. Ribosomes in chloroplasts and mitochondria of eukaryotic cells are more similar to prokaryotic ribosomes than to eukaryotic cytosolic ribosomes. Like bacterial ribosomes, chloroplast and mitochondrial ribosomes use a formylated tRNA. In addition, they are sensitive to many of the inhibitors of protein synthesis in bacteria.

67. The answer is e. *(Murray, pp 452–467. Scriver, pp 3–45. Sack, pp 1–40. Wilson, pp 101–120.)* For transfer RNAs, the 5′ end is often guanosine and is always phosphorylated, while the 3′ end is CCA. Although transfer (t) RNA molecules have many features in common, the primary feature that sets them apart is their specificity for different amino acids and the corresponding specific differences of their anticodons. Each tRNA is an L-shaped single chain composed of up to 93 ribonucleotides. Each contains up to 15 methylated bases, and about half of the nucleotides are base-paired into double helices. Activated amino acids attach to the terminal 3′-hydroxyl group of the adenosine.

68. The answer is c. *(Murray, pp 452–467. Scriver, pp 3–45. Sack, pp 1–40. Wilson, pp 101–120.)* Methionyl-tRNA is the special tRNA used in eukaryotes for initiation. Initiation of protein synthesis by bacterial, mitochondrial, and chloroplast ribosomes requires *N*-formylmethionyl-tRNA. The mitochondria of eukaryotic cells are similar to bacteria in the size of their ribosomal RNAs (23S and 16S) and their mechanisms for protein synthesis. Mitochondrial and prokaryotic ribosomes (including those of chloroplasts and bacteria) use formylmethionyl-tRNA for initiation of protein synthesis and are sensitive to inhibitors like streptomycin, tetracycline, and chloramphenicol that have little effect on eukaryotic cells. The latter drugs are useful as antibiotics in animals and humans since they inhibit bacteria but do not gain entry into mitochondria.

69. The answer is c. (*Murray, pp 452–467. Scriver, pp 3–45. Sack, pp 1–40. Wilson, pp 101–120.*) Signal recognition particles (SRPs) recognize the signal sequence on the N-terminal end of proteins destined for the lumen of the endoplasmic reticulum (ER). SRP binding arrests translation and an SRP receptor facilitates import of the SRP, ribosome, and nascent protein into the ER lumen. A signal peptidase removes the signal sequence from the protein, which may remain in the membrane or be routed for secretion. Common to both eukaryotic and prokaryotic protein synthesis is the requirement for ATP to activate amino acids. The activated aminoacyl-tRNAs then interact with ribosomes carrying mRNA. Peptidyl transferase catalyzes the formation of peptide bonds between the free amino group of activated aminoacyl-tRNA on the A site of the ribosome and the esterified carboxyl group of the peptidyl-rRNA on the P site; the liberated rRNA remains on the P site.

70. The answer is a. (*Murray, pp 452–467. Scriver, pp 5559–5628. Sack, pp 1–40. Wilson, pp 101–120.*) The decreased amount of AAT protein, its abnormal mobility, and the engorgement of liver ER suggest a mutant AAT that is inefficiently transported from the ER to serum. Since other serum protein abnormalities were not mentioned, general deficiencies of protein synthesis arising from defective energy metabolism or defective signal recognition particles are unlikely. A mutation affecting the N-terminal methionine of AAT or its signal sequence should drastically decrease its synthesis and import to the ER lumen. This would not explain the engorgement of liver ER. The usual binding of the signal recognition particle to the signal sequence of AAT, followed by import into the ER lumen, seems intact. An altered amino acid necessary for signal peptidase cleavage of the signal sequence of AAT might be invoked, but a general deficiency of the

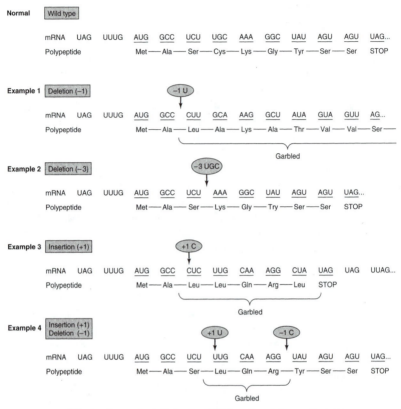

Effects of gene mutations on mRNA and protein products.
(Reproduced, with permission, from Murray RK, Granner DK, Mayes PA, Rodwell VW:
Harper's Biochemistry, 25/e. New York, McGraw-Hill, 2000: 458.)

signal peptidase should disrupt many secreted proteins and be an embryonic lethal mutation. AAT deficiency (107400) is a well-characterized autosomal dominant disease with common ZZ, SZ, and SS genotypes that can cause childhood liver disease and adult emphysema. The Z and S mutations alter AAT conformation and interfere with its secretion from ER to serum. Lack of AAT protection from proteases in lung is thought to cause the thinning of alveolar walls and dysfunctional "air sacs" of emphysema. The figure below illustrates how changes in the DNA code can effect protein products.

Gene Regulation

Questions

DIRECTIONS: Each item below contains a question or incomplete statement followed by suggested responses. Select the **one best** response to each question.

71. A patient suffers from adenosine deaminase (ADA) deficiency, an autosomal recessive immune deficiency in which bone marrow lymphoblasts cannot replicate to generate immunocompetent lymphocytes. The treatment option that would permanently cure the patient is

a. Germ-line gene therapy to replace one ADA gene copy
b. Germ-line gene therapy to replace both ADA gene copies
c. Somatic cell gene therapy to replace one ADA gene copy in circulating lymphocytes
d. Somatic cell gene therapy to replace both ADA gene copies in circulating lymphocytes
e. Somatic cell gene therapy to replace one ADA gene copy in bone marrow lymphoblasts

72. A major obstacle to gene therapy involves the difficulty of homologous gene replacement. Which of the following strategies addresses this issue?

a. A recombinant vector contains complementary DNA sequences that will facilitate site-specific recombination
b. A recombinant vector expresses antisense nucleotides that will hybridize with the targeted mRNA
c. A recombinant vector replaces inessential viral genes with a functional human gene
d. A recombinant vector transfects patient cells, which are returned to the patient
e. A recombinant vector contains DNA sequences that target its expressed protein to lysosomes

73. A family in which several individuals have arthritis and detached retina is diagnosed with Stickler syndrome. The locus for Stickler syndrome has been mapped near that for type II collagen on chromosome 12, and mutations in the COL2A1 gene have been described in Stickler syndrome. The family became interested in molecular diagnosis to distinguish normal from mildly affected individuals. Which of the results below would be expected in an individual with a promoter mutation at one COL2A1 gene locus?

a. Western blotting detects no type II collagen chains
b. Southern blotting using intronic restriction sites yields normal restriction fragment sizes
c. Reverse transcriptase–polymerase chain reaction (RT-PCR) detects one-half normal amounts of COL2A1 mRNA in affected individuals
d. Fluorescent in situ hybridization (FISH) analysis using a COL2A1 probe detects signals on only one chromosome 12
e. DNA sequencing reveals a single nucleotide difference between homologous COL2A1 exons

74. Gyrate atrophy (258870) is a rare autosomal recessive genetic disorder caused by a deficiency of ornithine aminotransferase. Affected individuals experience progressive chorioretinal degeneration. The gene for ornithine aminotransferase has been cloned, its structure has been determined, and mutations in affected individuals have been extensively studied. Which of the mutations listed below best fits with test results showing normal Southern blots with probes from all ornithine aminotransferase exons but absent enzymatic activity?

a. Duplication of entire gene
b. Two-kb deletion in coding region of gene
c. Two-kb insertion in coding region of gene
d. Deletion of entire gene
e. Missense mutation

75. A 5-year-old Egyptian boy receives a sulfonamide antibiotic as prophylaxis for recurrent urinary tract infections. Although he was previously healthy and well-nourished, he becomes progressively ill and presents to your office with pallor and irritability. A blood count shows that he is severely anemic with jaundice due to hemolysis of red blood cells. Which of the following would be the simplest test for diagnosis?

a. Northern blotting of red blood cell mRNA
b. Enzyme assay of red blood cell hemolysate
c. Western blotting of red blood cell hemolysates
d. Amplification of red blood cell DNA and hybridization with allele-specific oligonucleotides (PCR-ASOs)
e. Southern blot analysis for gene deletions

76. Hurler's syndrome (252800) is caused by a deficiency of L-iduronidase, an enzyme normally expressed in most human cell types. It was demonstrated by Neufeld that exogenous L-iduronidase could be taken up by deficient cells via a targeting signal that directed the enzyme to its normal lysosomal location. Which of the therapeutic strategies below would be the most realistic and efficient mode of therapy?

a. Germ-line gene therapy
b. Heterologous bone marrow transplant
c. Infection with a disabled adenovirus vector that carries the L-iduronidase gene
d. Injection with L-iduronidase purified from human liver
e. Autologous bone marrow transplant after transfection with a virus carrying the L-iduronidase gene

77. Which of the following mutations is most likely to be lethal?

a. Substitution of adenine for cytosine
b. Substitution of cytosine for guanine
c. Substitution of methylcytosine for cytosine
d. Deletion of three nucleotides
e. Insertion of one nucleotide

78. In the following partial sequence of mRNA, a mutation of the template DNA results in a change in codon 91 to UAA. What type of mutation is it?

88	89	90	91	92	93	94
GUC	GAC	CAG	UAG	GGC	UAA	CCG

a. Missense
b. Silent
c. Nonsense
d. Suppressor
e. Frame shift

79. Which one of the following causes a frame-shift mutation?

a. Transition
b. Transversion
c. Deletion
d. Substitution of purine for pyrimidine
e. Substitution of pyrimidine for purine

80. Most thalassemias are the result of mutations causing

a. Increased α chain synthesis
b. "Sticky" hemoglobin
c. RNA processing or production defects
d. Protein folding problems
e. Absence of both A and B hemoglobin

81. Which of the following would not be expected to result in a dysfunctional protein?

a. Mutation affecting the splice site of an intron
b. Substitution of glycine for alanine at the carboxyl terminus
c. Insertion of two bases in the code for the amino end
d. Nonsense mutation affecting the middle of a potential protein product
e. Deletion of a single base of a codon near the middle of a potential protein

82. Which of the following is a true statement about translation?

a. The genetic code can be overlapping
b. The first nucleotide in a codon has less specificity than the others
c. Only one group of nucleotides codes for each single amino acid
d. Every codon (three nucleotide bases) specifies an amino acid
e. Specific nucleotide sequences signal termination of peptide chains

83. Part of the triplet genetic code involving mRNA codon triplets that start with U is shown below.

5' End (Nucleotide 1)	Middle		3' End (Nucleotide 2)	(Nucleotide 3)
	U	C A	G	
	phe	ser tyr	cys	U
	phe	ser tyr	cys	C
U	leu	ser stop	stop	A
	leu	ser stop	stop	G

Using the portion of the genetic code shown, which of the following mutations in the 3' to 5' DNA coding segments corresponds to a nonsense mutation?

a. ACGACGACG to ACAAACACG
b. AGGAATATG to AGGAATATT
c. AGAATAACA to AAAATAACA
d. AAAATGAGC to AAAATAAGC
e. AACAACAAC to AACAAGAAC
f. AGAATCAAA to AGAATCAAA
g. AAAAAGAGG to ATAAAGAGG

84. Which of the following best describes the negatively controlled lactose operon in *Escherichia coli*?

a. An inducer (lactose) binds to the operator, enhancing simultaneous transcription and translation of β-galactosidase (z), permease (y), and transacetylase (a) genes

b. An inducer (lactose) alters the repressor protein and uncovers the operator and promoter, allowing simultaneous transcription and translation of β-galactosidase (z), permease (y), and transacetylase (a) genes

c. The repressor (lactose) alters the operator protein and uncovers the promoter, allowing simultaneous transcription and translation of β-galactosidase (z), permease (y), and transacetylase (a) genes

d. The repressor (lactose) alters the catabolite repression protein and uncovers the operator and promoter, allowing simultaneous transcription and translation of β-galactosidase (z), permease (y), and transacetylase (a) genes

e. An inducer (lactose) alters the repressor protein, uncovers the β-galactosidase (z) operator, and allows transcription. The inducer also uncovers separate operators for the permease (y) and transacetylase (a) genes

85. The lactose operon is negatively controlled by the lactose repressor and positively controlled by which of the following?

a. Increased concentrations of glucose and cyclic AMP (cAMP)

b. Decreased concentrations of glucose and cAMP

c. Increased concentrations of glucose, decreased concentration of cAMP

d. Decreased concentrations of glucose, increased concentration of cAMP

e. Increased concentrations of glucose and adenosine triphosphate (ATP)

86. Which of the following regulators are said to act in "*cis*"?

a. The *lac* repressor and mammalian transcription factors

b. The *lac* repressor and the *lac* operator

c. The *lac* operator and mammalian enhancers

d. The *lac* operator and mammalian transcription factors

e. Mammalian transcription factors and enhancers

87. Which of the structural domains of mammalian regulatory factors may be called intracellular receptors?

a. Response elements
b. Antirepressor domains
c. Transcription-activating domains
d. Ligand-binding domains
e. DNA-binding domains

88. The proopiomelanocortin (POMC) gene encodes several regulatory proteins that affect pituitary function. In different brain regions, proteins encoded by this gene have different carboxy-terminal peptides. Which of the following best explains the regulatory mechanism?

a. POMC transcription is regulated by different factors in different brain regions
b. POMC translation elongation is regulated by different factors in different brain regions
c. POMC transcription has different enhancers in different brain regions
d. POMC protein undergoes different protein processing in different brain regions
e. POMC protein forms different allosteric complexes in different brain regions

89. An Asian child has severe anemia with prominence of the forehead (frontal bossing) and cheeks. The red cell hemoglobin concentration is dramatically decreased, and it contains only β-globin chains with virtual deficiency of α-globin chains. Which of the following mechanisms is a potential explanation?

a. A transcription factor regulating the α-globin gene is mutated
b. A regulatory sequence element has been mutated adjacent to an α-globin gene
c. A transcription factor regulating the β-globin gene is mutated
d. A transcription factor regulating the α-globin and β-globin genes is deficient
e. A deletion has occurred surrounding an α-globin gene

90. Which of the following is involved in determining antibody class?

a. Different rearrangements of V-D-J and C segments in heavy chains
b. Different V-D-J rearrangements in heavy chains
c. Different V-J rearrangements in light chains
d. Alternative splicing to switch from κ to λ light chains
e. Alternative splicing to switch from membrane-bound to secreted antibody

91. Two boys with mental disability are found to have mutations in a gene on the X chromosome that has no homology with globin genes. Both are also noted to have deficiency of α-globin synthesis with α thalassemia. Which of the following is the best explanation for their phenotype?

a. The mutation disrupted an enhancer for an α-globin pseudogene
b. The mutation disrupted an X-encoded transcription factor that regulates the α-globin loci
c. There is a second mutation that disrupts an enhancer near the α-globin gene
d. There is a DNA rearrangement that joins the mutated X chromosome gene with an α-globin gene
e. There is a second mutation that disrupts the promoter of an α-globin gene

92. A middle-aged man presents with a markedly enlarged tonsil and recurrent infections with serum immunoglobulin deficiency. Chromosome analysis demonstrates a translocation between the immunuglobulin heavy chain locus on chromosome 14 and an unidentified gene on chromosome 8. Which of the following is the most likely cause of his phenotype?

a. The translocation has deleted constant chain exons on chromosome 14 and prevented heavy chain class switching
b. The translocation has deleted the interval containing diversity (D) and joining (J) regions
c. The translocation has activated a tumor-promoting gene on chromosome 8
d. The translocation has deleted the heavy chain constant chain Cμ so that virgin B cells cannot produce IgM on their membranes
e. The translocation has deleted an immunoglobulin transcription factor gene on chromosome 8

Gene Regulation

Answers

71. The answer is e. (*Murray, pp 468–487. Scriver, pp 175–192. Sack, pp 245–257. Wilson, pp 151–180.*) Gene therapy refers to a group of techniques by which gene structure or expression is altered to ameliorate a disease. Because of ethical and practical difficulties, germ-line therapy involving alterations of genes in primordial germ cells is not being explored in humans. Although germ-line genetic engineering is being performed in animals with the goals of improved breeding or agricultural yield, it alters the characteristics of offspring rather than the treated individuals. Somatic cell gene therapy is targeted to an affected tissue or group of tissues in the individual, and is most effective if stem cells such as bone marrow can be treated. Somatic cell gene therapy offers the hope of replacing damaged tissue without the rejection problems of transplantation. For autosomal recessive disorders, only one of the two defective alleles must be replaced or supplemented.

72. The answer is a. (*Murray, pp 468–487. Scriver, pp 175–192. Sack, pp 245–257. Wilson, pp 227–244.*) Challenges for gene therapy include the construction of recombinant viral genomes that can propagate the replacement gene (gene constructs or vectors), delivery of the altered gene to the appropriate tissues (gene targeting), and recombination at the appropriate locus so that replacement of the defective gene is achieved (site-specific recombination). The latter step positions DNA sequences in the vector so that the replacement gene pairs and recombines precisely with homologous DNA in the native gene. Ex vivo transfection (introduction of vector DNA into patient cells outside the body) is an ideal method for gene targeting if the engineered cells can repopulate the tissue/organ in question. Transfection of bone marrow stem cells with a functional adenosine deaminase gene, followed by bone marrow transplantation back to the patient, has been successful in restoring immunity to children with severe deficiency. Even when tissue targeting and precise gene replacement are feasible, mimicking the appropriate patterns of gene expression can be a substantial barrier to gene therapy. Injection of deficient enzymes into serum (enzyme therapy) has been successful in disorders such as Gaucher's disease [231000 (storage of lipids in the spleen and bone)], and takes advantage of cellular pathways that target enzymes to lysosomes.

73. The answer is c. (*Murray, pp 468–487. Scriver, pp 175–192. Sack, pp 245–257. Wilson, pp 151–180.*) After the locus responsible for a genetic disease is mapped to a particular chromosome region, "candidate" genes can be examined for molecular abnormalities in affected individuals. The connective tissue abnormalities in Stickler syndrome (108300) make the COL2A1 collagen locus an attractive candidate for disease mutations, prompting analysis of COL2A1 gene structure and expression. Western blotting detects gene alterations that interfere with protein expression, while use of the reverse transcriptase–polymerase chain reaction (RT-PCR) detects alterations in mRNA levels. Each analysis should detect one-half the respective amounts of COL2A1 protein or mRNA in the case of a promoter mutation that abolishes transcription of one COL2A1 allele. Southern blotting detects nucleotide changes that alter DNA restriction sites, but this is relatively insensitive unless large portions of the gene are deleted. Fluorescent in situ hybridization (FISH) analysis using DNA probes from the COL2A1 locus is a sensitive method for detecting deletions of the entire locus, and DNA sequencing of the entire gene provides the gold standard for detecting any alteration in the regulatory or coding sequences. Nucleotide sequence changes are still subject to interpretation, since they may represent polymorphisms that do not alter gene function. Population studies and/or in vitro studies of gene expression are often needed to discriminate DNA polymorphisms from mutations that disrupt gene function. For any autosomal locus, the interpretation of molecular analyses is complicated by the presence of two homologous copies of the gene.

74. The answer is e. (*Murray, pp 468–487. Scriver, pp 3–45. Sack, pp 245–257. Wilson, pp 151–180.*) Missense mutations, which cause the substitution of one amino acid for another, may significantly alter the function of the resultant protein without altering the size of DNA restriction fragments detected by Southern blotting. In this case, northern blot results would most likely also be normal. Single-base changes may also result in nonsense mutations. Large insertions or deletions in the exon or coding regions of the gene alter the Southern blot pattern and usually ablate the activity of one gene copy. In the case of an autosomal locus like that for ornithine aminotransferase, the homologous allele remains active and gives 50%

enzyme activity (heterozygote or carrier range with a normal phenotype). Similar effects on enzyme activity would be predicted from complete gene deletions at one locus, while a duplication might produce 150% or 50% of normal enzyme activity depending on the status of promoter sites.

75. The answer is b. (*Murray, pp 468–487. Scriver, pp 4517–4554. Sack, pp 245–257. Wilson, pp 151–180.*) Red cell hemolysis after drug exposure suggests a red cell enzyme defect, most easily confirmed by enzyme assay to demonstrate deficient activity. A likely diagnosis here is glucose-6-phosphate dehydrogenase (G6PD) deficiency (305900), probably the most common genetic disease (it affects 400 million people worldwide). Tropical African and Mediterranean peoples exhibit the highest prevalence because the disease, like sickle cell trait, confers resistance to malaria. DNA analysis is available to demonstrate particular alleles, but simple enzyme assay is sufficient for diagnosis. More than 400 types of abnormal G6PD alleles have been described, meaning that most affected individuals are compound heterozygotes. The phenotype of jaundice and red blood cell hemolysis with anemia is triggered by a variety of infections and drugs, including a dietary substance in fava beans. Sulfonamide and related antibiotics as well as antimalarial drugs are notorious for inducing hemolysis in G6PD-deficient individuals. G6PD deficiency exhibits X-linked recessive inheritance, explaining why male offspring but not the parents become ill when exposed to antimalarials.

76. The answer is b. (*Murray, pp 468–487. Scriver, pp 3421–3452. Sack, pp 245–257. Wilson, pp 151–180.*) All of the modes of therapy are theoretically possible, and enzyme therapy (i.e., injection of purified enzyme) has been successful in several lysosomal deficiencies, particularly those in which the central nervous system is not affected [i.e., Gaucher's disease (231000)]. Unfortunately, antibodies frequently develop to the injected enzyme and limit the term of successful enzyme delivery. Heterologous bone marrow transplant, preferably from a related donor, offers the most realistic and effective therapy since the graft provides a permanent source of enzyme. Bone marrow transplants do have a 10% mortality, however, and the enzyme diffuses poorly into the central nervous system. Somatic gene therapy (i.e., delivery of enzyme to somatic cells via viral vectors or transfected tissue) is now possible; however, targeting of the gene product to appropriate tissues and organelles is still a problem. Transfected autologous bone marrow transplant (i.e., marrow from the patient) has been used in a few cases of adenosine deaminase deficiency, an immune disorder affecting lymphocytes. Germ-line gene therapy requires the insertion of functional genes into gametes or blastomeres of early embryos prior to birth. The potential for embryonic damage, lack of knowledge regarding developmental gene control, and ethical controversies regarding selective breeding or embryo experimentation make germ-line therapy unrealistic at present.

77. The answer is e. *(Murray, pp 468–487. Scriver, pp 3–45. Sack, pp 245–257. Wilson, pp 151–180.)* Insertion of one extra nucleotide causes a frame-shift mutation and mistranslation of all the mRNA transcribed from beyond that point in the DNA. All the other mutations cited in the question usually cause an error in the identity of only one amino acid (choice a or b), removal of one amino acid from the sequence (choice d), or no error at all in the amino acid sequence (choice c). There is a chance that the mutations in choices a or b will give a "nonsense," or chain-terminator, mutation, and this is about as likely to be lethal as is a frame shift.

78. The answer is b. *(Murray, pp 452–467. Scriver, pp 3–45. Sack, pp 245–257. Wilson, pp 151–180.)* The replacement of the codon UAG with UAA would be a silent mutation since both codons are "stop" signals. Thus, transcription would cease when either triplet was reached. There are three termination codons in mRNA: UAG, UAA, and UGA. These are the only codons that do not specify an amino acid. A missense or a substitution mutation is the converting of a codon specifying one amino acid to another codon specifying a different amino acid. A nonsense mutation converts an amino acid codon to a termination codon. A suppression counteracts the effects of another mutation at another codon. The addition or deletion of nucleotides results in a frame-shift mutation.

79. The answer is c. *(Murray, pp 452–467. Scriver, pp 3–45. Sack, pp 245–257. Wilson, pp 151–180.)* Point mutations that are frame-shift mutations put the normal reading frame out of register by one base pair. The insertion of an extra base pair or the deletion of one or more base pairs falls into this category. Transitions and transversions are not frame-shift mutations; they are substitutions of one base pair for another. Substitutions are the most common type of mutation. In transitions, a purine is replaced by a purine or a pyrimidine by a pyrimidine. In transversions, a purine is replaced by a pyrimidine or vice versa. It has been suggested that transitions occur spontaneously owing to the tautomeric changes in base-hydrogen-bond locations. Transversions can be caused by defective DNA polymerases.

80. The answer is c. (*Murray, pp 468–487. Scriver, pp 3–45. Sack, pp 245–257. Wilson, pp 151–180.*) Thalassemias cause anemia due to genetically defective synthesis of either the α or β chains of hemoglobin. While many different types of mutations can cause thalassemias, mRNA production or processing is commonly affected. Premature termination of mRNA transcription leading to shorter-than-normal chains, frame-shift mutations leading to abnormal amino acid sequences in chains after the mutation (addition or deletion), and aberrant splicing are some of the RNA problems that can lead to dysfunctional or nonfunctional chains. In some thalassemias, one of the chains (α or β) may be missing completely. However, the absence of both chains is a lethal mutation that would not be seen in the population.

81. The answer is b. (*Murray, pp 452–467. Scriver, pp 3–45. Sack, pp 245–257. Wilson, pp 151–180.*) The structures of glycine and alanine are quite similar, with the $-H$ side group of glycine being replaced with the $-CH_3$ side group of alanine. Consequently, a mutation causing such a change is unlikely to produce a dysfunctional protein. In contrast, a mutation changing a splice site could result in either the abnormal exclusion of an exon or the inclusion of an intron in a protein, which would drastically change its properties. Likewise, frame-shift mutations caused by deletion or addition of one or two bases completely distort the remainder of the protein. The closer a frame shift is to the amino terminal that is synthesized first, the more garbled the protein. All nonsense mutations involve inserting a stop codon in place of whatever amino acid would have been coded. In the case given, only half the protein would be synthesized.

82. The answer is e. (*Murray, pp 452–467. Scriver, pp 3–45. Sack, pp 245–257. Wilson, pp 151–180.*) Chain termination is determined by three codons: UAA, UAG, and UGA. Aside from chain termination codons, each group of three bases in a sequence codes for an amino acid. The next three bases specify another amino acid. Thus, the genetic code is nonoverlapping. The triplet genetic code is degenerate, which is to say that for most amino acids there is more than one code word. The triplets of bases (codons) that specify the same amino acid usually differ only in the last base of the triplet.

83. The answer is b. (*Murray, pp 468–487. Scriver, pp 3–45. Sack, pp 245–257. Wilson, pp 151–180.*) The following mutations were shown in the DNA changes:

a. Missense (cys to leu)
b. Nonsense (tyr to stop)
c. Missense (ser to phe)
d. Harmless (tyr to tyr)
e. Missense (leu to phe)
f. No mutation
g. Missense (phe to tyr)

Most of the mutations shown result in a missense effect, with a different amino acid being incorporated into the same site in a protein. This may or may not have an effect depending upon its location. Some single-base mutations are harmless because of the degeneracy of the genetic code, whereby more than one triplet code exists for all amino acids except tryptophan and methionine. Choice a contains two mutations, one degenerate and the other missense.

DNA coding: 3'-ACGACGACG-5' to 3'-ACAAACACG-5'
mRNA: 5'-UGCUGCUGC-3' to 5'-UGUUUGUGC-3'
Protein: cys-cys-cys to cys-leu-cys

Nonsense mutations occur when the reading of the normal termination signal is changed. This can occur by mutation to a stop signal as in choice b, by deletions near a stop codon, or by insertions.

84. The answer is d. (*Murray, pp 468–487. Scriver, pp 3–45. Sack, pp 245–257. Wilson, pp 151–180.*) Several operons in *E. coli*, including the *lac* operon, are subject to catabolite repression. In the presence of glucose, there is decreased manufacture of cyclic AMP (cAMP) by adenylate cyclase. Low glucose levels increase production of cAMP, which binds to the catabolite activator protein (CAP). The cAMP-CAP complex binds to the promoters of several responsive operons at catabolite activator protein

(CAP) binding sites, greatly enhancing transcription of operon RNA. This positive control stimulates use of more exotic metabolites when glucose is not available and conserves energy when glucose is plentiful. High levels of glucose lower cAMP levels and direct metabolism toward constitutive glucose pathways such as glycolysis.

85. The answer is b. *(Murray, pp 468–487. Scriver, pp 3–45. Sack, pp 245–257. Wilson, pp 151–180.)* The lactose (*lac*) operon is a classic model for understanding gene regulation. It is negatively controlled through two regulatory genes—the *lac I* gene that constitutively (always) expresses a repressor protein and the operator (o) region to which the repressor binds. The *lac* operon is inducible by lactose and lactose analogues, inactivating the repressor and uncovering the operon and its neighboring promoter (p) sequence. RNA polymerase then transcribes the inducible, structural genes β-galactosidase (z), permease (y), and transacetylase (a). The RNA transcript is polycistronic, so that one regulatory site allows transcription of all three genes needed for the metabolism of lactose. The bacterial ribosomes immediately attach to the nascent RNA transcript, allowing for simultaneous transcription and translation. When all the lactose is metabolized, the repressor returns to its native conformation, binds to the operator, and shuts down *lac* operon transcription (see the figure below).

86. The answer is c. *(Murray, pp 468–487. Scriver, pp 3–45. Sack, pp 245–257. Wilson, pp 151–180.)* Certain regulatory elements act on genes on the same chromosome ("*cis*"), while others can regulate genes on the opposite chromosome ("*trans*"). The terminology makes analogy to carbon-carbon double bonds where two modifying groups may both be above or below the bond (*cis*) or opposite it (*trans*). *Cis* regulatory elements like the *lac* operator and promoter or mammalian enhancers are usually DNA sequences (regulatory sequences) adjoining or within the regulated gene. *Trans* regulatory elements like the *lac* repressor protein or mammalian transcription factors are usually diffusible proteins (regulatory factors) that can interact with adjoining target genes or with target genes on other chromosomes. Classification of bacterial elements as *cis* or *trans* requires mating experiments where portions of a second chromosome are introduced by transfection (with bacteriophage) or conjugation (with other bacteria). The distinction between *cis* and *trans* is fundamental for understanding how regulators work.

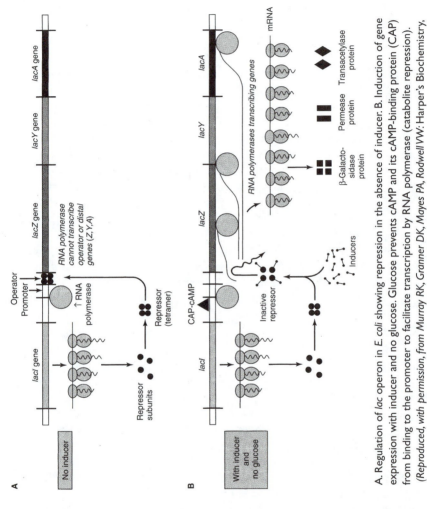

A. Regulation of *lac* operon in *E. coli* showing repression in the absence of inducer. B. Induction of gene expression with inducer and no glucose. Glucose prevents cAMP and its cAMP-binding protein (CAP) from binding to the promoter to facilitate transcription by RNA polymerase (catabolite repression). *(Reproduced, with permission, from Murray RK, Granner DK, Mayes PA, Rodwell VW: Harper's Biochemistry, 25/e. New York, McGraw-Hill, 2000: 471.)*

87. The answer is d. (*Murray, pp 468–487. Scriver, pp 3–45. Sack, pp 245–257. Wilson, pp 151–180.*) Mammalian regulatory factors are much more diverse than those of bacteria, possessing several types of structural domains. Activators of transcription, such as steroid hormones, may enter the cell and bind to regulatory factors at specific sites called ligand-binding domains; these intracellular "receptors" are analogous to G protein–linked membrane receptors that extend into the extracellular space. Response elements are not regulatory factors but DNA sequences near the transcription site for certain types of genes (e.g., steroid-responsive and heat shock–responsive genes). Regulatory factors interact with specific DNA sequences through their DNA-binding domains, and with other regulatory factors through transcription-activating domains. Some regulatory factors have antirepressor domains that counteract the inhibitory effects of chromatin proteins (histones and nonhistones).

88. The answer is d. (*Murray, pp 468–487. Scriver, pp 3–45. Sack, pp 245–257. Wilson, pp 151–180.*) The POMC gene provides a mammalian example in which several proteins are derived from the same RNA transcript. Unlike the polycistronic mRNA of the bacterial lactose operon, mammalian cells generate several mRNAs or proteins from the same gene by variable protein processing or by alternative splicing. Variable protein processing preserves the peptide products of some gene regions but degrades those from others. Alternative splicing would often produce proteins composed of different exon combinations with the same terminal exon and carboxy-terminal peptide, but could remove the terminal exon in some proteins and produce different C-terminal peptides. Different transcription factors or enhancers in different brain regions could regulate the total amounts of POMC gene transcript but not the types of protein produced. Elongation of protein synthesis involves GTP cleavage but is not differentially regulated in mammalian tissues.

89. The answer is a. (*Murray, pp 468–487. Scriver, pp 3–45. Sack, pp 245–257. Wilson, pp 151–180.*) Imbalance of globin chain synthesis occurs in the thalassemias. Deficiency of α-globin chains (α thalassemia) is common in Asian populations and may be associated with abnormal hemoglobins composed of four β-globin chains (hemoglobin H) or (in fetuses and newborns) of four γ-globin chains (hemoglobin Bart's). Mutation in a transcription factor necessary for expression of α-globin could ablate α-globin expression, since the same factor could act in *trans* on all four copies of the α-globin genes (two α-globin loci). Mutation of a regulatory sequence element that acts in *cis* would inactivate only one α-globin gene, leaving others to produce α-globin in reduced amounts (mild α thalassemia). Deletions of one α-globin would produce a similar mild phenotype, and deficiencies of transcription factors regulating α- and β-globin genes would not produce chain imbalance.

90. The answer is a. (*Murray, pp 746–751. Scriver, pp 3–45. Sack, pp 245–257. Wilson, pp 151–180.*) Antibody classes, called isotypes, are determined by the constant region of heavy chains. There are five isotypes that include IgM, IgD, IgG, IgE, and IgA. During B cell maturation, DNA rearrangements produce light chains with unique V-J segments and heavy chains with unique V-D-J segments. After activation, B cells can change their preferred DNA recombination to join the V-D-J segment to a different constant (C) segment. Different constant region exons are clustered downstream of the Cμ exon used for initial IgM synthesis by the activated B cell. Recombination at designated switch sites places another constant chain exon (e.g., Cγ for IgG) next to the V-D-J segment and allows the activated B cell to secrete a different antibody isotype (heavy chain class switching). Alternative splicing allows activated B cells to switch from membrane-bound to secreted IgM.

91. The answer is b. (*Murray, pp 468–487. Scriver, pp 3–45. Sack, pp 245–257. Wilson, pp 151–180.*) The boys have an X-linked recessive condition called α thalassemia/mental retardation or ATR-X syndrome (309510). The X-encoded gene has an unknown function in brain as well as being a factor that regulates α-globin gene transcription. In order to affect all four α-globin genes, the X-encoded gene must produce a *trans*-acting factor; second mutations altering enhancers or promoters would be *cis*-acting and affect only one α-globin gene. Pseudogenes are functionless gene copies, so altered expression would not influence α-globin chain synthesis.

92. The answer is c. (*Murray, pp 746–751. Scriver, pp 3–45. Sack, pp 245–257. Wilson, pp 151–180.*) This case is an example of Burkitt's lymphoma, which may affect the tonsils or other lymphoid tissues. The translocation places the *myc* oncogene on chromosome 8 downstream of the very active heavy chain locus on chromosome 14, activating *myc* gene expression in B cells and their derivatives. The translocation is likely an aberrant form of the normal DNA rearrangements that generate unique heavy chain genes in each B cell. The translocation joins one chromosome 8 to one chromosome 14, leaving their homologues unaffected. The cause for the phenotype must therefore be *trans*-acting, since *cis*-acting effects would pertain only to the translocated loci and not affect the homologous untranslocated loci. Activation of a tumor-promoting gene (oncogene) on chromosome 8 could produce an enlarged tonsil, while underactivity of immunoglobulin production due to one-half expression could decrease immune function but would not completely ablate the processes in choices a, b, d, and e. At the genetic level, *trans*-acting events are autosomal dominant in that one of the two homologous loci is abnormal and produces a phenotype. Mutations of *cis*-acting events must disrupt both homologous loci to produce phenotypes, making them autosomal recessive at the genetic level.

Acid-Base Equilibria, Amino Acids, and Protein Structure/Function

Acid-Base Equilibria, Amino Acids, and Protein Structure

Questions

DIRECTIONS: Each item below contains a question or incomplete statement followed by suggested responses. Select the **one best** response to each question.

93. A 2-day-old neonate becomes lethargic and uninterested in breast-feeding. Physical examination reveals tachypnea (rapid breathing) with a normal heartbeat and breath sounds. Initial blood chemistry values include normal glucose, sodium, potassium, chloride, and bicarbonate (HCO_3^-) levels; initial blood gas values reveal a pH of 7.53, partial pressure of oxygen (P_{O_2}) normal at 103 mmHg, and partial pressure of carbon dioxide (P_{CO_2}) decreased at 27 mmHg. Which of the following treatment strategies is indicated?

a. Administer alkali to treat metabolic acidosis
b. Administer alkali to treat respiratory acidosis
c. Decrease the respiratory rate to treat metabolic acidosis
d. Decrease the respiratory rate to treat respiratory alkalosis
e. Administer acid to treat metabolic alkalosis

94. A newborn with tachypnea and cyanosis (bluish color) is found to have a blood pH of 7.1. A serum bicarbonate is measured as 12 mM, but the blood gas machine that would determine the partial pressures of oxygen (PO_2) and carbon dioxide (PCO_2) is broken. Recall the pK_a of 6.1 for carbonic acid (reflecting the HCO_3^-/CO_2 equilibrium in blood) and the fact that the blood CO_2 concentration is equal to the PCO_2 in mmHg (normal value = 40 mmHg) multiplied by 0.03. Which of the following treatment strategies is indicated?

a. Administer oxygen to improve tissue perfusion and decrease metabolic acidosis
b. Administer oxygen to decrease respiratory acidosis
c. Increase the respiratory rate to treat respiratory acidosis
d. Decrease the respiratory rate to treat respiratory acidosis
e. Administer medicines to decrease renal hydrogen ion excretion

95. A 72-year-old male with diabetes mellitus is evaluated in the emergency room because of lethargy, disorientation, and long, deep breaths (Kussmaul respirations). Initial chemistries on venous blood demonstrate high glucose at 380 mg/dL (normal up to 120) and a pH of 7.3. Recalling the normal bicarbonate (22 to 28 mM) and PCO_2 (33 to 45 mmHg) values, which of the additional test results below would be consistent with the man's pH and breathing pattern?

a. A bicarbonate of 5 mM and PCO_2 of 10 mmHg
b. A bicarbonate of 15 mM and PCO_2 of 30 mmHg
c. A bicarbonate of 15 mM and PCO_2 of 40 mmHg
d. A bicarbonate of 20 mM and PCO_2 of 45 mmHg
e. A bicarbonate of 25 mM and PCO_2 of 50 mmHg

96. A diabetic teenager is found to have a pH of 7.1 and normal electrolyte levels (Na^+ = 140 mM, K^+ = 4 mM, Cl^- = 103 mM) except for a bicarbonate of 11 mM (normal 22 to 28 mM). The urine tests positive for ketone bodies, mostly due to acetoacetic acid and acetoacetate ($CH_3C=OCH_2COOH$ and $CH_3C=OCH_2COO^-$), which have a pK of 4.8. In this case, it is assumed that acetoacetate is the only significant anion in the blood besides chloride, and that each acetoacetate anion binds and removes one sodium cation during excretion by the kidney. Given that the patient has a normal glomerular filtration rate of about 7 L of blood per hour without any retention of acetoacetate/acetoacetic acid, the rates of sodium, acetoacetate, and acetoacetic acid loss will be

a. 10 mmol/h of each species
b. 50 mmol/h of sodium and acetoacetate, virtually no acetoacetic acid excretion
c. 100 mmol/h of sodium and acetoacetic acid, virtually no acetoacetate excretion
d. 200 mmol/h of sodium and acetoacetate, virtually no acetoacetic acid excretion
e. 300 mmol/h of each species

97. A solution of acid is prepared for cleaning surgical instruments by adding 0.5 L of 2 mM hydrochloric acid (HCl) to 0.5 L of pure water, which has a hydrogen ion concentration of 10^{-7} M. The initial pH of the pure water, then the pH after adding the HCl, are

a. 7, then 3
b. 7, then 4
c. 7, then 1
d. 14, then 3
e. 14, then 4

98. The greatest buffering capacity at physiologic pH would be provided by a protein rich in which of the following amino acids?

a. Lysine
b. Histidine
c. Aspartic acid
d. Valine
e. Leucine

99. The relationship between the ratio of acid to base in a solution and its pH is described by the Henderson-Hasselbalch equation

$$pH = pK + \log \text{[base]/[acid]}$$

The pK of acetic acid is 4.8. What is the approximate pH of an acetate solution containing 0.2 M acetic acid and 2 M acetate ion?

a. 0.48
b. 4.8
c. 5.8
d. 6.8
e. 10.8

100. Since the pK values for aspartic acid are 2.0, 3.9, and 10.0, it follows that the isoelectric point (pI) is

a. 3.0
b. 3.9
c. 5.9
d. 6.0
e. 7.0

101. A 0.22 M solution of lactic acid (pK_a 3.9) is found to contain 0.20 M in the dissociated form and 0.02 M undissociated. What is the pH of the solution?

a. 2.9
b. 3.3
c. 3.9
d. 4.9
e. 5.4

102. Which of the combinations of laboratory results below indicates compensated metabolic alkalosis?

a. Low P_{CO_2}, normal bicarbonate, high pH
b. Low P_{CO_2}, low bicarbonate, low pH
c. Normal P_{CO_2}, low bicarbonate, low pH
d. High P_{CO_2}, normal bicarbonate, low pH
e. High P_{CO_2}, high bicarbonate, high pH

103. The graph below shows a titration curve of a common biochemical compound. Which of the following statements about the graph is true?

a. The compound has one ionizable function
b. The compound has three ionizable side chains
c. The maximum buffering capacity of the compound is represented by points A and B on the graph
d. Point A could represent the range of ionization of an amino function
e. Points A and B represent the respective pKs of α and side chain carboxyl groups

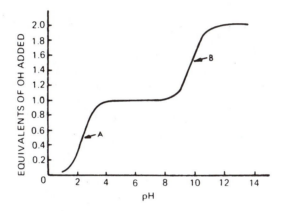

104. The pH of body fluids is stabilized by buffer systems. Which of the following compounds is the most effective buffer at physiologic pH?

a. Na_2HPO_4, pK_{a5} 12.32
b. NH_4OH, pK_{a5} 9.24
c. NaH_2PO_4, pK_{a5} 7.21
d. CH_3CO_2H, pK_{a5} 4.74
e. Citric acid, pK_{a5} 3.09

105. Water, which constitutes 70% of body weight, may be said to be the "cell solvent." The property of water that most contributes to its ability to dissolve compounds is the

a. Strong covalent bond formed between water and salts
b. Hydrogen bond formed between water and biochemical molecules
c. Hydrophobic bond formed between water and long-chain fatty acids
d. Absence of interacting forces
e. Fact that the freezing point of water is much lower than body temperature

106. A 5-year-old girl displays decreased appetite, increased urinary frequency, and thirst. Her physician suspects new-onset diabetes mellitus and confirms that she has elevated urine glucose ketones. Which of the following blood values would be most compatible with diabetic ketoacidosis?

	pH	Bicarbonate (mM)	Arterial P_{CO_2}
a.	7.05	16.0	52
b.	7.25	20.0	41
c.	7.40	24.5	39
d.	7.66	37.0	30
e.	7.33	12.0	21

107. A child presents with severe vomiting, dehydration, and fever. Initial blood studies show acidosis with a low bicarbonate and an anion gap (the sum of sodium plus potassium minus chloride plus bicarbonate is 40 and larger than the normal 20 to 25). Preliminary results from the blood amino acid screen show two elevated amino acids, both with nonpolar side chains. A titration curve performed on one of the elevated species shows two ionizable groups with approximate pKs of 2 and 9.5. The most likely pair of elevated amino acids consists of

a. Aspartic acid and glutamine
b. Glutamic acid and threonine
c. Histidine and valine
d. Leucine and isoleucine
e. Glutamine and isoleucine

108. Which of the hemoglobin designations below best describes the relationship of subunits in the quaternary structure of adult hemoglobin?

a. $(\alpha_1-\alpha_2)(\beta_1-\beta_2)$
b. $\alpha_1-\alpha_2-\alpha_3-\alpha_4$
c. $\beta-\beta-\beta-\alpha$
d. $(\beta_1-\beta_2-\beta_3-\alpha_1)$
e. $(\alpha_1-\beta_1)-(\alpha_2-\beta_2)$

109. Which of the following amino acids is most compatible with an α-helical structure?

a. Tryptophan
b. Alanine
c. Lysine
d. Proline
e. Cysteine

110. Blood is drawn from a child with severe anemia and the hemoglobin protein is degraded for peptide and amino acid analysis. Of the results below, which change in hemoglobin primary structure is most likely to correlate with the clinical phenotype of anemia?

a. ile-leu-val to ile-ile-val
b. leu-glu-ile to leu-val-ile
c. gly-ile-gly to gly-val-gly
d. gly-asp-gly to gly-glu-gly
e. val-val-val to val-leu-val

111. An adult with mild, chronic anemia does not respond to iron supplementation. Blood is drawn and the red cell hemoglobin is analyzed. Which of the following results is most likely if the patient has an altered hemoglobin molecule (hemoglobinopathy)?

a. Several proteins but only one red protein detected by high-performance liquid chromatography (HPLC)
b. Two proteins detected in normal amounts by western blotting
c. Several proteins and two red proteins separated by native gel electrophoresis
d. Two labeled bands a slight distance apart after SDS-gel electrophoresis and reaction with labeled antibody to α- and β-globin
e. A reddish mixture of proteins retained within a dialysis membrane

112. Which of the following statements about solutions of amino acids at physiologic pH is true?

a. All amino acids contain both positive and negative charges
b. All amino acids contain positively charged side chains
c. Some amino acids contain only positive charges
d. All amino acids contain negatively charged side chains
e. Some amino acids contain only negative charges

113. The highest concentration of cystine can be found in

a. Melanin
b. Chondroitin sulfate
c. Myosin
d. Keratin
e. Collagen

114. Parents bring in their 2-week-old child fearful that he has ingested a poison. They had delayed disposing one of the child's diapers, and noted a black discoloration where the urine had collected. Later, they realized that all of the child's diapers would turn black if stored as waste for a day or so. Knowing that phenol groups can complex to form colors, which amino acid pathways are implicated in this phenomenon?

a. The phenylalanine, tyrosine, and homogentisate pathway
b. The histidine pathway
c. The leucine, isoleucine, and valine pathway
d. The methionine and homocystine pathway
e. The arginine and citrulline pathway (urea cycle)

115. Certain amino acids are not part of the primary structure of proteins but are modified after translation. In scurvy, which amino acid that is normally part of collagen is not synthesized?

a. Hydroxytryptophan
b. Hydroxytyrosine
c. Hydroxyhistidine
d. Hydroxyalanine
e. Hydroxyproline

116. A newborn female has a large and distorted cranium, short and deformed limbs, and very blue scleras (whites of the eyes). Radiographs demonstrate multiple limb fractures and suggest a diagnosis of osteogenesis imperfecta (brittle bone disease). Analysis of type I collagen protein, a triple helix formed from two α_1 and one α_2 collagen chains, shows a 50% reduction in the amount of type I collagen in the baby's skin. DNA analysis demonstrates the presence of two normal α_1 alleles and one normal α_2 allele. These results are best explained by

a. Deficiency of α_1 collagen peptide synthesis
b. Inability of α_1 chains to incorporate into triple helix
c. Defective α_1 chains that interrupt triple helix formation
d. Incorporation of defective α_2 chains that cause instability and degradation of the triple helix
e. A missense mutation that alters the synthesis of α_1 chains

117. A child with tall stature, loose joints, and detached retinas is found to have a mutation in type II collagen. Recall that collagen consists of a repeating tripeptide motif where the first amino acid of each tripeptide is the same. Which of the following amino acids is the recurring amino acid most likely to be altered in mutations that distort collagen molecules?

a. Glycine
b. Hydroxyproline
c. Hydroxylysine
d. Tyrosine
e. Tryptophan

118. Immunoglobulin G molecules can be characterized by which of the following statements?

a. They are maintained at a constant level in the serum
b. They contain nucleic acids
c. They contain mostly carbohydrate
d. They can be separated into subunits with a reducing agent and urea
e. They can be separated into subunits with a proteolytic enzyme and urea

119. Which of the following techniques for purification of proteins can be made specific for a given protein?

a. Dialysis
b. Affinity chromatography
c. Gel filtration chromatography
d. Ion exchange chromatography
e. Electrophoresis

120. A solution of glutamic acid is titrated from pH 1.0 to 7.0 by the addition of 5 mL of a solution of 1 M NaOH. What is the approximate number of millimoles of amino acid in the sample ($pK_{a1} = 2.19$, $pK_{a2} = 4.25$, $pK_{a3} = 9.67$)?

a. 1.5
b. 3.0
c. 6.0
d. 12.0
e. 18.0

121. An adolescent presents with shortness of breath during exercise and is found to be anemic. A hemoglobin electrophoresis is performed that is depicted in the figure below. The adolescent's sample is run with controls including normal, sickle trait, and sickle cell anemia, and serum. The adolescent is determined to have an unknown hemoglobinopathy. Which one of the lanes contains the adolescent's sample?

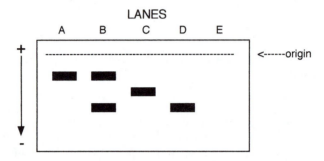

Electrophoretic Hemoglobin Patterns

a. Lane A
b. Lane B
c. Lane C
d. Lane D
e. Lane E

122. Which of the schematic drawings of protein configuration shown in the figure below represents the conformation of tropocollagen?

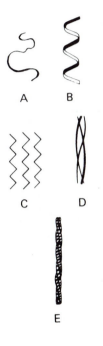

a. Drawing A
b. Drawing B
c. Drawing C
d. Drawing D
e. Drawing E

123. The specific activity of glycogen phosphorylase increases from 2.5 U/mg homogenate protein to 325.5 U/mg protein after being bound to and eluted from a cation exchange column at pH 2.7. What can you conclude from this information?

a. The yield of enzyme is greater than 80%
b. The enzyme is negatively charged at pH 2.7
c. The enzyme is purified over 100-fold
d. The enzyme is globular in structure
e. The enzyme is in an activated state

124. Which one of the following proteins is found in the thick filaments of skeletal muscle?

a. α-actinin
b. Myosin
c. Troponin
d. Tropomyosin
e. Actin

125. Which one of the following proteolytic enzymes is activated by acid hydrolysis of the proenzyme form?

a. Trypsin
b. Chymotrypsin
c. Elastase
d. Pepsin
e. Carboxypeptidase

126. Which one of the following structures may be classified as a hydrophobic amino acid at pH 7.0?

a. Isoleucine
b. Arginine
c. Aspartic acid
d. Lysine
e. Threonine

127. An immunoglobulin (see the figure below) is hydrolyzed by papain to form two A fragments and one B fragment. It is true of fragment A that it

a. Contains the constant regions
b. Is the heavy chain
c. Contains the light chain
d. Is not functional as an antibody-combining site
e. Cannot be further dissociated by mercaptoethanol

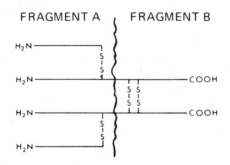

128. In comparing the secondary structure of proteins, which description applies to both the α helix and the β-pleated sheet?

a. All peptide bond components participate in hydrogen bonding
b. N-terminals of chains are together and parallel
c. The structure is composed of two or more segments of polypeptide chain
d. N-terminal and C-terminal ends of chains alternate in an antiparallel manner
e. The chains are almost fully extended

129. Which of the following amino acids is ionizable in proteins?

a. Leucine
b. Histidine
c. Valine
d. Alanine
e. Glycine

130. The oxygen carrier of muscle is the globular protein myoglobin. Which one of the following amino acids is highly likely to be localized within the interior of the molecule?

a. Arginine
b. Aspartic acid
c. Glutamic acid
d. Valine
e. Lysine

131. Which of the following statements concerning immunoglobulin is most accurate?

a. The distinctiveness of the light chains gives the different classes of immunoglobulins their unique biologic characteristics
b. IgE is the principal antibody in the serum
c. The heavy chains are similar in each class of immunoglobulin
d. The constant regions of the heavy chains are the same in each class of immunoglobulin
e. IgE is the major immunoglobulin found in external secretions

132. A child stops making developmental progress at age 2 years and develops coarse facial features with thick mucous drainage. Skeletal deformities appear over the next year, and the child regresses to a vegetative state by age 10 years. The child's urine tests positive for glycosaminoglycans that include which of the following molecules?

a. Collagen
b. γ-aminobutyric acid
c. Heparan sulfate
d. Glycogen
e. Fibrillin

133. Under normal conditions in blood, which of the following amino acid residues of albumin is neutral?

a. Arginine
b. Aspartate
c. Glutamine
d. Glutamate
e. Histidine

134. Which of the following statements correctly describes immunoglobulins?

a. Polypeptide chains composing immunoglobulins are held together by hydrogen bonds
b. Each immunoglobulin has two antigen-binding sites per molecule
c. Heavy immunoglobulin chains have constant N-terminal regions
d. Light immunoglobulin chains have variable C-terminal regions
e. Antigen-binding sites of all different antibodies are determined after encountering specific antigens

135. Which of the characteristics below apply to the amino acid glycine?

a. Optically inactive
b. Large molecular diameter interfering with α helix formation
c. Hydrophilic, basic, and charged
d. Hydrophobic
e. Hydrophilic, acidic, and charged

136. Which of the amino acids below is the uncharged derivative of an acidic amino acid?

a. Cystine
b. Arginine
c. Tyrosine
d. Glutamine
e. Proline
f. Serine
g. Leucine

137. Which of the substances below is primarily found in tendons?

a. Collagen
b. Troponin
c. Fibrillin
d. Fibrin
e. Fibronectin

138. Which of the substances below is primarily found in ground substance (extracellular matrix)?

a. Collagen
b. Troponin
c. Keratin
d. Fibrin
e. Proteoglycan

139. The presence of which of the following structural arrangements in a protein strongly suggests that it is a DNA-binding, regulatory protein?

a. β sheet
b. Triple helix
c. α helix
d. β bend
e. Zinc finger

140. During synthesis of mature collagen fiber, which one of the following steps would occur within the fibroblast?

a. Hydrolysis of procollagen to form collagen
b. Glycosylation of proline residues
c. Formation of a triple helix
d. Formation of covalent cross-links between molecules
e. Assembly of the collagen fiber

Acid-Base Equilibria, Amino Acids, and Protein Structure

Answers

93. The answer is d. (*Murray, pp 15–26.*) Tachypnea in term infants may result from brain injuries or metabolic diseases that irritate the respiratory center. The increased respiratory rate removes ("blows off") carbon dioxide from the lung alveoli and lowers blood CO_2, forcing a shift in the indicated equilibrium toward the left:

$$CO_2 + H_2O \rightleftharpoons H_2CO_2 \rightleftharpoons H^+ + HCO_3^-$$

Carbonic acid (H_2CO_2) can be ignored because negligible amounts are present at physiologic pH, leaving the equilibrium:

$$CO_2 + H_2O \rightleftharpoons H^+ + HCO_3^-$$

The leftward shift to replenish exhaled CO_2 decreases the hydrogen ion (H^+) concentration and increases the pH ($^-log_{10}[H^+]$) to produce alkalosis (blood pH above the physiologic norm of 7.4). This respiratory alkalosis is best treated by diminishing the respiratory rate to elevate the blood $[CO_2]$, force the above equilibrium to the right, elevate the $[H^+]$, and decrease the pH. The newborn does not have acidosis, defined as a blood pH below 7.4, either from excess blood acids (metabolic acidosis) or from increased $[CO_2]$ (respiratory acidosis). The baby also does not have metabolic alkalosis, caused by loss of hydrogen ion from the kidney (e.g., with defective tubular filtration) or stomach (e.g., with severe vomiting).

94. The answer is a. (*Murray, pp 15–26.*) The equilibrium between an acid and its conjugate base is defined by the Henderson-Hasselbalch equation:

$$pH = pK_a + \log \frac{[base]}{[acid]} \quad \text{or} \quad pH = 6.1 + \log \frac{[HCO_3^-]}{[CO_2]}$$

in the case of carbonic acid. Note that CO_2 is the effective acid and HCO_3^- the conjugate base for carbonic acid due to its complete dissociation in water.

Given a pH of 7.1 in the cyanotic newborn, then $7.1 - 6.1 = 1 = \log(10) = \log[HCO_3^-]/[CO_2] = \log[HCO_3^-]/0.03 \times P_{CO_2}$. Since the $[HCO_3^-]$ is 12 mM, the $P_{CO_2} \times 0.03$ must be 1.2 mM and the P_{CO_2} 40 mmHg. This normal calculated value for P_{CO_2} means that the baby must have metabolic acidosis, a common accompaniment of hypoxia (low P_{O_2}) that can be treated by providing oxygen or administering alkali to ameliorate the acidosis. If the baby had respiratory acidosis, the P_{CO_2} would be elevated; this would be treated by increasing the respiratory rate to blow off CO_2. Renal treatment of acidosis would require increasing acid excretion or alkali retention. The lungs compensate acidosis with increased breathing rates or tidal volumes to blow off CO_2 and increase pH, the kidneys by retaining HCO_3^-. The lungs can compensate alkalosis somewhat by decreasing breathing rates or volumes to retain CO_2 (and decrease oxygenation within limits), the kidneys by increasing excretion of HCO_3^-.

95. The answer is b. (*Murray, pp 298–307. Scriver, pp 1471–1488. Sack, pp 217–218. Wilson, pp 361–384.*) The man is acidotic as defined by the pH lower than the normal 7.4. His hyperventilation with Kussmaul respirations can be interpreted as compensation by the lungs to blow off CO_2, lower P_{CO_2}, increase $[HCO_3^-]/[CO_2]$ ratio, and raise pH. The correct answer therefore includes a low P_{CO_2}, eliminating choices c through e. Using the Henderson-Hasselbalch equation indicates that the pH minus the pK for carbonic acid ($7.3 - 6.1 = 1.2$) equals $\log[15]/[0.03 \times 30 \text{ mmHg}]$ or $\log[15/0.9]$. These values correspond to those in choice b. The man has compensated his metabolic acidosis (caused by the accumulation of ketone bodies such as acetoacetic acid) by increasing his respiratory rate and volume.

96. The answer is d. (*Murray, pp 298–307. Scriver, pp 1471–1488. Sack, pp 217–218. Wilson, pp 361–384.*) The sum of the major cations in blood (Na^+ plus K^+) minus the sum of the major anions (HCO_3^- plus Cl^-) is called the anion gap (filled by phosphate ions, negatively charged proteins, etc.). An anion gap over 20 suggests the presence of an abnormal anion, such as acetoacetate, which occurs in diabetics. The anion gap in this teenager is elevated at 30 (140 + 4) − (103 + 11). Assuming that all of the gap is made up by acetoacetate anion, then 7 L × 30 mmol/L = 210 mmol of acetoacetate and 210 mmol of sodium excreted per hour. Even with acidosis and a pH of 7.1, virtually all of the acetoacetic acid (pK 4.8) is present as acetoacetate and less than 1% is excreted as acetoacetic acid. To calculate the exact amount of acetoacetic acid present, the Henderson-Hasselbalch equation rearranges to (7.1 − 4.8) = 2.3 = log[base]/[acid]; $[CH_3C=OCH_2COO^-]/[CH_3C=OCH_2COOH]$ = antilog 2.3 = 102. Less than 0.3 mmol of acetoacetic acid is excreted for each liter of blood filtered through the kidney.

97. The answer is b. (*Murray, pp 15–26.*) The dissociation of acids in water can be described by the equilibium $HA + H_2O \rightleftharpoons H_3O+ + A^-$, or, more simply, $HA \rightleftharpoons H^+ + A^-$. The ratio of $[H^+] [A^-]/[HA]$ is constant (called the dissociation constant K_a or K_a') for each acid. The resulting equation of $[H^+] [A^-]/[HA] = K_a$ can be rearranged to $[H^+] = K_a [HA]/[A^-]$ or $1/[H^+] = 1/K_a + [A^-]/[HA]$. Taking logarithms of both sides, and noting that pH is defined as $-\log [H^+]$, one derives the Henderson-Hasselbalch equation of pH = $-\log K$ (pK) + log $[A^-]/[HA]$. Strong acids dissociate completely in water, so that $[H^+]$ and $[A^-]$ are equivalent to the amount of HA added to solution (K_a becomes infinite and meaningless). Since pure water has an $[H^+]$ concentration of 1.0×10^{-7} M, pH = $-\log 10^{-7}$ = $-(-7)$ = 7.0. For hydrochloric acid, the dissociation of $HCl \rightleftharpoons H^+ + Cl^-$ in water is shifted entirely to the right, leaving virtually no HCl. The dilution of 2 mM hydrochloric acid with an equal volume of water produces an $[H^+]$ concentration of 1.0×10^{-3} M and a pH of 3. Note that the preexisting 10^{-7} $[H^+]$ of water is negligible compared to that resulting from the addition of HCl.

98. The answer is b. (*Murray, pp 15–26.*) Proteins can be effective buffers of body and intracellular fluids. Buffering capacity is dependent upon the presence of amino acids having ionizable side chains with pKs near physiologic pH. In the example given, only histidine has an ionizable imidazolium group that has a pK close to neutrality (pK = 6.0). Valine and leucine are amino acids with uncharged, branched side chains. Lysine has a very basic amino group (pK = 10.5) on its aliphatic side chain that is positively charged at physiologic pH, and aspartic acid has a side chain carboxyl (pK = 3.8) that is negative at pH 7.

99. The answer is c. *(Murray, pp 15–26.)* The calculation of pH requires substitution of the concentrations of acid and base into the the Henderson-Hasselbalch equation. For the given ratio of acetate and acetic acid, the pH equals the pK of 4.8 plus the log of the concentration of base/acid (2 *M* acetate/0.2-*M* acetic acid). This simplifies to:

$$pH = 4.8 + \log 10 = 4.8 + 1 = 5.8$$

100. The answer is a. *(Murray, pp 15–26.)* The isoelectric point (p*I*) of an amino acid is that pH at which the net charge is zero. Since pK values denote the pH at which a given α-COOH, α-NH₃, or R side chain group is dissociated, it is possible to calculate the p*I*. For amino acids with uncharged side groups, the p*I* is simply the halfway point between the α-COOH (pK_1) and the α-NH₃ (pK_2) = (pK_1 + pK_2)/2. For basic amino acids, the p*I* is the average of the α-NH₃ and the side chain group. If the side chain group is designated as pK_3, then p*I* = (pK_2 + pK_3)/2. For acidic amino acids, the p*I* is halfway between the α-COOH and the side chain group: (pK_1 + pK_3)/2. For aspartate, (2.0 + 3.9)/2 = 3.0.

101. The answer is d. *(Murray, pp 15–26.)* According to the Henderson-Hasselbalch equation, pH = pK_a + log [base]/[acid]. (A useful mnemonic is that you need your "b/a" to remember it.) In the case of 0.2 *M* lactate and 0.02 *M* lactic acid, as presented in the question, pH = 3.9 + log 10 = 4.9.

102. The answer is e. *(Murray, pp 15–26.)* Pure metabolic acidosis (choice c) or pure metabolic alkalosis exhibits abnormal bicarbonate and normal lung function. Pure respiratory acidosis (choice d) or alkalosis (choice a) is associated with normal renal function (and normal blood acids) with a normal bicarbonate and abnormal PCO_2. Thus choices b and e must involve compensation, since both the PCO_2 and bicarbonate are abnormal. Choice e must represent compensated metabolic alkalosis since the PCO_2 is high—if it were compensated respiratory acidosis with a high PCO_2, the pH would be low.

103. The answer is c. *(Murray, pp 15–26.)* The figure in the question shows the titration curve of glycine, an amino acid with two dissociable protons—one from the α-carboxyl group and the other from the α-amino group. The maximum buffering capacity of any ionizable function is at the pH equivalent to the pK_a of the dissociation, as represented by points A and B on the graph. The curve clearly demonstrates two ionizable functions, one that ionizes at high pH (~9) that would be atypical of α or side chain carboxyl groups. Point A would suggest the ionization of a relatively strong acid like a carboxyl group rather than of a base like the α-amino group.

104. The answer is c. *(Murray, pp 15–26.)* In any fluid, maximum buffering action is achieved by the acid whose pK_a most nearly approximates the pH of the fluid. Physiologic pH is about 7.4, so that among those buffers listed in the question, NaH_2PO_4 is the most effective.

105. The answer is b. *(Murray, pp 15–26.)* Water molecules have a dipole nature and dissolve salts because of attractions between the water dipoles and the ions that exceed the force of attraction between the oppositely charged ions of the salt. In addition, the latter force is weakened by the high dielectric constant of water. Nonionic but polar compounds are dissolved in water because of hydrogen bonding between water molecules and groups such as alcohols, aldehydes, and ketones.

106. The answer is e. *(Murray, pp 298–307. Scriver, pp 1471–1488. Sack, pp 217–218. Wilson, pp 361–384.)* In the presence of insulin deficiency, a shift to fatty acid oxidation produces the ketones such as acetoacetate that cause metabolic acidosis. The pH and bicarbonate are low, and there is frequently some respiratory compensation (hyperventilation with deep breaths) to lower the P_{CO_2}, as in choice e. A low pH with high P_{CO_2} would represent respiratory acidosis (choices a and b—the low-normal bicarbonate values in these choices indicate partial compensation). Choice d represents respiratory alkalosis as would occur with anxious hyperventilation (high pH and low P_{CO_2}, partial compensation with high bicarbonate). Choice c illustrates normal values.

107. The answer is d. *(Murray, pp 313–322. Scriver, pp 1971–2006. Sack, pp 121–138. Wilson, pp 298–305.)* Leucine and isoleucine have nonpolar methyl groups as side chains. As for any amino acid, titration curves obtained by noting the change in pH over the range of 1 to 14 would show a pK of about 2 for the primary carboxyl group and about 9.5 for the primary amino group; there would be no additional pK for an ionizable side chain. Recall that the pK is the point of maximal buffering capacity when the amounts of charged and uncharged species are equal (see answer to question 104). Aspartic and glutamic acids (second carboxyl group), histidine (imino group), and glutamine (second amino group) all have ionizable side chains that would give an additional pK on the titration curve. The likely diagnosis here is maple syrup urine disease, which involves elevated isoleucine, leucine, and valine together with their ketoacid derivatives. The ketoacid derivatives cause the acidosis, and the fever suggests that the metabolic imbalance was worsened by an infection.

108. The answer is e. (*Murray, pp 48–62. Scriver, pp 3–45. Sack, pp 1–3. Wilson, pp 101–120.*) Adult hemoglobin, or hemoglobin A, is composed of four polypeptide chains. Two of the chains are α chains and two are β chains. The chains are held together by noncovalent interactions. The hemoglobin tetramer can best be represented as being composed of two dimers, each containing the two different polypeptides. Thus the designation $(\alpha_1\text{-}\beta_1)(\alpha_2\text{-}\beta_2)$, which refer to dimers 1 and 2, respectively, is the most correct way to refer to the quaternary structure of adult hemoglobin. Hydrophobic interactions are thought to be the main noncovalent interactions holding all four polypeptides together.

109. The answer is b. (*Murray, pp 27–36. Scriver, pp 3–45. Sack, pp 1–3. Wilson, pp 101–120.*) The α-helical segments of proteins represent one of the most common secondary structures of proteins. The helical structure is composed of a spiraled polypeptide backbone core with the side chains of component amino acids extending outward from the central axis in order to avoid interfering sterically or electrostatically with each other. All the peptide bond carbonyl oxygens are hydrogen-bonded to a peptide linkage that is four residues ahead in the polypeptide. This leads to 3.6 amino acids per turn, spatially held together in the α-helical structure. Since the configuration of the α helix is compatible with being in the interior of proteins, amino acids with nonpolar, hydrophobic side chains predominate. Conversely, amino acids that are charged or have bulky side chains may interfere with the α-helical structure if present in large enough amounts. Proline and hydroxyproline are not at all compatible with the right-handed spiral of the α-helix. They insert a kink in the chain. Likewise, large numbers of charged amino acids such as lysine or histidine disrupt the helix by forming electrostatic bonds or by ionically repelling one another. In addition, amino acids with bulky side chains, such as tryptophan or isoleucine, also tend to disrupt the configuration of the α helix.

110. The answer is b. *(Murray, pp 27–36. Scriver, pp 3–45. Sack, pp 1–3. Wilson, pp 101–120.)* Primary protein structures denote the sequence of amino acids held together by peptide bonds (carboxyl groups joined to amino groups to form amide bonds). The types of amino acids then determine the secondary structure of peptide regions within the protein, sometimes forming spiral α helices or flat pleated sheets. These regional peptide secondary structures then determine the overall three-dimensional tertiary structure of a protein, which is vital for its function. Amino acid substitutions that alter the charge of an amino acid side chain, like the change from glutamic acid (charged carboxyl group) to valine (nonpolar methyl groups) in choice b, are most likely to change the secondary and tertiary protein structure. A change in hemoglobin structure can cause instability, decreased mean cellular hemoglobin concentration (MCHC), and anemia. A change from glutamic acid to valine at position 6 in the β-hemoglobin chain is the mutation responsible for sickle cell anemia.

111. The answer is c. *(Murray, pp 48–62. Scriver, pp 3–45. Sack, pp 1–3. Wilson, pp 101–120.)* In the technique of polyacrylamide gel electrophoresis (PAGE), the distance that a protein is moved by an electrical current is proportional to its charge and inversely proportional to its size. Patients with normal hemoglobin A have two α-globin and two β-globin chains, each encoded by a pair of normal globin alleles. Mutation in one α- or β-globin allele alters the primary amino acid sequence of the encoded globin peptide. If the amino acid change alters the charge of the peptide, then the hemoglobin tetramer assembled with the mutant globin peptide has a different charge and electrophoretic migration than the normal hemoglobin tetramer. The electrophoresis of native (undenatured) hemoglobin therefore produces two species (two bands) rather than one, each retaining its heme molecule and red color. If the hemoglobins were first denatured into their α-globin and β-globin chains as with SDS-polyacrylamide gel electrophoresis, then the similar size of the α- or β-globin peptides would cause them to move closely together as two colorless bands. Identification of these peptides as globin would require use of labeled antibody specific for globin (western blotting). Since the sodium dodecyl sulfate (SDS) detergent covers the protein surface and causes all proteins to be negatively charged, the distance migrated is solely dependent (inversely proportional) to protein size. High-performance liquid chromatography (HPLC) uses ionic resins to separate proteins by charge. The columns are run under high pressure, rapidly producing a series of proteins that are separated from most negative to most positive (or vice versa, depending on the charge of the ionic resin). A mutant hemoglobin with altered charge should produce a second red protein in the pattern. In dialysis, semipermeable membranes allow smaller proteins to diffuse into the outer fluid, but not larger proteins such as hemoglobin.

112. The answer is a. (*Murray, pp 27–36. Scriver, pp 3–45. Sack, pp 1–3. Wilson, pp 101–120.*) At neutral pH, amino acids in solution are zwitterions (i.e., dipolar ions) containing both a protonated amino group (pK approximately 9.5) and a dissociated carboxyl group (pK approximately 2). At pH 7.4, the pH − pK from the Henderson-Hasselbalch equation is ~5 for the carboxy group, predicting a ratio of base (carboxyl anion) to acid (carboxylic acid) of 10^5. Similarly, the pH − pK for the amino group is about −2, predicting a ratio of base (amino group) to acid (protonated ammonium ion) of less than 10^{-2}. Amino acids with ionizable side chains may have charges in addition to those of the amino and carboxyl groups.

113. The answer is d. (*Murray, pp 48–62. Scriver, pp 3–45. Sack, pp 1–3. Wilson, pp 101–120.*) Keratins are a type of intermediate filament that comprises a large portion of many epithelial cells. The characteristics of skin, nails, and hair are all due to keratins. Keratins contain a large amount of the disulfide amino acid cystine. Approximately 14% of the protein composing human hair is cystine. This is the chemical basis of depilatory creams, which are reducing agents that render keratins soluble by breaking the disulfide bridges of these insoluble proteins. The basic structure of intermediate filament proteins is a two- or three-stranded α-helical core 300 amino acids in length.

114. The answer is a. (*Murray, pp 313–322. Scriver, pp 1971–2006. Sack, pp 121–138. Wilson, pp 298–305.*) Lack of the enzyme homogentisate oxidase causes the accumulation of homogentisic acid, a metabolite in the pathway of degradation of phenylalanine and tyrosine. Homogentisate, like tyrosine, contains a phenol group. It is excreted in the urine, where it oxidizes and is polymerized to a dark substance upon standing. Under normal conditions, phenylalanine is degraded to tyrosine, which is broken down through a series of steps to fumarate and acetoacetate. The dark pigment melanin is another end product of this pathway. Deficiency of homogentisate oxidase is called alkaptonuria (black urine), a mild disease discovered by Sir Archibald Garrod, the pioneer of biochemical genetics. Garrod's geneticist colleague, William Bateson, recognized that alkaptonuria, like nearly all enzyme deficiencies, exhibits autosomal recessive inheritance.

115. The answer is e. *(Murray, pp 48–62. Scriver, pp 3–45. Sack, pp 1–3. Wilson, pp 101–120.)* Hydroxyproline and hydroxylysine are not present in newly synthesized collagen. Proline and lysine residues are modified by hydroxylation in a reaction requiring the reducing agent ascorbic acid (vitamin C). The enzymes catalyzing the reactions are prolyl hydroxylase and lysyl hydroxylase. In scurvy, which results from a deficiency of vitamin C, insufficient hydroxylation of collagen causes abnormal collagen fibrils. The weakened collagen in teeth, bone, and blood vessels causes tooth loss, brittle bones with fractures, and bleeding tendencies with bruising and bleeding gums.

116. The answer is d. *(Murray, pp 48–62. Scriver, pp 3–45. Sack, pp 1–3. Wilson, pp 101–120.)* Collagen peptides assemble into helical tertiary structures that form quaternary triple helices. The triple helices in turn assemble end to end to form collagen fibrils that are essential for connective tissue strength. Over 15 types of collagen contribute to the connective tissue of various organs, including the contribution of type I collagen to eyes, bones, and skin. The fact that only one of two α_2 alleles is normal in this case implies that a mutant α_2 allele could be responsible for the disease (even if the α_2 locus is on the X chromosome, since the baby is female with two X chromosomes). The mutant α_2 collagen peptide would be incorporated into half of the type I collagen triple helices, causing a 50% reduction in normal type I collagen. (A mutant α_1 collagen peptide would distort 75% of the molecules since two α_1 peptides go into each triple helix). The ability of one abnormal collagen peptide allele to alter triple helix structure with subsequent degradation is well documented and colorfully named protein suicide or, more properly, a dominant-negative mutation.

117. The answer is a. *(Murray, pp 48–62. Scriver, pp 3–45. Sack, pp 1–3. Wilson, pp 101–120.)* The primary structure of collagen peptides consists of repeating tripeptides with a gly-X-Y motif, where gly is glycine and X and Y are any amino acid. The small CH_2 group connecting the amino and carboxyl groups of glycine contrasts with the larger connecting groups and side chains of other amino acids. The small volume of glycine molecules is crucial for the α helix secondary structure of collagen peptides. This in turn is necessary for their tertiary helical structure and their assembly into quaternary tripeptide, triple-helix structures. The most severe clinical phenotypes caused by amino acid substitutions in collagen peptides are those affecting glycine that prevent α helix formation. The child has a disorder called Stickler syndrome (108300) that exhibits autosomal dominant inheritance.

118. The answer is d. (*Murray, pp 745–761. Scriver, pp 3–45. Sack, pp 1–3. Wilson, pp 101–120.*) Immunoglobulin G is composed of pairs of light chains and heavy chains attached by disulfide bridges. If the reducing agent mercaptoethanol is used to break the disulfide bridges and urea is used to disrupt noncovalent interactions, two identical light subunits (25 kd) and two identical heavy chains (50 kd) per protein can be resolved with electrophoresis. A small amount of carbohydrate is also present. In contrast, the proteolytic enzyme papain cleaves the heavy chains, which results in two Fab molecules consisting of the entire light chain attached to the amino terminal half of each heavy chain and two Fc molecules consisting of the carboxyl terminal half of each heavy chain. Other proteolytic enzymes are nonspecific. Levels rise and fall in the serum dependent upon specific induction by antigen.

119. The answer is b. (*Murray, pp 48–62. Scriver, pp 3–45. Sack, pp 1–3. Wilson, pp 101–120.*) Each of the techniques listed separates proteins from each other and from other biologic molecules based upon characteristics such as size, solubility, and charge. However, only affinity chromatography can use the high affinity of proteins for specific chemical groups or the specificity of immobilized antibodies for unique proteins. In affinity chromatography, a specific compound that binds to the desired protein—such as an antibody, a polypeptide receptor, or a substrate—is covalently bound to the column material. A mixture of proteins is added to the column under conditions ideal for binding the protein desired, and the column is then washed with buffer to remove unbound proteins. The protein is eluted either by adding a high concentration of the original binding material or by making the conditions unfavorable for binding (e.g., changing the pH). The other techniques are less specific than affinity binding for isolating proteins. Dialysis separates large proteins from small molecules. Ion exchange chromatography separates proteins with an overall charge of one sort from proteins with an opposite charge (e.g., negative from positive). Gel filtration chromatography separates on the basis of size. Electrophoresis separates proteins on the principle that net charge influences the rate of migration in an electric field.

120. The answer is b. (*Murray, pp 15–26.*) To reach pH 7.0, approximately 100% of the α-carboxyl group (pK_{a1} = 2.19) and 90% of the γ-carboxyl group (pK_{a2} = 4.25) of glutamic acid must be dissociated. At that pH, approximately twice the amount of NaOH as glutamic acid molecules has been utilized to titrate the two carboxyl groups. Since each milliliter of a 1 M NaOH solution contains 1 mmol of OH⁻ ion, about 3 mmol of the amino acid is present.

121. The answer is c. (*Murray, pp 48–62. Scriver, pp 3–45. Sack, pp 1–3. Wilson, pp 101–120.*) Protein electrophoresis is an important laboratory technique for investigating red cell proteins such as hemoglobin or plasma proteins such as the immunoglobulins. The proteins are dissolved in a buffer of low pH where the amino groups of amino acid side chains are positively charged, causing most proteins to migrate toward the negative electrode (anode). Red cell hemolysates are used for hemoglobin electrophoresis, plasma (blood supernatant with unhemolyzed red cells removed) for plasma proteins. Serum (blood supernatant after clotting) would not contain red cells but would contain many blood enzymes and proteins. In sickle cell anemia, the hemoglobin S contains a valine substitution for the glutamic acid at position 6 in hemoglobin A. Hemoglobin S thus loses two negative charges (loss of a glutamic acid carboxyl group on each of two β-globin chains) compared to hemoglobin A. Hemoglobin S is thus more positively charged and migrates more rapidly toward the anode than hemoglobin A. Lane B must represent the heterozygote with sickle cell trait (hemoglobins S and A), establishing lane A as the normal and lane D as the sickle cell anemia sample. The hemoglobin in lane C migrates differently from normal and hemoglobin S, as would befit an abnormal hemoglobin that is different from S.

122. The answer is d. (*Murray, pp 48–62. Scriver, pp 3–45. Sack, pp 1–3. Wilson, pp 101–120.*) In drawing D, a triple helix is represented. Tropocollagen has the structure of a triple helix because its many proline and hydroxyproline residues prevent the hydrogen bond formation necessary for an α helix like that in drawing B. Tropocollagen is the basic unit of collagen fibrils and is obtained through extraction of insoluble collagen with dilute acid.

123. The answer is c. (*Murray, pp 48–62. Scriver, pp 3–45. Sack, pp 1–3. Wilson, pp 101–120.*) Proteins can be separated on the basis of their overall charge at a given pH by ion exchange chromatography. At low pH all proteins have an overall positive charge because carboxyl groups are protonated. Thus, proteins tend to bind to a cation exchange column that has immobilized the negative charges. Usually negatively charged sulfonic polystyrene resin is used, and Na charges are exchanged for the positively charged protein groups. Once binding has occurred, the pH and NaCl concentration of the eluting medium are increased, and proteins that have a low density of net negative charge emerge first, with those having a higher density of negative charge following. The only information that can be obtained from the information given in the question is that the enzyme has been purified over 100-fold. The turnover rate of the enzyme cannot be deduced. Likewise, the yield, which is the amount of original enzyme protein recovered, cannot be determined. The structure of the enzyme is not revealed by the information given.

124. The answer is b. (*Murray, pp 48–62. Scriver, pp 3–45. Sack, pp 1–3. Wilson, pp 101–120.*) Two kinds of interacting protein filaments are found in skeletal muscle. Thick filaments 15 nm in diameter contain primarily myosin. Thin filaments 7 nm in diameter are composed of actin, troponin, and tropomyosin. The thick and thin filaments slide past one another during muscle contraction. Myosin is an ATPase that binds to thin filaments during contraction. α-actinin can be found in the Z line.

125. The answer is d. (*Murray, pp 48–62. Scriver, pp 3–45. Sack, pp 1–3. Wilson, pp 101–120.*) Pepsin is secreted in a proenzyme form in the stomach. Unlike the majority of proenzymes, it is not activated by protease hydrolysis. Instead, spontaneous acid hydrolysis at pH 2 or lower converts pepsinogen to pepsin. Hydrochloric acid secreted by the stomach lining creates the acid environment. All the enzymes secreted by the pancreas are activated at the same time upon entrance into the duodenum. This is accomplished by trypsin hydrolysis of the inactive proenzymes trypsinogen, chymotrypsinogen, procarboxypeptidase, and proelastase. Primer amounts of trypsin are derived from trypsinogen by the action of enteropeptidase secreted by the cells of the duodenum.

126. The answer is a. *(Murray, pp 27–36. Scriver, pp 3–45. Sack, pp 1–3. Wilson, pp 101–120.)* The carbon next to a carboxyl (C=O) group may be designated as the α carbon, with subsequent carbons as β, γ, δ, etc. α-amino acids contain an amino group on their α carbon, as distinguished from compounds like γ-aminobutyric acid, in which the amino group is two carbons down (γ-carbon). In α-amino acids the amino acid, carboxylic acid, and the side chain or R group are all bound to the central α-carbon, which is thus asymmetric (except when R is hydrogen, as for glycine). Amino acids are classified as acidic, neutral hydrophobic, neutral hydrophilic, or basic, depending on the charge or partial charge on the R group at pH 7.0. Hydrophobic (water-hating) groups are carbon-hydrogen chains like those of leucine, isoleucine, glycine, or valine. Basic R groups, such as those of lysine and arginine, carry a positive charge at physiologic pH owing to protonated amide groups, while acidic R groups, such as glutamic acid, carry a negative charge owing to ionized carboxyl groups. Threonine with its hydroxyl side chain is neutral at physiologic pH. Neutral hydrophilic side chains have uncharged but polar or partially charged groups.

127. The answer is c. *(Murray, pp 48–62. Scriver, pp 3–45. Sack, pp 1–3. Wilson, pp 101–120.)* The light chain and part of the heavy chain at the amino terminal contain the antibody-combining site in the "hypervariable regions." These regions are all contained in fragment A, which is known as Fab. Fragment B is known as Fc. The Fc fragment contains a site for binding of complement. The Fab fragments mediate complement fixation. Each of the fragments can be further dissociated into two subunits by breaking its disulfide bridge with mercaptoethanol or some other reducing agent.

128. The answer is a. *(Murray, pp 48–62. Scriver, pp 3–45. Sack, pp 1–3. Wilson, pp 101–120.)* Regular arrangements of groups of amino acids located near each other in the linear sequence of a polypeptide are the secondary structure of a protein. The α helix, β sheet, and β bend are the secondary structures usually observed in proteins. In both the α helix and the β sheet, all the peptide bond components participate in hydrogen bonding. That is, the oxygen components of the peptide bond form hydrogen bonds with the amide hydrogens. In the case of the α helix, all hydrogen bonding is intrachain and stabilizes the helix. In the case of β sheets, the bonds are interchain when formed between the polypeptide backbones of separate polypeptide chains and intrachain when the β sheet is formed by a single polypeptide chain folding back on itself. While the spiral of the α helix prevents the chain from being fully extended, the chains of β sheets are almost fully extended and relatively flat. The chains of β sheets can be either parallel or antiparallel. When the N-terminals of chains run together, the chain or segment is considered parallel. In contrast, when N-terminal and C-terminal ends of the chains alternate, the β strand is considered antiparallel.

129. The answer is b. (*Murray, pp 27–36. Scriver, pp 3–45. Sack, pp 1–3. Wilson, pp 101–120.*) Except for terminal amino acids, all α-amino groups and all α-carboxyl groups are utilized in peptide bonds. Thus only amino acids with side chains may be considered. Of these, 7 of the 20 common amino acids have easily ionizable side chains. These are the basic amino acids lysine, arginine, and histidine; the acidic amino acids aspartate and glutamate; and tyrosine and cysteine. Leucine, valine, and alanine have hydrocarbon side chains.

130. The answer is d. (*Murray, pp 48–62. Scriver, pp 3–45. Sack, pp 1–3. Wilson, pp 101–120.*) The structure of myoglobin is illustrative of most water-soluble proteins. Globular proteins tend to fold into compact configurations with nonpolar cores. The interior of myoglobin is composed almost exclusively of nonpolar, hydrophobic amino acids like valine, leucine, phenylalanine, and methionine. In contrast, polar hydrophilic residues such as arginine, aspartic acid, glutamic acid, and lysine are found mostly on the surface of the water-soluble protein.

131. The answer is d. (*Murray, pp 746–751. Scriver, pp 3–45. Sack, pp 1–3. Wilson, pp 101–120.*) Five classes of immunoglobulins are known: IgG, IgA, IgM, IgD, and IgE. The difference between each class is due to the variations in the constant chains from one class to another. The respective heavy chains corresponding to each class of immunoglobulin are γ and IgG; α and IgA; μ and IgM; δ and IgD; and ε and IgE. In contrast, the light chains are the same in each class: either κ or λ. The different biologic characteristics are due to the unique heavy chains. IgM is the first class of antibodies to be observed in the plasma following antigenic stimulation. IgG is the major antibody produced in serum at 10 days following antigenic stimulation. IgA acts against bacteria and viruses and is observed in external secretions such as mucus, tears, and saliva. While the undesirable effects of IgE in allergic reactions are known, its possible benefits are not understood. Likewise, the role of IgD is not known.

132. The answer is c. *(Murray, pp 48–62. Scriver, pp 3–45. Sack, pp 1–3. Wilson, pp 101–120.)* Glycosaminoglycans (mucopolysaccharides) are polysaccharide chains that may be bound to proteins as proteoglycans. Each proteoglycan is a complex molecule with a core protein that is covalently bound to glycosaminoglycans—repeating units of disaccharides. The amino sugars forming the disaccharides contain negatively charged sulfate or carboxylate groups. The primary glycosaminoglycans found in mammals are hyaluronic acid, heparin, heparan sulfate, chondroitin sulfate, and keratan sulfate. Inborn errors of glycosaminoglycan degradation cause neurodegeneration and physical stigmata described by the outmoded term "gargoylism." Glycogen is a polysaccharide of glucose used for energy storage, and has no sulfate groups. Collagen and fibrillin are important proteins in connective tissue. γ-aminobutyric acid is a γ-amino acid involved in neurotransmission.

133. The answer is c. *(Murray, pp 48–62. Scriver, pp 3–45. Sack, pp 1–3. Wilson, pp 101–120.)* In blood and other solutions at physiologic pH (approximately 7.0), only terminal carboxyl groups, terminal amino groups, and ionizable side chains of amino acid residues in proteins have charges. The basic amino acids lysine, arginine, and histidine have positive charges (protonated amines). The acidic amino acids aspartate and glutamate have negative charges (ionized carboxyls). Glutamine possesses an uncharged but hydrophilic side chain.

134. The answer is b. *(Murray, pp 48–62. Scriver, pp 3–45. Sack, pp 1–3. Wilson, pp 101–120.)* There are two antigen-binding sites per antibody molecule, each defined by the N-terminals of the light and heavy chain from one subunit. Each of the two subunits have one light chain and one heavy chain, and all are held together by intra- or interchain disulfide linkages. The N-terminal peptides of heavy and light chains comprise the variable regions that recognize many different antigens, whereas the C-terminal peptides comprise the constant region that triggers responses to antigen-antibody complexes. Antigen-binding sites are determined prior to encounter of specific antigens. A large repertoire of virgin B cells are produced after differentiation from stem and pre-B cells. Each virgin B cell carries a unique immunoglobulin M (IgM) molecule on its surface. The surface IgM is determined by one DNA rearrangement of variable-joining-constant (V-J-C) segments to produce a unique light chain and two DNA rearrangements of variable-diversity-joining-constant (V-D-J-C) segments to produce a unique heavy chain. Those unique virgin B cells that do not encounter antigens die, while those that do encounter antigens become activated as plasma (immunoglobulin-producing) or memory B (immunity) cells. A spectrum of cells with specific antibodies are thus made before antigen is contacted, allowing antigen experience to guide the clonal selection process and determine immunoglobulin production/immune status. Note that some mature antibodies have multiple subunits, like the five subunits in IgM. Mature IgM antibodies thus have 10 binding sites in total.

135. The answer is a. (*Murray, pp 27–36. Scriver, pp 3–45. Sack, pp 1–3. Wilson, pp 101–120.*) All α-amino acids have an asymmetric α-carbon atom to which an α-carboxyl group, an α-amino group, and an α-side chain are attached. Levorotary (L) isomers of amino acids compose proteins in nature. Because glycine has a hydrogen as its side chain, with two hydrogens, an amino group, and a carboxyl group on the α-carbon, it is the only optically inactive amino acid. Side chains contribute the distinctive properties at physiological pH to each amino acid (and hence proteins), which include: basic (positive); acidic (negative); neutral polar; neutral nonpolar; sulfur-containing (thiol); hydroxyl-containing; aromatic; hydrophobic; hydrophilic; branched; or straight-chained.

136. The answer is d. (*Murray, pp 27–36. Scriver, pp 3–45. Sack, pp 1–3. Wilson, pp 101–120.*) Each of the 20 unique amino acids coded for by DNA is composed of an α-carbon atom bonded to a hydrogen, a carboxyl group, an amino group, and a side chain R group. The α-carbon is so named because it is adjacent to the carboxyl group. The distinctive side chains of each different amino acid allow variation in charge, shape, size, and reactivity. Although glutamine is often referred to as an acidic amino acid, in fact it is an uncharged polar amino acid with no ionizable group. It is an amide derivative of glutamate, which is an acidic amino acid with an ionizable carboxyl group.

Aliphatic amino acids with large side chains, such as leucine, isoleucine, and valine, are hydrophobic in nature. Their hydrophobicity forces them to sequester together away from water in the interior of proteins. The three-dimensional structure of proteins is highly dependent on the hydrophobic side chains of aliphatic amino acids forming the interior of proteins. In contrast to aliphatic amino acids, which have no ionizable side chains, basic amino acids have ionizable amino groups that are positively charged at neutral pH. These include lysine and arginine, which have a pK of pH 10 and pH 12, respectively, and histidine, with an ionizable imidazole ring and a pK of 6.5. The different characteristics of the side chains of amino acids are responsible for the different qualities of the proteins into which they are incorporated.

137. The answer is a. (*Murray, pp 48–62. Scriver, pp 3–45. Sack, pp 1–3. Wilson, pp 101–120.*) Collagens are insoluble proteins that have great tensile strength. They are the main fibers composing the connective tissue elements of skin, bone, teeth, tendons, and cartilage. Collagen is composed of tropocollagen, a triple-stranded helical rod rich in glycine, proline, and hydroxyproline residues. Troponin is found in muscle, fibrillin in heart valves, blood vessels, and ligaments [it is defective in Marfan's syndrome (154700)]. Fibrin is a component of blood clots and fibronectin is a component of extracellular matrix.

138. The answer is e. (*Murray, pp 48–62. Scriver, pp 3–45. Sack, pp 1–3. Wilson, pp 101–120.*) The major macromolecular components of ground substance are proteoglycans, which are made up of polysaccharide chains attached to core proteins. The polysaccharide chains are made up of repeats of negatively charged disaccharide units. This polyanionic quality of proteoglycans allows them to bind water and cations and thus determines the viscoelastic properties of connective tissues. Collagen is the other major component of connective tissue besides ground substance. The cornified layer of epidermis derives its toughness and waterproof nature from keratin. Keratins are disulfide-rich proteins that compose the cytoskeletal elements known as intermediate filaments. Hair and animal horns are also composed of keratin. Troponin is a component of muscle and fibrin of blood clots.

139. The answer is e. *(Murray, pp 48–62. Scriver, pp 3–45. Sack, pp 1–3. Wilson, pp 101–120.)* Regulatory proteins must bind with great specificity and high affinity to the correct portion of DNA. Several structural motifs have been discovered in DNA-regulatory proteins: the zinc finger, the leucine zipper, and the helix-turn-helix (found in homeotic proteins). Due to the uniqueness of these structural arrangements, their presence in a protein indicates that the protein might bind to DNA. The β sheet, β bend, and α helix are secondary structures found in polypeptide chains, and the triple helix is a tertiary structure composed of three polypeptides as in collagen.

140. The answer is c. *(Murray, pp 48–62. Scriver, pp 3–45. Sack, pp 1–3. Wilson, pp 101–120.)* The connective tissue fiber collagen is synthesized by fibroblasts. However, because the length of the finished collagen fibers is many times greater than that of the cell of origin, a portion of assembly occurs extracellularly. The intracellular formation of the biosynthetic precursor of collagen, procollagen peptides pro-α_1(I) and pro-α_2, occurs in the following steps: (1) synthesis of polypeptides, (2) hydroxylation of proline and lysine residues, (3) glycosylation of lysine residues (proline residues are not glycosylated), (4) formation of the triple helix, and (5) secretion. Once outside the fibroblasts, procollagen molecules are activated by fibroblast-specific procollagen peptidases. Before specific proteolytic cleavage of procollagen, tropocollagen bundles do not assemble into collagen fibers. Once the collagen fibers are formed, aldo cross-links between lysine residues and histidine-aldo cross-links are formed. These cross-links covalently bind the collagen chains to one another. The extent and type of cross-linking determines the flexibility and strength of the collagen mass formed.

Protein Structure/Function

Questions

DIRECTIONS: Each item below contains a question or incomplete statement followed by suggested responses. Select the **one best** response to each question.

141. A 72-year-old woman with emphysema presents to the emergency room with fatigue and respiratory distress. Which set of arterial blood gas values below would represent her condition and reflect a shift of the hemoglobin oxygen dissociation curve to the right?

a. pH 7.05, bicarbonate 15 mM, P_{CO_2} 60, P_{O_2} 88
b. pH 7.15, bicarbonate 10 mM, P_{CO_2} 30, P_{O_2} 88
c. pH 7.25, bicarbonate 15 mM, P_{CO_2} 30, P_{O_2} 88
d. pH 7.40, bicarbonate 24 mM, P_{CO_2} 60, P_{O_2} 88
e. pH 7.45, bicarbonate 15 mM, P_{CO_2} 60, P_{O_2} 88

142. The ability of hemoglobin to serve as an effective transporter of oxygen and carbon dioxide between lungs and tissues is explained by which of the following properties?

a. The isolated heme group with ferrous iron binds oxygen much more avidly than carbon dioxide
b. The α- and β-globin chains of hemoglobin have very different primary structures than myoglobin
c. Hemoglobin utilizes oxidized ferric iron to bind oxygen, in contrast to the ferrous ion of myoglobin
d. In contrast to myoglobin, hemoglobin exhibits greater changes in secondary and tertiary structure after oxygen binding
e. Hemoglobin binds proportionately more oxygen at low oxygen tension than does myoglobin

143. A 65-year-old obese male presents with severe indigestion and chest pain after a spicy meal. A lactate dehydrogenase (LDH) level obtained to evaluate possible myocardial infarction is normal, but the laboratory recommends that LDH isozymes be performed. The managing physician knows that lactate dehydrogenase is composed of two different polypeptide chains arranged in the form of a tetramer. Assuming that all possible combinations of the different polypeptide chains occur, how many isozyme forms of lactate dehydrogenase must be measured?

a. Two
b. Three
c. Four
d. Five
e. Six

144. Contraction of skeletal muscle is initiated by the binding of calcium to

a. Tropomyosin
b. Troponin
c. Myosin
d. Actomyosin
e. Actin

145. Which one of the following statements correctly describes transport of O_2 by hemoglobin?

a. O_2 binds to hemoglobin more avidly than does CO
b. The binding of O_2 to hemoglobin causes a valence change in the iron of the heme moiety
c. Each of the four heme moieties binds O_2 independently
d. The plot of percentage of O_2 bound versus O_2 pressure is sigmoidal in shape
e. Increased CO_2 concentrations increase O_2 affinity

146. The oxygen dissociation curve of normal adult hemoglobin shown below is most effectively shifted to the right by
a. Mixing with fetal hemoglobin
b. Increased 2,3-bisphosphoglycerate (BPG)
c. Cooperative binding of oxygen
d. Increased pH
e. Decreased CO_2

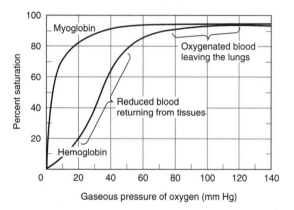

Oxygen binding curves of myoglobin and hemoglobin. Note the reduced hemoglobin saturation at low oxygen pressure that allows better delivery of oxygen to peripheral tissues.

[Reproduced, with permission, from Murray RK, Granner DK, Mayes PA, Rodwell VW: Harper's Biochemistry, 25/e. New York: McGraw-Hill, 2000, as modified from Scriver CR et al (eds): The Molecular and Metabolic Basis of Inherited Disease, 7/e. New York, McGraw-Hill, 1995.]

147. A young man with hypercholesterolemia is rushed to the hospital with crushing chest pain radiating to his left arm and a probable heart attack. Which of the following treatments should be considered?
a. A platelet transfusion
b. Heparin infusion
c. Thrombin infusion
d. Fibrinogen infusion
e. Tissue plasminogen activator infusion

148. Which of the following mutations would produce a severe thalassemia?

a. Deletion of one α-globin locus
b. Deletion of one β-globin locus
c. Oxidation of heme groups to produce methemoglobin
d. Altered RNA processing at both β-globin loci
e. Sickle cell anemia

149. The substitution of valine for glutamate at position 6 on the two β chains in sickle cell hemoglobin causes which of the following?

a. Increased electrophoretic mobility at pH 7.0
b. Increased solubility of deoxyhemoglobin
c. Decreased polymerization of deoxyhemoglobin
d. Unchanged primary structure
e. More flexible red blood cells

150. An increased affinity of hemoglobin for O_2 may result from which of the following?

a. Initial binding of O_2 to one of the four sites available in each deoxyhemoglobin molecule
b. High pH
c. High CO_2 levels
d. High 2,3-bisphosphoglycerate (BPG) levels within erythrocytes
e. Acidosis

151. The specific activity of an enzyme would be reported in which of the following units of measure?

a. Millimoles per liter
b. Units of activity per milligram of protein
c. Micromoles per minute
d. Units of activity per minute
e. Milligrams per micromole

152. The functions of many enzymes, membrane transporters, and other proteins can be quickly activated or deactivated by phosphorylation of specific amino acid residues catalyzed by enzymes called

a. Cyclases
b. Kinases
c. Phosphatases
d. Proteases
e. Zymogens

153. The chemotherapy drug fluorouracil undergoes a series of chemical changes in vivo that result in a covalent complex such that it is bound to both thymidylate synthase and methylene-tetrahydrofolate. The inhibition of deoxythymidilate formation and subsequent blockage of cell division is due to

a. Allosteric inhibition
b. Competitive inhibition
c. Irreversible inhibition
d. Noncovalent inhibition
e. Noncatalytic inhibition

154. The Lineweaver-Burk plot of the reciprocal of the Michaelis-Menten equation is shown below. It is used to graphically determine K_m and V_{max}. When V is the reaction velocity at substrate concentration S, the y axis experimental data are expressed as

a. V
b. $1/V$
c. S
d. $1/S$
e. V/K_m

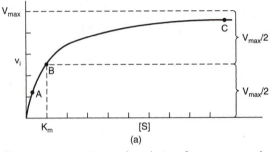

a. Effect of substrate concentration on the velocity of an enzyme-catalyzed reaction. *(From Murray, p. 94, with permission.)*

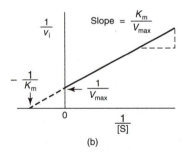

b. Lineweaver-Burk plot. *(From Murray, p. 96, with permission.)*

155. The V_{max} of an enzyme with the kinetic data shown in panel B of the figure in question 154 is

a. Reciprocal of the absolute value of the intercept of the curve with the x axis
b. Reciprocal of the absolute value of the intercept of the curve with the y axis
c. Absolute value of the intercept of the curve with the x axis
d. Slope of the curve
e. Point of inflection of the curve

156. In the study of enzymes, a sigmoidal plot of substrate concentration ($[S]$) versus reaction velocity (V) may indicate

a. Michaelis-Menten kinetics
b. Myoglobin binding to oxygen
c. Cooperative binding
d. Competitive inhibition
e. Noncompetitive inhibition

157. A noncompetitive inhibitor of an enzyme

a. Increases K_m with no or little change in V_{max}
b. Decreases K_m and decreases V_{max}
c. Decreases V_{max}
d. Increases V_{max}
e. Increases K_m and increases V_{max}

158. The velocity-substrate curve below characterizes an allosteric enzyme system. The curve demonstrates that

a. A modifier changes the binding constant for the substrate but not the velocity of the reaction
b. A modifier binding to the allosteric site can also affect the catalytic site
c. Binding of the substrate is independent of its concentration
d. Binding of the modifier is independent of its concentration
e. Binding of substrate to the allosteric site displaces modifier

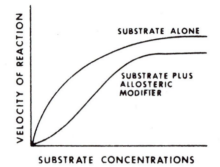

159. Which one of the following statements correctly describes allosteric enzymes?

a. Effectors may enhance or inhibit substrate binding
b. They are not usually controlled by feedback inhibition
c. The regulatory site may be the catalytic site
d. Michaelis-Menten kinetics describe their activity
e. Positive cooperativity occurs in all allosteric molecules except hemoglobin

160. Which one of the following enzymes is regulated primarily through allosteric interaction?

a. Chymotrypsin
b. Pyruvate dehydrogenase
c. Glycogen phosphorylase
d. Glycogen synthase
e. Aspartate transcarbamoylase

161. Which one of the following statements correctly describes allosteric enzymes?

a. Regulatory molecules bind the active site
b. Regulatory molecules alter equilibrium but not activity
c. Regulatory molecules do not affect activity or equilibrium
d. Hyperbolic plots are obtained when reaction velocity is plotted against substrate concentration
e. Binding of substrate to one site can affect other sites

162. Of the six curves labeled in the Lineweaver-Burk graph below, three represent the effects of 0 mM, 5 mM, and 15 mM of a competitive inhibitor on a hypothetical enzyme. Which of the curves most likely represents the 15-mM concentration of the competitive inhibitor?

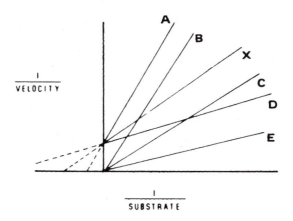

163. Which of the following enzymes exhibits a hyberbolic curve when initial reaction velocity is plotted against substrate concentration?

a. Aspartate transcarbamoylase
b. Phosphofructokinase
c. Hexokinase
d. Pyruvate kinase
e. Lactate dehydrogenase

Protein Structure/Function

Answers

141. The answer is a. (*Murray, pp 48–73. Scriver, pp 4571–4636. Sack, pp 3–17. Wilson, pp 101–120.*) The woman would exhibit respiratory acidosis due to shortness of breath and decreased efficiency of gas exchange in the lungs. Emphysema involves dilated and dysfunctional alveoli from alveolar tissue damage, usually secondary to cigarette smoking. The hypoxia leads to tissue deoxygenation and acidosis, exacerbated by the hypercarbia (CO_2 accumulation) that distinguishes respiratory acidosis (higher bicarbonate than expected) from metabolic acidosis (very low bicarbonate, usually with low P_{CO_2} due to compensatory hyperventilation). Choice a shows the only set of values indicating acidosis (pH lower than 7.4), hypoxia (P_{O_2} lower than 95), and hypercarbia (P_{CO_2} greater than 44).

The tetrameric structure of hemoglobin allows cooperative binding of oxygen in that binding of oxygen to the heme molecule of the first subunit facilitates binding to the other three. This enhanced binding is due to allosteric changes of the hemoglobin molecule, accounting for its S-shaped oxygen saturation curve as compared with that of myoglobin (see the figure in question 146). At the lower oxygen saturations in peripheral tissues (P_{O_2} 30 to 40), hemoglobin releases much more oxygen (up to 50% desaturated) than myoglobin with its single polypeptide structure. The amount of oxygen released (and CO_2 absorbed as carboxyhemoglobin) is further increased by the Bohr effect—increasing hydrogen ion (H^+) concentration (lowering pH) and increasing CO_2 partial pressure (P_{CO_2}) shift the sigmoidal-shaped oxygen binding curve for hemoglobin further to the right.

142. The answer is d. (*Murray, pp 48–73. Scriver, pp 4571–4636. Sack, pp 3–17. Wilson, pp 101–120.*) After binding of the first oxygen, hemoglobin shifts from a taut (T) state toward a relaxed (R) state with the ferrous iron in plane with the four planar pyrrole groups of heme. Binding of subsequent oxygen atoms requires less change of secondary, tertiary, and quaternary structure, producing the cooperative kinetics reflected in the sigmoidal oxygen binding curve (see the figure in answer 141 above). Besides accounting for allosteric changes during oxygen binding, the tertiary folding of each hemoglobin chain and its quaternary (four-chain) structure produce preferred binding of oxygen due to steric restraint. Isolated heme binds carbon dioxide 25,000 times more strongly than oxygen, but in myoglobin and each hemoglobin chain, a histidine group interferes with the preferred mode of carbon dioxide binding such that oxygen is favored. The myoglobin molecule is virtually identical to the β-globin chain of hemoglobin, emphasizing again that the quaternary structure of four subunits in hemoglobin produces its sigmoidal oxygen binding curve, which provides for lung oxygen saturation and tissue desaturation with CO_2 loading. Because of this sigmoidal curve, hemoglobin binds proportionately less oxygen at low oxygen tension (low Po_2) than does myoglobin. Oxidation of the ferrous iron in myoglobin or hemoglobin to ferric ion abolishes oxygen binding, in contrast to the case with other proteins like cytochromes or catalase, where oxidation/reduction of iron modulates their function.

143. The answer is d. *(Murray, pp 48–73. Scriver, pp 4571–4636. Sack, pp 3–17. Wilson, pp 101–120.)* Isozymes are multiple forms of a given enzyme that occur within a given species. Since isozymes are composed of different proteins, analysis by electrophoretic separation can be done. Lactate dehydrogenase is a tetramer composed of any combination of two different polypeptides, H and M. Thus the possible combinations are H4, H3M1, H2M2, H1M3, and M4. Although each combination is found in most tissues, M4 predominates in the liver and skeletal muscle while H4 is the predominant form in the heart. White and red blood cells as well as brain cells contain primarily intermediate forms. The M4 forms of the isozyme seem to have a higher affinity for pyruvate compared with the H4 form. Following a myocardial infarction, the H4 (LDH1) type of lactate dehydrogenase rises and reaches a peak approximately 36 h later. Elevated LDH1 levels may signal myocardial disease even when the total lactate dehydrogenase level is normal.

144. The answer is b. *(Murray, pp 48–73. Scriver, pp 4571–4636. Sack, pp 3–17. Wilson, pp 101–120.)* Calcium ions are the regulators of contraction of skeletal muscle. Calcium is actively sequestered in sarcoplasmic reticulum by an ATP pump during relaxation of muscle. Nervous stimulation leads to the release of calcium into the cytosol and raises the concentration from less than 1 mM to about 10 mM. The calcium binds to troponin C. The calcium-troponin complex undergoes a conformational change, which is transmitted to tropomyosin and causes tropomyosin to shift position. The shift of tropomyosin allows actin to interact with myosin and contraction to proceed.

145. The answer is d. (*Murray, pp 48–73. Scriver, pp 4571–4636. Sack, pp 3–17. Wilson, pp 101–120.*) Hemoglobin is a tetrameric hemoprotein whose oxygen saturation curves exhibit sigmoidal kinetics because of cooperative interactions among the four binding sites. Oxygen is bound to hemoglobin without changing the redox state of the iron from the ferrous state. Carbon monoxide and cyanide both bind to hemoglobin more tightly than does oxygen itself. O_2 is released to tissues and exchanged with CO_2 since increased CO_2 levels in capillaries lead to decreased affinity of hemoglobin for O_2.

146. The answer is b. (*Murray, pp 48–73. Scriver, pp 4571–4636. Sack, pp 3–17. Wilson, pp 101–120.*) In the oxygen dissociation curve, percent saturation of hemoglobin with oxygen on the y axis is plotted against the amount of oxygen present in solution [the partial pressure of oxygen (PO_2)]. Hemoglobin saturation varies from 0 to 100%. The O_2 pressure can vary from no oxygen in solution to high PO_2 levels. 2,3-bisphosphoglycerate (BPG) is present in concentrations similar to those of hemoglobin in red blood cells. BPG cross-links deoxyhemoglobin and lowers its affinity for oxygen, aiding the unloading of oxygen in capillaries. Thus, increased BPG shifts the oxygen dissociation curve to the right. Similarly, increased H^+ ions and CO_2 enhance the release of O_2 from hemoglobin and shift the curve to the right. Conversely, the lower H^+ levels with increasing pH and decreasing CO_2 shift the curve leftward. Fetal hemoglobin has a greater affinity for O_2 under all conditions. Mixing of fetal with adult hemoglobin increases O_2 affinity and shifts the curve to the left.

147. The answer is e. (*Murray, pp 48–73. Scriver, pp 2863–2914. Sack, pp 3–17. Wilson, pp 361–370.*) Many enzymes interact to regulate blood clotting. Plasmin is activated by proteolytic cleavage of its zymogen, plasminogen. The activating protease is called tissue plasminogen activator (tPA). Plasmin hydrolyzes fibrin clots to form soluble products, and is used to dissolve clots in coronary arteries that cause myocardial infarction. Platelets, thrombin, and fibrinogen promote clotting through the intrinsic pathway and would be contraindicated in myocardial infarction. Platelets form a plug at the site of bleeding and bind prothrombin to facilitate its conversion to thrombin. Fibrinogen is the substrate acted upon by thrombin to yield the fibrin mesh of blood clots. Heparin is a mucopolysaccharide that terminates clot formation by interfering with a number of steps in the coagulation cascade. Heparin inhibits the formation of clots, but cannot dissolve clots that have already formed.

148. The answer is d. (*Murray, pp 48–73. Scriver, pp 4571–4636. Sack, pp 3–17. Wilson, pp 101–120.*) Mutations that alter the balance of α- and β-globin synthesis from their respective loci on chromosomes 16 and 11 produce thalassemias. Since these loci are autosomal, mutations at both homologous loci are required to produce severe thalassemia, as with the β thalassemias that involved altered RNA splicing at both β-globin loci. Methemoglobin is hemoglobin with the iron oxidized from the ferrous (Fe^{++}) to the ferric (Fe^{+++}) state. Methemoglobin cannot bind oxygen, so there is a specific enzyme (methemoglobin reductase) and reducing substances like glutathione in red cells that maintain hemoglobin iron in its reduced state. Point mutations that cause amino acid substitutions produce an abnormal hemoglobin rather than imbalance chain synthesis. Sickle cell anemia (141900) is one example, in which both β-globin chains have a valine replacing glutamine. The mutant β-globin chains in hemoglobin S have a "sticky patch" on their surface that is particularly adhesive when hemoglobin S is deoxygenated. For this reason, individuals with sickle cell anemia are prone to thrombotic crises (strokes, heart attacks, ischemic extremities) when they become dehydrated (increased hemoglobin concentration) or hypoxic (more deoxyhemoglobin S). There are also mutant hemoglobins (hemoglobin M, etc.) that predispose to oxidation of the iron group in heme, producing higher concentrations of methemoglobin and cyanosis (bluish color of the lips and fingertips).

149. The answer is a. (*Murray, pp 48–73. Scriver, pp 4571–4636. Sack, pp 3–17. Wilson, pp 101–120.*) The carboxyl of glutamate at position 6 on the β chain of normal hemoglobin is dissociated and negatively charged at pH 7.0. Substitution of uncharged valine for glutamate by mutation produces sickle cell hemoglobin, which is less negatively charged and has an increased electrophoretic mobility. Polymerization of the deoxygenated form of sickle hemoglobin occurs owing to the alteration of primary structure caused by the valine substitution. The insoluble, polymerized hemoglobin causes the erythrocyte to lose flexibility and to become rigid and sickle-shaped. The brittle cells produce anemia and block capillaries.

150. The answer is a. (*Murray, pp 48–73. Scriver, pp 4571–4636. Sack, pp 3–17. Wilson, pp 287–317.*) In addition to its function as a carrier of O_2 and CO_2, hemoglobin buffers sudden additions of acid or base to the blood by virtue of the histidine 146 on each β chain. However, protonation of the imidazole of histidine causes deoxygenation of hemoglobin. Thus, decreased binding of O_2 occurs in the high-pH conditions of acidosis. 2,3-bisphosphoglycerate (BPG) binds specifically to deoxyhemoglobin; that is, BPG cross-links positively charged residues on the β chain, thereby decreasing oxygen affinity and stabilizing the deoxygenated form of hemoglobin. The addition of each O_2 molecule to deoxyhemoglobin requires the breakage of salt links, such as those formed by 2,3-BPG. Each subsequent O_2 molecule requires the breakage of fewer salt links. Thus, initial O_2 binding actually results in an increased affinity for subsequent O_2 binding, which in turn results in a cooperative allosteric binding mechanism. CO_2 reacts reversibly with the amino acid terminals of hemoglobin to create carbaminohemoglobin, which is negatively charged and which forms salt bridges stabilizing deoxyhemoglobin. Hence, CO_2 binding lowers the affinity of hemoglobin for O_2.

151. The answer is b. (*Murray, pp 48–73. Scriver, pp 4571–4636. Sack, pp 3–17. Wilson, pp 287–317.*) Substrate concentrations are usually expressed in terms of molarity, e.g., M = moles per liter, mM = millimoles per liter, μM = micromoles per liter. K_m, the Michaelis constant, is expressed in terms of substrate concentration. Each unit of enzyme activity is described as the amount of enzyme that converts a specific amount of substrate to a product within a given time. The standard units of activity are micromoles of substrate per minute. Specific activity relates the units of enzyme activity to the amount of protein present in the reaction, expressed as units of enzyme activity per milligram of protein. If the enzyme is pure (no proteins except the assayed enzyme are present), then the specific activity is maximal and constant for that particular enzyme (units of activity per milligram of enzyme). The specific activity is a useful measure of enzyme purity that should increase during enzyme purification.

152. The answer is b. *(Murray, pp 48–73. Scriver, pp 4571–4636. Sack, pp 3–17. Wilson, pp 287–317.)* A variety of highly regulated protein kinases can cause activation or deactivation of certain key regulatory proteins by covalent modification of specific serine, threonine, or tyrosine hydroxyl residues by phosphorylation. For example, skeletal muscle glycogen phosphorylase b is activated by phosphorylation of a single serine residue (serine 14) in each subunit of the dimers composing the enzyme. The phosphorylation reaction itself is catalyzed by phosphorylase kinase. Protein phosphatases can quickly reverse such effects. Activated muscle glycogen phosphorylase a is deactivated by a specific phosphatase that hydrolyzes the phosphoryl group off of serine 14. Whether the phosphorylated or dephosphorylated form of a protein predominates depends upon the relative activities of the kinase versus the phosphatase.

153. The answer is c. *(Murray, pp 48–73. Scriver, pp 4571–4636. Sack, pp 3–17. Wilson, pp 287–317.)* Since rapidly multiplying cancer cells are dependent upon the synthesis of deoxythymidilate (dTMP) from deoxyuridylate (dUMP), a prime target in cancer therapy has been inhibition of dTMP synthesis. The anticancer drug fluorouracil is converted in vivo to fluorodeoxyuridylate (FdUMP), which is an analogue of dUMP. FdUMP irreversibly forms a covalent complex with the enzyme thymidylate synthase and its substrate N5,N10-methylene-tetrahydrofolate. This is a case of suicide inhibition, where an enzyme actually participates in the change of a substrate into a covalently linked inhibitor that irreversibly inhibits its catalytic activity.

154. The answer is b. *(Murray, pp 48–73. Scriver, pp 4571–4636. Sack, pp 3–17. Wilson, pp 287–317.)* The Michaelis-Menten equation is:

$$V = V_{max} \, [S]/[S] + K_m$$

The Lineweaver-Burk equation is the reciprocal of the Michaelis-Menten equation:

$$1/V = K_m/V_{max}[1/S] + [1/V_{max}]$$

In the Lineweaver-Burk plot, the reciprocal of velocity $1/V$ is plotted on the y axis against the reciprocal of substrate concentration $1/S$ on the x axis. Direct graphic determination of V_{max} is made by measuring the y intercept ($= 1/V_{max}$ when $1/S = 0$). Direct graphic measurement of the K_m is made by measuring the x intercept ($= -1/K_m$ when $1/V = 0$). The slope is K_m/V_{max}.

155. The answer is b. (*Murray, pp 48–73. Scriver, pp 4571–4636. Sack, pp 3–17. Wilson, pp 287–317.*) When an enzyme obeys classic Michaelis-Menten kinetics as seen in the figure presented in question 154, the Michaelis constant (K_m) and the maximal rate (V_{max}) can be readily derived. By plotting a reciprocal of the Michaelis-Menten equation, a straight-line Lineweaver-Burk plot is produced. The y intercept is $1/V_{max}$, while the x intercept is $-1/K_m$. Thus, a reciprocal of these absolute values yields V_{max} and K_m.

156. The answer is c. (*Murray, pp 48–73. Scriver, pp 4571–4636. Sack, pp 3–17. Wilson, pp 287–317.*) Allosteric enzymes, unlike simpler enzymes, do not obey Michaelis-Menten kinetics. Often, one active site of an allosteric enzyme molecule can positively affect another active site in the same molecule. This leads to cooperativity and sigmoidal enzyme kinetics in a plot of [S] versus V. The terms *competitive inhibition* and *noncompetitive inhibition* apply to Michaelis-Menten kinetics and not to allosteric enzymes.

157. The answer is c. (*Murray, pp 48–73. Scriver, pp 4571–4636. Sack, pp 3–17. Wilson, pp 287–317.*) In contrast to competitive inhibitors, noncompetitive inhibitors are not structural analogues of the substrate. Consequently, noncompetitive inhibitors bind to enzymes in locations remote from the active site. For this reason, the degree of inhibition is based solely upon the concentration of inhibitor and increasing the substrate concentrations do not compete with or change the inhibition. Therefore, unlike the increase in K_m seen with competitive inhibition, in noncompetitive inhibition V_{max} increases while K_m usually remains the same. While competitive inhibitors can be overcome at sufficiently high concentration of substrate, noncompetitive inhibition is irreversible.

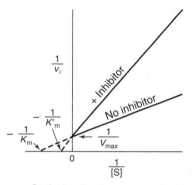

a. Lineweaver-Burk plot showing competitive inhibition.

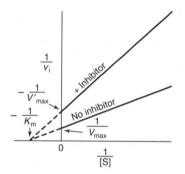

b. Lineweaver-Burk plot showing noncompetitive inhibition.
(Reproduced, with permission, from Murray RK, Granner DK, Mayes PA, Rodwell VW:
Harper's Biochemistry, 25/e. New York, McGraw-Hill, 2000: 98, 99.)

158. The answer is b. *(Murray, pp 48–73. Scriver, pp 4571–4636. Sack, pp 3–17. Wilson, pp 287–317.)* When a modifier binds at the allosteric site, it affects the active site by altering V_{max} and K_m. The substrate binds to the active, or catalytic, site, where it is modified. Binding of both substrate and modifier is, of course, concentration-dependent. The velocity of an allosteric enzyme reaction depends on the concentration of both the substrate and the modifier.

159. The answer is a. *(Murray, pp 48–73. Scriver, pp 4571–4636. Sack, pp 3–17. Wilson, pp 287–317.)* The binding of an effector to the regulatory subunit of an allosteric enzyme causes a conformational change that either increases or decreases the activity of the enzyme's separate catalytic site. Only in some allosteric molecules, such as hemoglobin, does positive cooperativity occur. A positive effector increases substrate binding. This is the case with cyclic AMP–dependent protein kinase of the glycogen phosphorylase cascade. Cyclic AMP binds the regulatory subunit that dissociates from the catalytic subunit and thereby activates it. In the absence of cyclic AMP, the regulatory subunit tightly binds the catalytic subunit and inactivates the enzymes. Many allosteric enzymes are often placed at the first, or committed, step of a metabolic pathway. The end product of the pathway then acts as a negative effector of the enzyme. This is called feedback inhibition. An allosteric enzyme does not obey Michaelis-Menten kinetics.

160. The answer is e. *(Murray, pp 48–73. Scriver, pp 4571–4636. Sack, pp 3–17. Wilson, pp 287–317.)* Aspartate transcarbamoylase, which controls the rate of pyrimidine synthesis in mammals, is negatively inhibited by the allosteric effector cytidine triphosphate, an end product of pyrimidine synthesis. The allosteric modulation occurs via the binding of effectors at the regulatory site of the enzyme. Noncovalent bonds are formed during the binding between effector and enzyme. In contrast, all the other enzymes are activated or deactivated by covalent modification. Chymotrypsinogen is secreted as an inactive proenzyme (zymogen) in pancreatic juice and is irreversibly activated by trypsin cleavage of a specific peptide bond. Glycogen phosphorylase is reversibly activated by phosphorylation of a specific serine residue. At the same time, glycogen synthase is reversibly deactivated by phosphorylation of a specific serine residue, thereby preventing a futile cycle of breakdown and resynthesis of glycogen. Pyruvate dehydrogenase also is reversibly inactivated by phosphorylation of a specific serine residue. In all four enzymes, a single, discrete, covalent modification leads to conformational changes that allow the switching on or off of enzyme activity.

161. The answer is e. *(Murray, pp 48–73. Scriver, pp 4571–4636. Sack, pp 3–17. Wilson, pp 287–317.)* Unlike Michaelis-Menten enzymes, allosteric enzymes exhibit sigmoidal plots when reaction velocity is plotted against substrate concentrations. The enzyme contains both a catalytic site and a regulatory site. The binding of regulatory molecules to the regulatory site alters enzyme activity. The binding of one substrate molecule can affect the binding of substrate to other catalytic sites.

162. The answer is a. (*Murray, pp 48–73. Scriver, pp 4571–4636. Sack, pp 3–17. Wilson, pp 287–317.*) Competitive inhibitors resemble the structure of the substrate and compete with the substrate to bind to the active site of the enzyme. For this reason, K_m increases with increasing inhibitor concentration, while V_{max} remains the same. That is, V_{max} can be reached at substrate concentrations sufficiently high to overcome the inhibitor. Since the x axis intercept represents $-1/K_m$ and the y axis intercept represents $1/V_{max}$, only curves A, X, and D show changes in K_m with no changes in V_{max}. When $-1/K_m$ is interpreted properly, the highest K_m value is given by curve A.

163. The answer is e. (*Murray, pp 48–73. Scriver, pp 4571–4636. Sack, pp 3–17. Wilson, pp 287–317.*) Nonregulatory enzymes, such as lactate dehydrogenase, typically exhibit a hyperbolic saturation curve when initial velocity is plotted against substrate concentration (see the figure in question 154). Enzymes at key points in metabolic pathways are typically allosteric—their velocities at a given substrate concentration may be altered due to effects of metabolites in the pathway. Allosteric enzymes typically exhibit sigmoidal kinetics. Examples of allosteric enzymes include aspartate transcarbamoylase, which is inhibited by cytidine triphosphate (CTP); phosphofructokinase, which is inhibited by adenosine triphosphate (ATP) and activated by fructose 2,6-bisphosphate; hexokinase, which is inhibited by glucose-6-phosphate; and pyruvate kinase, which is inhibited by ATP. Allosteric enzymes produce sigmoidal kinetics when substrate concentration is plotted against reaction velocity. In contrast, hyperbolic plots are observed with Michaelis-Menten enzymes. The binding of effector molecules, such as end products or second messengers, to regulatory subunits of allosteric enzymes can either positively or negatively regulate catalytic subunits.

Intermediary Metabolism

Carbohydrate Metabolism

Questions

DIRECTIONS: Each item below contains a question or incomplete statement followed by suggested responses. Select the **one best** response to each question.

164. Structure 2 in panel (a) of the figure below is referred to as

a. α-D-glucopyranose
b. β-D-glucopyranose
c. α-D-glucofuranose
d. β-L-glucofuranose
e. α-D-fructofuranose

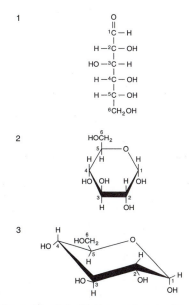

a. D-glucose drawn in the straight chain (1), Hayworth projection (2), and chair (3) forms. *(Reproduced, with permission, from Murray RK, Granner DK, Mayes PA, Rodwell VW: Harper's Biochemistry, 25/e. New York, McGraw-Hill, 2000: 150.)*

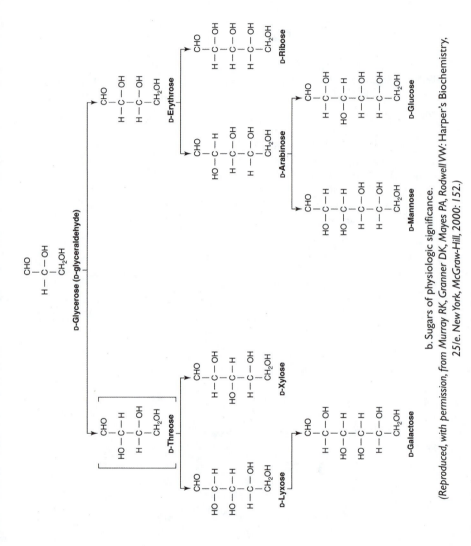

b. Sugars of physiologic significance.

(Reproduced, with permission, from Murray RK, Granner DK, Mayes PA, Rodwell VW: Harper's Biochemistry, 25/e. New York, McGraw-Hill, 2000: 152.)

165. A child develops chronic diarrhea and liver inflammation in early infancy when the mother begins using formula that includes corn syrup. Evaluation of the child demonstrates sensitivity to fructose in the diet. Which of the following glycosides contains fructose and therefore should be avoided when feeding or treating this infant?

a. Sucrose
b. Oaubain
c. Lactose
d. Maltose
e. Streptomycin

166. Which of the following carbohydrates would be most abundant in the diet of strict vegetarians?

a. Amylose
b. Lactose
c. Cellulose
d. Maltose
e. Glycogen

167. The major metabolic product produced under normal circumstances by erythrocytes and by muscle cells during intense exercise is recycled through the liver in the Cori cycle. The metabolite is

a. Oxaloacetate
b. Glycerol
c. Alanine
d. Pyruvate
e. Lactate

168. Chronic alcoholics require more ethanol than do nondrinkers to become intoxicated because of a higher level of specific enzyme. However, independent of specific enzyme levels, the availability of what other substance is rate-limiting in the clearance of ethanol?

a. NADH
b. NAD$^+$
c. FADH
d. FAD$^+$
e. NADPH

169. In lung diseases such as emphysema or chronic bronchitis, there is chronic hypoxia that is particularly obvious in vascular tissues such as the lips or nail beds (cyanosis). Poorly perfused areas exposed to chronic hypoxia have decreased metabolic energy for tissue maintenance and repair. An important reason for this is

a. Increased hexokinase activity owing to increased oxidative phosphorylation
b. Increased ethanol formation from pyruvate on changing from anaerobic to aerobic metabolism
c. Increased glucose utilization via the pentose phosphate pathway on changing from anaerobic to aerobic metabolism
d. Decreased ATP generation and increased glucose utilization on changing from aerobic to anaerobic metabolism
e. Decreased respiratory quotient on changing from carbohydrate to fat as the major metabolic fuel

170. Following a fad diet meal of skim milk and yogurt, an adult female patient experiences abdominal distention, nausea, cramping, and pain followed by a watery diarrhea. This set of symptoms is observed each time the meal is consumed. A likely diagnosis is

a. Steatorrhea
b. Lactase deficiency
c. Maltose deficiency
d. Sialidase deficiency
e. Lipoprotein lipase deficiency

171. Asians and Native Americans may flush and feel ill after drinking small amounts of ethanol in alcoholic beverages. This reaction is due to genetic variation in an enzyme that metabolizes the liver metabolite of alcohol, which is

a. Methanol
b. Acetone
c. Acetaldehyde
d. Hydrogen peroxide
e. Glycerol

172. Which one of the following enzymes catalyzes high-energy phosphorylation of substrates during glycolysis?

a. Pyruvate kinase
b. Phosphoglycerate kinase
c. Triose phosphate isomerase
d. Aldolase
e. Glyceraldehyde-3-phosphate dehydrogenase

173. Which one of the following enzymes is common to both glycolysis and gluconeogenesis?

a. Pyruvate kinase
b. Pyruvate carboxylase
c. Hexokinase
d. Phosphoglycerate kinase
e. Fructose-1,6-bisphosphatase

174. During the first week of a diet of 1500 calories per day, the oxidation of glucose via glycolysis in the liver of a normal 59-kg (130-lb) woman is inhibited by the lowering of which one of the following?

a. Citrate
b. ATP
c. Fatty acyl CoA
d. Ketone bodies
e. Fructose-2,6-bisphosphate

175. Familial fructokinase deficiency causes no symptoms because

a. Hexokinase can phosphorylate fructose
b. Most tissues utilize fructose
c. Liver fructose-1-P aldolase is still active
d. Excess fructose does not escape into the urine
e. Excess fructose spills into the bowel and is eliminated in feces

176. A newborn begins vomiting after feeding, becomes severely jaundiced, and has liver disease. Treatment for possible sepsis is initiated, and the urine is found to have reducing substances. A blood screen for galactosemia is positive, and lactose-containing substances are removed from the diet. Lactose is toxic in this case because

a. Excess glucose accumulates in the blood
b. Galactose is converted to the toxic substance galactitol (dulcitol)
c. Galactose competes for glucose during hepatic glycogen synthesis
d. Galactose is itself toxic in even small amounts
e. Glucose metabolism is shut down by excess galactose

177. Which one of the following enzymes catalyzes phosphorylation with the use of inorganic phosphate?

a. Hexokinase
b. Phosphofructokinase
c. Glyceraldehyde-3-phosphate dehydrogenase
d. Phosphoglycerate kinase
e. Pyruvate kinase

178. After a well-rounded breakfast, which of the following would be expected to occur?

a. Increased activity of pyruvate carboxylase
b. Decreased activity of acetyl CoA carboxylase
c. Decreased rate of glycogenolysis
d. Decreased rate of protein synthesis
e. Increased activity of phosphoenolpyruvate carboxykinase

179. Which of the following metabolites is involved in glycogenolysis, glycolysis, and gluconeogenesis?

a. Galactose-1-phosphate
b. Glucose-6-phosphate
c. Uridine diphosphoglucose
d. Fructose-6-phosphate
e. Uridine diphosphogalactose

180. Which of the following is an allosteric effector that enhances activity of phosphofructokinase of the glycolytic pathway?

a. Adenosine monophosphate (AMP)
b. Citric acid
c. Adenosine triphosphate (ATP)
d. Glucose-6-phosphate
e. Glucose

181. Which of the following hormones stimulates gluconeogenesis?

a. Progesterone
b. Glucagon
c. Aldosterone
d. Epinephrine
e. Thyroxine
f. Growth hormone
g. Insulin
h. Glucocorticoids

182. The key regulatory enzyme of the pentose phosphate pathway is positively regulated by

a. Reduced nicotinamide dinucleotide (NADH)
b. Adenosine diphosphate (ADP)
c. Guanosine triphosphate (GTP)
d. Nicotinamide dinucleotide phosphate (NADP$^+$)
e. Reduced flavine adenine dinucleotide (FADH)

183. The activity of pyruvate carboxylase is dependent upon the positive allosteric effector

a. Succinate
b. AMP
c. Isocitrate
d. Citrate
e. Acetyl CoA

184. Which of the following explains why individuals with hyperlipi-demia and/or gout should minimize their intake of sucrose and high-fructose syrups?

a. Fructose is initially phosphorylated by liver fructokinase
b. After initial modification, fructose is cleaved by a specific enolase
c. Fructose is converted to UDP-fructose
d. Fructose is ultimately converted to galactose
e. Fructose can be phosphorylated by hexokinase in adipose cells

185. Glycogen synthetase, the enzyme involved in the biosynthesis of glycogen, may

a. Be activated by the phosphorylation of a specific serine residue
b. Be activated by increased calcium levels
c. Be more specifically defined as UDP-glucose-glycogen glucosyl transferase
d. Synthesize glycogen without a polymer primer
e. Employ UDP-D-glucose as a glucosyl donor in both plants and animals

186. Which one of the following activities is simultaneously stimulated by epinephrine in muscle and inhibited by epinephrine in the liver?

a. Fatty acid oxidation
b. Glycogenolysis
c. Cyclic AMP synthesis
d. Glycolysis
e. Activation of phosphorylase

187. Which one of the following compounds is common to both the oxidative branch and the nonoxidative branch of the pentose phosphate pathway?

a. Xylulose-5-phosphate
b. Glucose-6-phosphate
c. Glyceraldehyde-3-phosphate
d. Fructose-6-phosphate
e. Ribulose-5-phosphate

188. A Nigerian medical student studying in the United States develops hemolytic anemia after taking the oxidizing antimalarial drug pamaquine. This severe reaction is most likely due to

a. Glucose-6-phosphate dehydrogenase deficiency
b. Concomitant scurvy
c. Vitamin C deficiency
d. Diabetes
e. Glycogen phosphorylase deficiency

189. Which of the following events occurs during formation of phospho-enolpyruvate from pyruvate during gluconeogenesis?

a. CO_2 is consumed
b. Inorganic phosphate is consumed
c. Acetyl CoA is utilized
d. ATP is generated
e. GTP is generated

190. Among the many molecules of high-energy phosphate compounds formed as a result of the functioning of the citric acid cycle, one molecule is synthesized at the substrate level. In which of the following reactions does this occur?

a. Citrate → α-ketoglutarate
b. α-ketoglutarate → succinate
c. Succinate → fumarate
d. Fumarate → malate
e. Malate → oxaloacetate

191. After alcohol ingestion, which of the following intermediates accumulates in liver that is not typical of glycolysis or the citric acid cycle?

a. Acetyl CoA
b. Lactate
c. Acetaldehyde
d. Citrate
e. Oxaloacetate

192. Citrate has a positive allosteric effect on which one of the following enzymes?

a. Pyruvate kinase
b. Acetyl CoA carboxylase
c. Phosphofructokinase
d. Fatty acid synthetase
e. Enolase

193. Reduction of which one of the following substrates leads to a reducing equivalent in a step of the citric acid cycle?

a. Succinyl CoA
b. Malate
c. Fumarate
d. Oxaloacetate
e. Citrate

194. The entry point into the citric acid cycle for isoleucine, valine, and the product of odd-chain fatty acids is

a. Fumarate
b. Pyruvate
c. Oxaloacetate
d. Citrate
e. Succinyl CoA

195. A child has ingested cyanide from her parents' garage and is rushed to the emergency room. Which of the following components of the citric acid cycle will be depleted first in this child?

a. NAD^+ cofactor
b. Citrate synthase
c. Aconitase
d. Citrate production
e. Acetyl coenzyme A (CoA) production

196. Which of the following statements correctly describes ketone bodies?

a. They accumulate in children with fatty acid oxidation disorders
b. They accumulate in diabetes mellitus after insulin therapy
c. They are produced by muscle but not by liver
d. They include β-hydroxybutyrate and acetone
e. They are found in blood but not in urine

197. Oxidative degradation of acetyl coenzyme A (CoA) in the citric acid cycle gives a net yield of which of the following chemicals?

a. Flavin adenine dinucleotide (FAD^+)
b. Nicotinamide adenine dinucleotide (NAD^+)
c. Adenosine triphosphate (ATP)
d. Guanosine diphosphate (GDP)
e. Carbon dioxide (CO_2)

198. The citric acid cycle is inhibited by which of the following?

a. Fluoroacetate
b. Fluorouracil
c. Aerobic conditions
d. Arsenic
e. Malic acid

199. In the pathway leading to biosynthesis of acetoacetate from acetyl CoA in the liver, the immediate precursor of acetoacetate is which of the following substances?

a. 3-hydroxybutyrate
b. Acetoacetyl CoA
c. 3-hydroxybutyryl CoA
d. Mevalonic acid
e. 3-hydroxy-3-methylglutaryl CoA

200. A child presents with low blood glucose (hypoglycemia), enlarged liver (hepatomegaly), and excess fat deposition in the cheeks (cherubic facies). A liver biopsy reveals excess glycogen in hepatocytes. Deficiency of which of the following enzymes might explain this phenotype?

a. α-1,1-glucosidase
b. α-1,1-galactosidase
c. α-1,4-glucosidase
d. α-1,4-galactosidase
e. α-1,6-galactosidase

201. Which of the following statements about glycogen metabolism is true?

a. Cyclic AMP–activated protein kinase stimulates glycogen synthase
b. Phosphorylase kinase is activated by phosphorylation
c. Phosphorylase b is inactivated by phosphorylation
d. Cyclic AMP levels are lowered by epinephrine and glucagon stimulation of adenylate cyclase
e. Glycogen synthesis is stimulated by glucagon

202. A man goes on a hunger strike and confines himself to a liquid diet with minimal calories. Which of the following would occur after 4 to 5 h?

a. Decreased cyclic AMP and increased liver glycogen synthesis
b. Increased cyclic AMP and increased liver glycogenolysis
c. Decreased epinephrine levels and increased liver glycogenolysis
d. Increased Ca^{++} in muscle and decreased glycogenolysis
e. Decreased Ca^{++} in muscle and decreased glycogenolysis

203. After a meal, blood glucose enters cells and is stored as glycogen, particularly in the liver. Which of the following is the donor of new glucose molecules in glycogen?

a. UDP-glucose-1-phosphate
b. UDP-glucose
c. UDP-glucose-6-phosphate
d. glucose-6-phosphate
e. glucose-1-phosphate

204. Which of the following statements about the structure of glycogen is true?

a. Glycogen is a copolymer of glucose and galactose
b. There are more branch residues than residues in straight chains
c. Branch points contain α-1,4 glycosidic linkages
d. New glucose molecules are added to the C1 aldehyde group of chain termini, forming a hemiacetal
e. The monosaccharide residues alternate between D- and L-glucose

205. Which of the following steps is involved in the generation of glucose from lipolysis?

a. Glycerol from lipolysis is converted to triglycerides
b. Fatty acids from lipolysis are oxidized, producing NADH and stimulating gluconeogenesis
c. Glycerol from lipolysis is phosphorylated, converted to fructose-1,6-bisphosphate, and eventually converted to glucose
d. Fatty acids from lipolysis stimulate the citric acid cycle
e. Glycerol from lipolysis is taken up by liver cells and dimerized to fructose

206. McArdle's disease causes muscle cramps and muscle fatigue with increased muscle glycogen. Which of the following enzymes is deficient?

a. Hepatic hexokinase
b. Muscle glycogen synthetase
c. Muscle phosphorylase
d. Muscle hexokinase
e. Muscle debranching enzyme

207. Which of the following enzymes is associated with glycogen synthesis?

a. Amylo-$(1,4 \rightarrow 1,6)$-transglycosylase
b. Phosphorylase
c. Phosphorylase kinase
d. Amylo-1,6-glucosidase
e. Glucose-6-phosphatase

Carbohydrate Metabolism

Answers

164. The answer is a. *(Murray, pp 190–198. Scriver, pp 1521–1552. Sack, pp 121–138. Wilson, pp 287–317.)* Hexose (six-carbon) and pentose (five-carbon) sugars have first carbons (C1) with aldehyde groups and fifth or sixth carbons with alcohol groups. All but the initial and terminal carbons are optically active, meaning that glucose has four optically active carbons and 2^4 or 16 stereoisomers with the same structural formula, including galactose and mannose (epimers). By convention, the position of the hydroxyl to the right or left of the carbon next to the alcohol group (C5 in glucose) determines whether it is the D (to right) or L (to left) form. Other carbohydrates such as D-glycerol (hydroxyl on C2 to right) or D-fructose (hydroxyl on C4 to right) are named relative to D-glucose. In aqueous solutions, the C4 of hexoses (C3 of pentoses) binds to the C1 aldehyde to form a hemiacetal pyranose (six-membered) ring structure (depicted as a Hayworth formula). Less favorable for hexoses are the furanose (five-membered) rings formed by bonding C1 aldehyde to the C3 hydroxyl. The C1 hydroxyl formed by hemiacetal formation can extend above (β) or below (α) the ring. In D-glucose, the α and β forms (anomers) are free to interconvert. When joined with other carbohydrates to form α or β polysaccharides, they are fixed. As with most stereoisomers, biological systems exhibit strong preferences for certain isomers of hexoses (e.g., glucose, fructose), pentoses (e.g., ribose), or glycosides (e.g., α-glycosides in linear glycogen and β-oriented cardiac glycosides).

165. The answer is a. *(Murray, pp 190–198. Scriver, pp 1521–1552. Sack, pp 121–138. Wilson, pp 287–317.)* Glycosides are formed by condensation of the aldehyde or ketone group of a carbohydrate with a hydroxyl group of another compound. Other linked groups (aglycones) include steroids with hydroxyl groups (e.g., cardiac glycosides such as digitalis or ouabain) or other chemicals (e.g., antibiotics such as steptomycin). Sucrose (α-D-glucose-β-1 $\rightarrow$ 2-D-fructose), maltose (α-D-glucose-α-1 $\rightarrow$ 4-D-glucose), and lactose (α-D-galactose-β-1 $\rightarrow$ 4-D-glucose) are important disaccharides. Fructose is among several carbohydrate groups known as ketoses because it possesses a ketone group. The ketone group is at carbon 2 in fructose, and its alcohol group at carbon 1 (also at carbon 6) allows ketal formation to produce pyranose and furanose rings as with glucose. Most of the fructose found in the diet of North Americans is derived from the disaccharide sucrose (common table sugar). Sucrose is cleaved into equimolar amounts of glucose and fructose in the small intestine by the action of the pancreatic enzyme sucrase. Deficiency of sucrase can also cause chronic diarrhea. Hereditary fructose intolerance (229600) is caused by deficiency of the liver enzyme aldolase B, which hydrolyzes fructose-1-phosphate.

166. The answer is c. *(Murray, pp 190–198. Scriver, pp 1521–1552. Sack, pp 121–138. Wilson, pp 287–317.)* Cellulose, the most abundant compound known, is the structural fiber of plants and bacterial walls. It is a polysaccharide consisting of chains of glucose residues linked by β $1\rightarrow 4$ bonds. Since humans do not have intestinal hydrolases that attack β $1\rightarrow 4$ linkages, cellulose cannot be digested but forms an important source of "bulk" in the diet. Lactose is a disaccharide of glucose and galactose found in milk. Amylose is an unbranched polymer of glucose residues in α-1,4 linkages. Glycogen is a branched polymer of glucose with both α-1,4 and α-1,6 linkages. Maltose is a disaccharide of glucose, which is usually the breakdown product of amylose.

167. The answer is e. *(Murray, pp 190–198. Scriver, pp 1521–1552. Sack, pp 121–138. Wilson, pp 287–317.)* Under circumstances of intense muscular contraction, the rate of formation of NADH by glycolysis exceeds the capacity of mitochondria to reoxidize it. Consequently, pyruvate produced by glycolysis is reduced to lactate, thereby regenerating NAD^+. Since erythrocytes have no mitochondria, accumulation of lactate occurs normally. Lactate goes to the liver via the blood, is formed into glucose by gluconeogenesis, and then reenters the bloodstream to be reutilized by erythrocytes or muscle. This recycling of lactate to glucose is called the Cori cycle. A somewhat similar phenomenon using alanine generated by muscles during starvation is called the glucose-alanine cycle. All of the other substances listed— oxaloacetate, glycerol, and pyruvate—can be made into glucose by the liver.

168. The answer is b. *(Murray, pp 190–198. Scriver, pp 1521–1552. Sack, pp 121–138. Wilson, pp 287–317.)* In humans, ethanol is cleared from the body by oxidation catalyzed by two NAD$^+$-linked enzymes: alcohol dehydrogenase and acetaldehyde dehydrogenase. These enzymes act mainly in the liver to convert alcohol to acetaldehyde and acetate, respectively. In chronic alcoholics, alcohol dehydrogenase may be elevated somewhat. The NADH level is significantly increased in the liver during oxidation of alcohol, owing to the consumption of NAD$^+$. This leads to a swamping of the normal means of regenerating NAD$^+$. Thus, NAD$^+$ becomes the rate-limiting factor in oxidation of excess alcohol.

169. The answer is d. (*Murray, pp 190–198. Scriver, pp 1521–1552. Sack, pp 121–138. Wilson, pp 287–317.*) The exposure of tissues to chronic hypoxia makes them rely more on anaerobic metabolism for the generation of energy as ATP and other high-energy phosphates. Most tissues except for red blood cells can metabolize glucose under anaerobic or aerobic conditions (red blood cells do not have mitochondria for electron transport and must rely on other tissues to generate glucose back from lactate). In most tissues, a switch from aerobic to anaerobic metabolism greatly increases glucose utilization and decreases energy production. (A reduction of glucose utilization under anaerobic conditions in bacteria is known as the Pasteur effect after its discoverer). Under aerobic conditions, the cell can produce a net gain in moles of ATP formed per mole of glucose utilized that can be as high as 18 times that produced under anaerobic conditions. Thus the cell generates more energy and requires less glucose under aerobic conditions. Such increased ATP concentrations, together with the release of citrate from the citric acid cycle under aerobic conditions, allosterically inhibit the key regulatory enzyme of the glycolytic pathway, phosphofructokinase. Decreased phosphofructokinase activity decreases metabolism of glucose by glycolysis.

170. The answer is b. (*Murray, pp 190–198. Scriver, pp 1521–1552. Sack, pp 121–138. Wilson, pp 287–317.*) In many populations, a majority of adults are deficient in lactase and hence intolerant to the lactose in milk. In all populations, at least some adults have lactase deficiency (223000). Since virtually all children are able to digest lactose, this deficiency obviously develops in adulthood. In lactase-deficient adults, lactose accumulates in the small intestine because no transports exist for the disaccharide. An outflow of water into the gut owing to the osmotic effect of the milk sugar causes the clinical symptoms. Steatorrhea, or fatty stools, is caused by unabsorbed fat, which can occur following a fatty meal in persons with a deficiency of lipoprotein lipase (238600). Sialidase deficiency (256550) causes accumulation of sialic acid–containing proteoglycans and neurodegeneration.

171. The answer is c. *(Murray, pp 190–198. Scriver, pp 1521–1552. Sack, pp 121–138. Wilson, pp 287–317.)* The principal pathway for hepatic metabolism of ethanol is thought to be oxidation to acetaldehyde in the cytoplasm by alcohol dehydrogenase. Acetaldehyde is then oxidized, chiefly by acetaldehyde dehydrogenase within the mitochondrion, to yield acetate. Acetone, methanol, hydrogen peroxide, and glycerol do not appear in this biodegradation pathway. The genetic variations of acetaldehyde dehydrogenase have few phenotypic effects aside from sensitivity to alcoholic beverages, and are extremely common in the affected populations. These characteristics qualify acetaldehyde dehydrogenase variation as an example of enzyme polymorphism.

172. The answer is e. *(Murray, pp 190–198. Scriver, pp 1521–1552. Sack, pp 121–138. Wilson, pp 287–317.)* High-energy phosphate bonds are added to the substrates of glycolysis at three steps in the pathway. Hexokinase—or, in the case of liver, glucokinase—adds phosphate from ATP to glucose to form glucose-6-phosphate. Strictly speaking, this is not always considered a step of the glycolytic pathway. Phosphofructokinase uses ATP to convert fructose-6-phosphate to fructose-1,6-phosphate. Using NAD⁺ in an oxidation-reduction reaction, inorganic phosphate is added to glyceraldehyde-3-phosphate by the enzyme glyceraldehyde-3-phosphate dehydrogenase to form 1,3-diphosphoglycerate. The enzymes phosphoglycerate kinase and pyruvate kinase transfer substrate high-energy phosphate groups to ADP to form ATP.

173. The answer is d. *(Murray, pp 208–218. Scriver, pp 1521–1552. Sack, pp 121–138. Wilson, pp 287–317.)* All the enzymes listed are specific to either glycolysis or gluconeogenesis, except for phosphoglycerate kinase. It is one of seven enzymes common to both glycolysis and gluconeogenesis. The enzymes hexokinase, phosphofructokinase, and pyruvate kinase catalyze irreversible reactions unique to glycolysis. In order for gluconeogenesis to occur, the three irreversible reactions must be replaced. Pyruvate is synthesized into phosphoenolpyruvate by a two-step reaction. First, oxaloacetate is formed by carboxylation in the presence of pyruvate carboxylase. Then, phosphoenolpyruvate carboxykinase decarboxylates and phosphorylates oxaloacetate in the presence of GTP. The next irreversible step to be bypassed in gluconeogenesis requires fructose-6-phosphate to be produced by the action of fructose-1,6-phosphatase on fructose-1,6-phosphate. When glucose-6-phosphate is finally produced during gluconeogenesis, it is converted to glucose by glucose-6-phosphatase, an enzyme unique to the endoplasmic reticulum. The free glucose may then diffuse from the liver into the bloodstream. Of the enzymes given as possible answers, only phosphoglycerate kinase catalyzes a reversible reaction common to both glycolysis and gluconeogenesis.

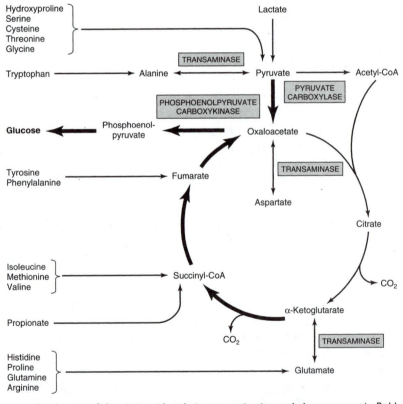

Involvment of the citric acid cycle in transamination and gluconeogenesis. Bold arrows indicate the main pathway of gluconeogenesis.
(Reproduced, with permission, from Murray RK, Granner DK, Mayes PA, Rodwell VW: Harper's Biochemistry, 25/e. New York, McGraw-Hill, 2000: 187.)

174. The answer is e. *(Murray, pp 208–218. Scriver, pp 1521–1552. Sack, pp 121–138. Wilson, pp 287–317.)* The main control of glycolysis is through the enzyme phosphofructokinase. This enzyme is controlled by a high level of ATP, which inhibits it, or a high level of fructose-2,6-bisphosphate (F-2,6-BP), which activates it. The inhibitory effect of ATP is potentiated by citrate, while high AMP levels reverse it. During fasting, when blood glucose levels are low, a glucagon-signaled increase of liver cyclic AMP leads to the activation of a phosphatase that hydrolyzes the 2-phosphoryl group from F-2,6-BP. The same glucagon-stimulated cascade deactivates the kinase that phosphorylates fructose-6-phosphate. The subsequent lowering of F-2,6-BP inactivates phosphofructokinase.

175. The answer is a. *(Murray, pp 190–198. Scriver, pp 1521–1552. Sack, pp 121–138. Wilson, pp 287–317.)* While most tissues cannot utilize fructose, the liver, kidneys, intestine, and adipose tissue can. Genetic fructokinase deficiency (229650) causes no symptoms. It can be detected by urine measurements of fructose that spills over into the urine. Unless care is taken, this could be misinterpreted as glucosuria, like that seen in diabetes, since both fructose and glucose are positive for a reducing-sugar test. Liver hexokinase rarely phosphorylates fructose to fructose-6-phosphate because the liver enzyme has a much greater affinity for glucose. However, adipose tissue hexokinase produces fructose-6-phosphate, which then can be acted upon by fructose-1-phosphate aldolase, which splits it into dihydroxyacetone phosphate and glyceraldehyde. Glyceraldehyde and dihydroxyacetone phosphate proceed through glycolysis or gluconeogenesis through the action of triose kinase. Under normal circumstances, liver fructokinase phosphorylates fructose to fructose-1-phosphate, and fructose-1-phosphate aldolase acts upon it.

176. The answer is b. *(Murray, pp 190–198. Scriver, pp 1553–1588. Sack, pp 121–138. Wilson, pp 287–317.)* Lactose in breast milk and infant formula is converted by intestinal lactase to glucose and galactose that are efficiently absorbed. In galactosemia (230400), deficiency of galactose-1-phosphate uridyl transferase prevents the conversion of galactose into glucose-6-phosphate by the liver or erythrocytes. Most other organs do not metabolize galactose. The severe symptoms of galactosemia are caused by the reduction of galactose to galactitol (dulcitol) in the presence of the enzyme aldose reductase. High levels of galactitol cause cataracts, the accumulation of galactose-1-phosphate contributes to liver disease, and the accumulation of galactose metabolites in urine can be measured as reducing substances by the Clinitest method. Any carbohydrate, including glucose, with a C1 aldehyde registers as a reducing substance by Clinitest, so a Dextrostix (glucose only) test is often performed as a control. In normal children, galactose is first phosphorylated by ATP to produce galactose-1-phosphate in the presence of galactokinase. Next, galactose-1-phosphate uridyl transferase transfers UDP from UDP-glucose to form UDP-galactose and glucose-1-phosphate. Under the action of UDP-galactose-4-epimerase, UDP-galactose is epimerized to UDP-glucose. Finally, glucose-1-phosphate is isomerized to glucose-6-phosphate by phosphoglucomutase. Infants with suspected galactosemia (230400) must be withdrawn from breast-feeding or lactose formulas and placed on nonlactose formulas such as Isomil.

177. The answer is c. (*Murray, pp 190–198. Scriver, pp 1521–1552. Sack, pp 121–138. Wilson, pp 287–317.*) All the enzymes named are glycolytic enzymes that carry out phosphorylation of glucose-derived substrates or of ADP to form ATP. However, only the reaction catalyzed by glyceraldehyde-3-phosphate dehydrogenase is a phosphorylation reaction coupled to oxidation that uses inorganic phosphate. In this reaction, glyceraldehyde-3-phosphate is converted to 1,3-bisphosphoglycerate by the addition of inorganic phosphate and the oxidation of glyceraldehyde-3-phosphate with the concomitant reduction of NAD^+ to $NADH + H^+$. This reaction is an example of a high-energy phosphate compound being produced by an oxidation-reduction reaction. The oxidation of the aldehyde group at C1 of glyceraldehyde-3-phosphate provides the energy for the reaction. The 1,3-bisphosphoglycerate can then be utilized to phosphorylate ADP to ATP through the action of phosphoglycerate kinase, which is the next step in the glycolytic pathway.

178. The answer is c. (*Murray, pp 199–207. Scriver, pp 1521–1552. Sack, pp 121–138. Wilson, pp 287–317.*) During an overnight fast, glycogenolysis and gluconeogenesis occur to some degree. Following a well-rounded breakfast, amino acids are available for protein synthesis, glycogen synthesis occurs from excess glucose, gluconeogenesis decreases, and fatty acid synthesis occurs from excess acetyl CoA produced from dietary sources. Thus, the activity of enzymes of gluconeogenesis (pyruvate carboxylase and phosphoenolpyruvate carboxykinase) decreases, while the activity of enzymes of fatty acid synthesis (acetyl CoA carboxylase) increases.

179. The answer is b. *(Murray, pp 190–198. Scriver, pp 1521–1552. Sack, pp 121–138. Wilson, pp 287–317.)* Glucose-6-phosphate is a pivotal compound in many pathways. Immediately upon entering cells, blood glucose is phosphorylated to glucose-6-phosphate by hexokinase in most cells and by glucokinase in the liver. Glucose may only leave a cell in the dephosphorylated form produced by glucose-6-phosphatase, which is only found in liver. Glucose-6-phosphate may be the starting point of glycolysis, glycogen synthesis, and the pentose phosphate pathway. It can be considered the end point or switching point of glycogenolysis and gluconeogenesis. Uridine-diphosphoglucose (UDP-glucose) and UDP-galactose are high-energy forms of their respective sugars that are involved in converting galactose-1-phosphate to glucose-1-phosphate (the block in galactosemia) and in donating sugar groups to polysaccharides such as glycogen or glycosaminoglycans. Fructose-6-phosphate is involved in glycolysis and gluconeogenesis.

180. The answer is a. *(Murray, pp 190–198. Scriver, pp 1521–1552. Sack, pp 121–138. Wilson, pp 287–317.)* The glycolytic pathway has three key irreversible enzymes: hexokinase, phosphofructose kinase, and pyruvate kinase. Under conditions of limiting cellular energy (low-energy charge), ADP and AMP accumulate and positively regulate phosphofructokinase. Under conditions of cellular "plenty," ATP and citrate, both negative effectors of phosphofructokinase, accumulate. When phosphofructokinase is inhibited, glucose-6-phosphate accumulates and shuts off hexokinase ATP, inhibiting the regulatory enzymes of glycolysis, while a lower energy charge actually stimulates glycolysis.

181. The answer is b. *(Murray, pp 208–218. Scriver, pp 1521–1552. Sack, pp 121–138. Wilson, pp 287–317.)* The balance and integration of the metabolism of fats and carbohydrates are mediated by the hormones insulin, glucagon, epinephrine, and norepinephrine. All of these hormones exercise acute effects upon metabolism. Glucagon stimulates gluconeogenesis and blocks glycolysis. When blood sugar levels get low, the α cells of the pancreas release glucagon. The main targets of glucagon are the liver and adipose tissue. In the liver, glucagon stimulates the cyclic AMP–mediated cascade that causes phosphorylation of phosphorylase and glycogen synthesis. This effectively turns off glycogen synthase and turns on glycogen phosphorylase, thereby causing a breakdown of glycogen and a production of glucose in liver, which ultimately raises blood glucose levels. Insulin and glucagon are two antagonistic hormones that maintain the balance of sugar and fatty acids in blood. Insulin is produced by the β cells of the pancreas and its release is stimulated by high levels of glucose in the blood. It has a number of effects, but its major effect is to allow the entry of glucose into cells. Insulin also allows the dephosphorylation of key regulatory enzymes. The consequence of these actions is to allow glycogen synthesis and storage in both muscle and liver, suppression of gluconeogenesis, acceleration of glycolysis, promotion of the synthesis of fatty acids, and promotion of the uptake and synthesis of amino acids into protein. All in all, insulin acts to promote anabolism.

182. The answer is d. (*Murray, pp 219–229. Scriver, pp 1521–1552. Sack, pp 121–138. Wilson, pp 287–317.*) The pentose phosphate pathway (hexose monophosphate shunt) functions to generate NADPH for reductive synthesis of compounds such as fatty acids or steroids, and to generate ribose for nucleotide and nucleic acid synthesis. As is the case with many pathways, the first step in the pentose phosphate pathway is regulated. This irreversible step is catalyzed by glucose-6-phosphate dehydrogenase, which is stimulated by increasing levels of $NADP^+$ and competitively inhibited by $NADP^+$. The dehydrogenation (oxidation) of glucose-6-phosphate produces 6-phosphoglucono-δ-lactone and reduced nicotinamide dinucleotide phosphate (NADPH). NAD^+, $NADP^+$, FAD^+, and flavin adenine mononucleotide (FMN^+) function as oxidizing agents for many biochemical reactions. The removal of positive hydrogen ions (H^+) from a substrate AH_2 effectively removes electrons (oxidizes it) to form A, simultaneously adding H^+ ions and reducing (adding electrons) to form the reduced cofactors NADH/NADPH/FADH/FMNH. The reduced cofactors are oxidized back to $NAD^+/NADP^+/FAD^+/FMN^+$ through chemical reactions driven by high-energy phosphates (anaerobic conditions) or by molecular oxygen during electron transport (aerobic conditions).

183. The answer is e. (*Murray, pp 182–189. Scriver, pp 1521–1552. Sack, pp 121–138. Wilson, pp 287–317.*) The enzyme controlling the first step in gluconeogenesis is pyruvate carboxylase. It catalyzes the conversion of pyruvate to oxaloacetate. Pyruvate is absolutely dependent upon the presence of the allosteric effector acetyl CoA or a closely related acyl CoA for its function. Under conditions of high-energy charge and high levels of acetyl CoA, oxaloacetate is utilized for gluconeogenesis. If low amounts of ATP are present, oxaloacetate is consumed in the citric acid cycle.

184. The answer is a. (*Murray, pp 190–198. Scriver, pp 1521–1552. Sack, pp 121–138. Wilson, pp 287–317.*) Fructose is taken in by humans as sucrose, sucrose-containing syrups, and the free sugar. Fructose is mainly phosphorylated to fructose-1-phosphate by liver fructokinase. Aldol cleavage by fructose-1-phosphate-specific aldolase, not enolase, yields glyceraldehyde and dihydroxyacetone phosphate. The glyceraldehyde is phosphorylated to glyceraldehyde-3-phosphate by triose kinase, and both triose phosphates can enter glycolysis. Excess fructose from commercial foods can exercise adverse effects by raising blood lipids and uric acid. Fructose phosphorylation bypasses phosphofructokinase, a regulatory enzyme of glycolysis, and provides excess glycerol metabolites and excess triglyceride/lipid biosynthesis. Fructose phosphorylation can also deplete liver cell ATP, lessening its inhibition of adenine nucleotide degradation and increasing production of uric acid. In adipocytes, fructose can be alternatively phosphorylated by hexokinase to fructose-6-phosphate. However, this reaction is competitively inhibited by appreciable amounts of glucose, as it is in other tissues.

185. The answer is c. (*Murray, pp 199–207. Scriver, pp 1521–1552. Sack, pp 121–138. Wilson, pp 287–317.*) Glycogen synthetase is an enzyme that transfers glucosyl moieties from UDP-glucose to a glycogen polymer primer. In plants, ADP-glucose plays a part similar to that of UDP-glucose in animals. The enzyme exists in two forms: an active, dephosphorylated form and an inactive, phosphorylated form. It is inactivated by phosphorylation of a specific serine residue. Glycogen breakdown, not synthesis, is positively affected by increased calcium levels.

186. The answer is d. (*Murray, pp 199–207. Scriver, pp 1521–1552. Sack, pp 121–138. Wilson, pp 287–317.*) Epinephrine stimulates both muscle and liver adenylate cyclase to produce cyclic AMP. In the liver, the increased cyclic AMP levels activate a phosphatase that dephosphorylates fructose-2,6-bisphosphate (F-2,6-BP) while deactivating a kinase that produces

F-2,6-BP. Thus, F-2,6-BP levels are decreased and phosphofructokinase activity is decreased. In liver and muscle, F-2,6-BP is the major allosteric activator of phosphofructokinase. In skeletal muscle, however, the kinase responsible for the synthesis of F-2,6-BP is activated, not inhibited, by cyclic AMP. Thus, muscle sees an increase in glycolysis following epinephrine stimulation, while the liver experiences a decrease in glycolytic activity. In both tissues, glycogen phosphorylase is activated and glycogenolysis occurs. Under these conditions, glucose is utilized in muscle for ATP production relative to contractile activity, while the liver produces glucose for export to the blood.

187. The answer is e. *(Murray, pp 219–229. Scriver, pp 1521–1552. Sack, pp 121–138. Wilson, pp 287–317.)* The pentose phosphate pathway generates reducing power in the form of NADPH in the oxidative branch of the pathway and synthesizes five-carbon sugars in the nonoxidative branch of the pathway. The pentose phosphate pathway also carries out the interconversion of three-, four-, five-, six-, and seven-carbon sugars in the nonoxidative reactions. The final sugar product of the oxidative branch of the pathway is ribulose-5-phosphate. The first step of the nonoxidative branch of the pathway is the conversion of ribulose-5-phosphate to ribose-5-phosphate or xylulose-5-phosphate in the presence of the enzymes phosphopentose isomerase and phosphopentose epimerase, respectively. Thus ribulose-5-phosphate is a key intermediate that is common to both the oxidative and nonoxidative branches of the pentose phosphate pathway.

188. The answer is a. *(Murray, pp 190–198. Scriver, pp 4517–4554. Sack, pp 121–138. Wilson, pp 287–317.)* One of the world's most common enzyme deficiencies is glucose-6-phosphate-dehydrogenase deficiency (305900). This deficiency in erythrocytes is particularly prevalent among African and Mediterranean males. A deficiency in glucose-6-phosphate dehydrogenase blocks the pentose phosphate pathway and NADPH production. Without NADPH to maintain glutathione in its reduced form, erythrocytes have no protection from oxidizing agents. This X-linked recessive deficiency is often diagnosed when patients develop hemolytic anemia after receiving oxidizing drugs such as pamaquine or after eating oxidizing substances such as fava beans.

189. The answer is a. *(Murray, pp 190–198. Scriver, pp 1521–1552. Sack, pp 121–138. Wilson, pp 287–317.)* In the formation of phosphoenolpyruvate during gluconeogenesis, oxaloacetate is an intermediate. In the first step, catalyzed by pyruvate carboxylase, pyruvate is carboxylated with the utilization of one high-energy ATP phosphate bond:

$$\text{pyruvate} + \text{ATP} + CO_2 \rightarrow \text{oxaloacetate} + \text{ADP} + P_i$$

In the second step, catalyzed by phosphoenolpyruvate carboxykinase, a high-energy phosphate bond of GTP drives the decarboxylation of oxaloacetate:

$$\text{oxaloacetate} + \text{GTP} \rightarrow \text{phosphoenolpyruvate} + \text{GDP} + CO_2$$

In contrast to gluconeogenesis, the formation of pyruvate from phosphoenolpyruvate during glycolysis requires only pyruvate kinase, and ATP is made.

190. The answer is b. *(Murray, pp 190–198. Scriver, pp 1521–1552. Sack, pp 121–138. Wilson, pp 287–317.)* A molecule of guanosine triphosphate is synthesized from guanosine diphosphate and phosphate at the cost of hydrolyzing succinyl CoA to succinate and CoA. This constitutes substrate-level phosphorylation, and, in contrast to oxidative phosphorylation, this is the only reaction in the citric acid cycle that directly yields a high-energy phosphate bond. The sequence of reactions from α-ketoglutarate to succinate is catalyzed by the α-ketoglutarate dehydrogenase complex and succinyl-CoA synthetase, respectively.

$$\alpha\text{-ketoglutarate} + \text{NAD}^+ + \text{acetyl CoA} \rightarrow \text{succinyl CoA} + CO_2 + \text{NADH}$$
$$\text{succinyl CoA} + P_i + \text{GDP} \rightarrow \text{succinate} + \text{GTP} + \text{acetyl CoA}$$

191. The answer is c. *(Murray, pp 190–198. Scriver, pp 1521–1552. Sack, pp 121–138. Wilson, pp 287–317.)* During alcohol ingestion by humans, liver alcohol dehydrogenase converts ethanol to acetaldehyde. The acetaldehyde can be metabolized to acetate by acetaldehyde dehydrogenase, then to acetyl CoA. The alcohol and acetaldehyde dehydrogenases both generate NADH, increasing the NADH/NAD⁺ ratio and stimulating lipid synthesis. The increased lipid synthesis with chronic ethanol ingestion contributes to the fatty liver of alcoholism. In normal glycolysis, three-carbon metabolites such as glyceraldehyde are metabolized to pyruvate. In the liver and in resting muscle, almost all pyruvate produced is converted to acetyl CoA for oxidation in the citric acid cycle. In actively contracting muscle, when oxygen is limited, lactate accumulates. No acetate is converted to acetaldehyde since the acetaldehyde dehydrogenase is irreversible. This reverse pathway is utilized by yeast to produce ethanol during fermentation of grapes or other plant products. Yeast converts pyruvate to acetaldehyde, then acetaldehyde to ethanol.

192. The answer is b. *(Murray, pp 182–189. Scriver, pp 1521–1552. Sack, pp 121–138. Wilson, pp 287–317.)* Under conditions in which the entry charge of liver cells is high, intermediates of the citric acid cycle are abundant. Citrate, an early intermediate in the cycle, readily diffuses across the inner membrane of mitochondria and out into the cytosol. Citrate allosterically inhibits phosphofructokinase and, conversely, stimulates fructose-1,6-diphosphatase. Thus, when the energy level of hepatocytes is low and biosynthetic precursors are not abundant, phosphofructokinase is stimulated and glycolysis is favored. When the energy level is high, citrate inhibits phosphofructokinase, stimulates the diphosphatase, and thereby promotes gluconeogenesis. The diffusion of high levels of citrate into the cytosol also stimulates synthesis of fatty acids. Citrate activates acetyl CoA carboxylase, the first step in the synthesis of fatty acids, as well as provides its substrates, acetyl CoA and NADPH. However, citrate does not allosterically activate fatty acid synthetase. Enolase, an enzyme of the glycolytic pathway, is not regulated.

193. The answer is b. *(Murray, pp 182–189. Scriver, pp 1521–1552. Sack, pp 121–138. Wilson, pp 287–317.)* Reducing equivalents are produced at four sites in the citric acid cycle. NADH is produced by the isocitrate dehydrogenase–catalyzed conversion of α-ketoglutarate to succinyl CoA and by the malate dehydrogenase–catalyzed conversion of malate to oxaloacetate. $FADH_2$ is produced by the succinate dehydrogenase–catalyzed conversion of succinate to fumarate. Succinyl CoA synthetase catalyzes the formation of succinate from succinyl CoA, with the concomitant phosphorylation of GDP to GTP.

194. The answer is e. (*Murray, pp 182–189. Scriver, pp 1521–1552. Sack, pp 121–138. Wilson, pp 287–317.*) The final thiolytic cleavage in β-oxidation of odd-chain fatty acids yields propionyl CoA. Propionyl CoA is also formed during the breakdown of methionine and isoleucine. It is carboxylated to form D-methylmalonyl CoA, which is in equilibrium with 1-methylmalonyl CoA. Valine forms methylmalonyl CoA during its degradation. The 1-isomer of methylmalonyl CoA is converted to succinyl CoA through the action of the B_{12} coenzyme–containing methylmalonyl CoA mutase. Thus, succinyl CoA serves as the entry point into the citric acid cycle for three amino acids and the last three carbons of odd-chain fatty acids. The amino acids and fatty acid carbons introduced in this manner may either be catabolized in the cycle for energy production or utilized for gluconeogenesis.

195. The answer is a. (*Murray, pp 182–189. Scriver, pp 1521–1552. Sack, pp 121–138. Wilson, pp 287–317.*) Cyanide blocks respiration by displacing oxygen from hemoglobin. Oxidative phosphorylation in the mitochondria cannot proceed because cyanide cannot oxidize (remove electrons) from reduced cofactors like NADH. The citric acid cycle is the major pathway for generating ATP and reducing equivalents (NADH, H⁺) from catabolism of carbohydrates, amino acids, and lipids. Inability to regenerate NAD⁺ from NADH through mitochondrial oxidative phosphorylation depletes the cell of NAD⁺ and inhibits the citric acid cycle. Failure to generate ATP by oxidative phosphorylation using NADH from the citric acid cycle depletes the cell of energy and leads to cell and tissue death (organ failure). Enzymes (citrate synthase, aconitase) and intermediates of the citric acid cycle (citrate, acetyl coenzyme A) need only be present in trace amounts because they are not consumed.

196. The answer is d. (*Murray, pp 190–198. Scriver, pp 1521–1552. Sack, pp 121–138. Wilson, pp 287–317.*) Ketone bodies include acetoacetic acid and β-hydroxybutyrate, which are formed in the liver, and acetone, which is spontaneously formed from excess acetoacetate in the blood. Starvation results in glycogen depletion and deficiency of carbohydrates, causing increased use of lipids as energy sources. Increased oxidation of fatty acids produces acetyl coenzyme A (CoA) and acetoacetyl CoA, a precursor of ketone bodies. Although the liver synthesizes ketone bodies from excess acetyl CoA produced by β-oxidation of fatty acids, it cannot use ketone bodies as fuel for energy. Insulin deficiency in diabetes mellitus, like starvation, depletes carbohydrate energy sources because glucose cannot enter cells. Increased oxidation of fatty acids again results, with increased production of ketone bodies by the liver. Children with inherited blocks in fatty acid oxidation such as medium chain CoA dehydrogenase deficiency [MCAD (201450)] cannot switch to fatty oxidation when illness or overnight fasting causes carbohydrate depletion. They often present with low blood glucose (hypoglycemia) and without the expected ketone bodies (nonketonic hypoglycemia). The unavailability of fatty acid oxidation as an alternative energy source may lead to energy depletion, organ failure, and unexpected "sudden death" in an otherwise healthy child.

197. The answer is e. *(Murray, pp 182–189. Scriver, pp 1521–1552. Sack, pp 121–138. Wilson, pp 287–317.)* The net result of the citric acid cycle's oxidation of acetyl CoA is shown below:

$$\text{acetyl CoA} + \text{FAD} + 3\ \text{NAD}^+ + \text{GDP} + 2\ H_2O + P_i \rightarrow$$
$$2\ CO_2 + \text{CoA} + \text{FADH}_2 + 3\ \text{NADH} + \text{GTP} + 2\ H^+$$

The cycle produces reducing equivalents (NADH, $FADH_2$) and carbon dioxide directly, but not ATP. The reducing equivalents are used to produce ATP by mitochondrial oxidative phosphorylation. Two carbon atoms enter the cycle as acetyl CoA, with an immediate loss of CoA as citrate is formed from oxaloacetate. Two carbon atoms leave the cycle at the level of isocitrate dehydrogenase and α-ketoglutarate dehydrogenase. The two carbons that leave as CO_2 are actually not the original acetyl CoA carbons. Two NAD^+ molecules are reduced by isocitrate dehydrogenase and then α-ketoglutarate dehydrogenase. One FAD is reduced during the oxidation of succinate, and one NAD^+ is reduced when malate is oxidized. GTP is formed from GDP by utilization of the high-energy thioester linkage of succinyl CoA.

198. The answer is a. *(Murray, pp 182–189. Scriver, pp 1521–1552. Sack, pp 121–138. Wilson, pp 287–317.)* Fluoracetate can be converted to fluorocitrate, which is an inhibitor of aconitase. Arsenic is not a direct inhibitor, but arsenite is an inhibitor of lipoic acid–containing enzymes such as α-ketoglutarate dehydrogenase. Malonate, not malic acid, is an inhibitor of succinate dehydrogenase. The citric acid cycle requires oxygen and would be inhibited by anaerobic, not aerobic, conditions. Fluorouracil is a suicide inhibitor of thymidylate synthase and blocks deoxythymidylate synthesis.

199. The answer is e. *(Murray, pp 190–198. Scriver, pp 1521–1552. Sack, pp 121–138. Wilson, pp 287–317.)* The major fate of acetoacetyl CoA formed from condensation of acetyl CoA in the liver is the formation of 3-hydroxy-3-methylglutaryl CoA (HMG CoA). Under normal postabsorptive conditions, HMG CoA production occurs in the cytoplasm of hepatocytes as part of the overall process of cholesterol biosynthesis. However, in fasting or starving persons, as well as in patients with uncontrolled diabetes mellitus, HMG CoA production occurs in liver mitochondria as part of ketone body synthesis. In this process, HMG CoA is cleaved by HMG CoA lyase to yield acetoacetate and acetyl CoA. The NADH-dependent enzyme β-hydroxybutyrate dehydrogenase converts most of the acetoacetate to β-hydroxybutyrate. These two ketone bodies, acetoacetate and β-hydroxybutyrate, diffuse into the blood and are transported to peripheral tissues.

200. The answer is c. *(Murray, pp 199–207. Scriver, pp 1521–1552. Sack, pp 121–138. Wilson, pp 287–317.)* The child has symptoms of glycogen storage disease. Glycogen is a glucose polymer with linear regions linked through the C1 aldehyde of one glucose to the C4 alcohol of the next (α-1,4-glucoside linkage). There are also branches from the linear glycogen polymer that have α-1,6-glucoside linkages. Glycogen is synthesized during times of carbohydrate and energy surplus, but must be degraded during fasting to provide energy. Separate enzymes for breakdown include phosphylases (α-1,4-glucosidases) that cleave linear regions of glycogen and debranching enzymes (α-1,6-glucosidases) that cleave branch points. Glucose-6-phosphatase is needed in the liver to liberate free glucose from glucose-6-phosphate, providing fuel for other organs. There is no glucose-6-phosphatase in muscle, and muscle glycogenolysis provides energy just for muscle with production of lactate. Deficiencies of more than eight enzymes involved in glycogenolysis, including those mentioned, can produce glycogen storage disease.

201. The answer is b. *(Murray, pp 199–207. Scriver, pp 1521–1552. Sack, pp 121–138. Wilson, pp 287–317.)* The sequential cleavage of the α-1,4-

glycosidic bonds of glycogen to release successive glucose-1-phosphate residues is known as glycogenolysis. The enzyme catalyzing this reaction is glycogen phosphorylase a, an active, phosphorylated tetramer formed by covalent modification of phosphorylase b, an inactive dimer. In glycogenesis or glycogen synthesis, activated glycogen synthase adds the glucose of uridine diphosphate (UDP)-glucose units to a growing glycogen polymer by forming α-1,4 linkages. In contrast to phosphorylase, glycogen synthase is inactivated by covalent phosphate binding. The same enzyme that inactivates glycogen synthase by catalyzing its phosphorylation activates another enzyme, phosphorylase kinase, which activates glycogen phosphorylase by phosphorylation.

202. The answer is b. (*Murray, pp 199–207. Scriver, pp 1521–1552. Sack, pp 121–138. Wilson, pp 287–317.*) In the presence of low blood glucose, epinephrine or norepinephrine interacts with specific receptors to stimulate adenylate cyclase production of cyclic AMP. Cyclic AMP activates protein kinase, which catalyzes phosphorylation and activation of phosphorylase kinase. Activated phosphorylase kinase activates glycogen phosphorylase, which catalyzes the breakdown of glycogen. Phosphorylase kinase can be activated in two ways. Phosphorylation leads to complete activation of phosphorylase kinase. Alternatively, in muscle, the transient increases in levels of Ca^{++} associated with contraction lead to a partial activation of phosphorylase kinase. Ca^{++} binds to calmodulin, which is a subunit of phosphorylase kinase. Calmodulin regulates many enzymes in mammalian cells through Ca^{++} binding.

203. The answer is c. (*Murray, pp 199–207. Scriver, pp 1521–1552. Sack, pp 121–138. Wilson, pp 287–317.*) Blood glucose is rapidly converted to glucose-6-phosphate upon entering cells by hexokinase or, in the case of the liver, by glucokinase. Glucose-6-phosphate is in equilibrium with glucose-1-phosphate via the action of phosphoglucomutase. Glucose-1-phosphate is activated by UTP to form UDP-glucose, which is added to glycogen by an α-1,4 linkage in the presence of glycogen synthase. To increase the solubility of glycogen and to increase the number of terminal residues, glycogen-branching enzyme transfers a block of about 7 residues from a chain at least 11 residues long to a branch point at least 4 residues from the last branch point. The branch is attached by an α-1,6 linkage.

204. The answer is d. *(Murray, pp 199–207. Scriver, pp 1521–1552. Sack, pp 121–138. Wilson, pp 287–317.)* Glycogen is a highly branched polymer of α-D-glucose residues joined by α-1,4-glycosidic linkage. Under the influence of glycogen synthase, the C4 alcohol of a new glucose is added to the C1 aldehyde group of the chain terminus. The branched chains occur about every 10 residues and are joined in α-1,6-glycosidic linkages. Large amounts of glycogen are stored as 100- to 400-Å granules in the cytoplasm of liver and muscle cells. The enzymes responsible for making or breaking the α-1,4-glycosidic bonds are contained within the granules. Thus glycogen is a readily mobilized form of glucose.

205. The answer is c. *(Murray, pp 238–249. Scriver, pp 1521–1552. Sack, pp 121–138. Wilson, pp 287–317.)* Lipolysis in adipose tissue leads to increased blood levels of fatty acids and glycerol. Since most tissues have little glycerol kinase, the liver takes up most of the free glycerol, phosphorylates it using glycerol kinase, and oxidizes it to dihydroxyacetone phosphate (DHAP) using a dehydrogenase:

$$\text{glycerol} + \text{ATP} \rightarrow \text{glycerol-3-P} + \text{ADP}$$
$$\text{glycerol-3-P} + \text{NAD}^+ \rightarrow \text{DHAP} + \text{NADH} + \text{H}^+$$

Aldolase allows both of the triose phosphates DHAP and glyceraldehyde-3-phosphate to condense and form fructose-1,6-bisphosphate. In this manner, aldolase allows adipocyte glycerol to enter hepatic gluconeogenesis.

206. The answer is c. *(Murray, pp 199–207. Scriver, pp 1521–1552. Sack, pp 121–138. Wilson, pp 287–317.)* Muscle phosphorylase deficiency leads to a glycogen storage disease [McArdle's disease (232600)] and, in young adults, an inability to do strenuous physical work because of muscular cramps resulting from ischemia. The compromised phosphorylation of muscle glycogen characteristic of McArdle's disease compels the muscles to rely on auxiliary energy sources such as free fatty acids and ambient glucose.

207. The answer is a. *(Murray, pp 199–207. Scriver, pp 1521–1552. Sack, pp 121–138. Wilson, pp 287–317.)* Amylo-(1,4 → 1,6)-transglycosylase (also known as the branching enzyme) functions in glycogen synthesis. The other enzymes listed are involved in glycogenolysis. Deficiencies in these enzymes lead to glycogen storage with enlarged liver and hypoglycemia. Mobilization of glycogen stores to produce glucose in the liver requires phosphorolysis of the glycogen chain by the enzyme phosphorylase, which is phosphorylated by phosphorylase kinase. Also needed are the hydrolysis of α-1,6-glycosidic bonds by amylo-1,6-glucosidase (also known as the debranching enzyme) and the hydrolysis of glucose-6-phosphate derived from glucose-1-phosphate (a product of phosphorylase) by glucose-6-phosphatase to produce glucose for export into the blood.

Bioenergetics and Energy Metabolism

Questions

DIRECTIONS: Each item below contains a question or incomplete statement followed by suggested responses. Select the **one best** response to each question.

208. Which of the following occurs in nonshivering thermogenesis?

a. Glucose is oxidized to lactate
b. Fatty acids uncouple oxidative phosphorylation
c. Ethanol is formed
d. ATP is burned for heat production
e. Adipose tissue is functionally absent

209. Transfer of H^+/e^- pairs to electron transport carriers, decarboxylation, and substrate-level phosphorylation occur at some of the steps shown in the following diagram of the citric acid cycle. All three of these events occur at which step?

a. Step A
b. Step B
c. Step C
d. Step D
e. Step E

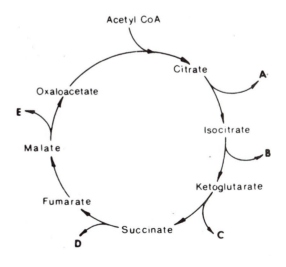

210. A comatose laboratory technician is rushed into the emergency room. She dies while you are examining her. Her most dramatic symptom is that her body is literally hot to your touch, indicating an extremely high fever. You learn that her lab has been working on metabolic inhibitors and that there is a high likelihood that she accidentally ingested one. Which one of the following is the most likely culprit?

a. Barbiturates
b. Piericidin A
c. Dimercaprol
d. Dinitrophenol
e. Cyanide

211. Which of the following statements about flavoproteins is true?

a. They are not oxidized by coenzyme Q
b. They receive electrons from cytochrome P450 in liver mitochondria
c. They do not participate in oxidation of NADH dehydrogenases
d. They can be associated with sulfur and nonheme iron
e. They cannot produce hydrogen peroxide

212. As electrons are received and passed down the transport chain shown below, the various carriers are first reduced with acceptance of the electron and then oxidized with loss of the electron. A patient poisoned by which of the following compounds has the most highly reduced state of most of the respiratory chain carriers?

a. Antimycin A
b. Rotenone
c. Carbon monoxide
d. Puromycin
e. Chloramphenicol

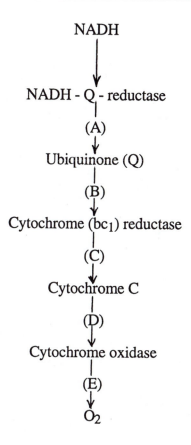

NADH

↓

NADH - Q - reductase

(A)
↓
Ubiquinone (Q)

(B)
↓
Cytochrome (bc₁) reductase

(C)
↓
Cytochrome C

(D)
↓
Cytochrome oxidase

(E)
↓
O₂

213. A step in the tricarboxylic acid cycle is described by which of the following?

a. Produces 3 mol of ATP equivalents for each cytoplasmic NADH produced
b. Carries protons across the inner mitochondrial membrane
c. Determines the rate of oxidative phosphorylation
d. Yields 2 mol of ATP for each cytoplasmic NADH
e. Is utilized by hibernating animals to produce heat
f. Requires inorganic phosphate
g. Defines respiratory quotient (RQ)

214. Which of the following compounds is a member of the electron transport chain?

a. Octanoyl carnitine
b. Cytochrome c
c. Reduced nicotinamide adenine dinucleotide (NADH)
d. Palmitoyl carnitine
e. Carnitine

215. Given that the standard free energy change ($\Delta G^{\circ\prime}$) for the hydrolysis of ATP is -7.3 kcal/mol and that for the hydrolysis of glucose-6-phosphate is -3.3 kcal/mol, what is the $\Delta G^{\circ\prime}$ for the phosphorylation of glucose?

$$\text{glucose} + \text{ATP} \rightarrow \text{glucose-6-phosphate} + \text{ADP}$$

a. -10.6 kcal/mol
b. -7.3 kcal/mol
c. -4.0 kcal/mol
d. $+4.0$ kcal/mol
e. $+10.6$ kcal/mol

216. All known effects of cyclic AMP in eukaryotic cells result from

a. Activation of the catalytic unit of adenylate cyclase
b. Activation of synthetases
c. Activation of protein kinase
d. Phosphorylation of G protein
e. Stimulation of Ca^{++} release from endoplasmic reticulum

217. The connection between oxidation phosphorylation and electron transport is best described by

a. Existence of a higher pH in the cisternae of the endoplasmic reticulum than in the cytosol
b. Synthesis of ATP as protons flow into the mitochondrial matrix along a proton gradient that exists across the inner mitochondrial membrane
c. Symmetric distribution of the ATPase of the inner membrane of the mitochondria
d. Dissociation of electron transport and oxidative phosphorylation
e. Absence of ATPase in the inner membrane of the mitochondria

218. If all potential sources of ATP production are taken into account, the net number of ATP molecules formed per molecule of glucose in aerobic glycolysis is

a. 2
b. 6
c. 18
d. 36
e. 54

219. In the figure below, which letter designates an enzyme that has an extremely low K_m in most but not all tissues?

a. Letter A
b. Letter B
c. Letter C
d. Letter D
e. Letter E

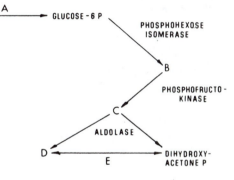

220. Which of the following reactions generates ATP?

a. Glucose-6-phosphate to fructose-6-phosphate
b. Glucose to glucose-6-phosphate
c. Fructose-6-phosphate to fructose-1,6-diphosphate
d. Phosphoenolpyruvate to pyruvate
e. Pyruvate to lactate

221. Which one of the following enzymes catalyzes high-energy phosphorylation of substrates during glycolysis?

a. Pyruvate kinase
b. Phosphoglycerate kinase
c. Triose phosphate isomerase
d. Aldolase
e. Glyceraldehyde-3-phosphate dehydrogenase

222. Which one of the following products of triacylglycerol breakdown and subsequent β oxidation may undergo gluconeogenesis?

a. Propionyl CoA
b. Acetyl CoA
c. All ketone bodies
d. Some amino acids
e. β-hydroxybutyrate

223. Which of the following regulates lipolysis in adipocytes?

a. Activation of fatty acid synthesis mediated by cyclic AMP
b. Activation of triglyceride lipase as a result of hormone-stimulated increases in cyclic AMP levels
c. Glycerol phosphorylation to prevent futile esterification of fatty acids
d. Activation of cyclic AMP production by insulin
e. Hormone-sensitive lipoprotein lipase

224. Inhibition of the synthesis of ATP during oxidative phosphorylation by oligomycin is thought to be due to

a. Blocking of the proton gradient between NADH-Q reductase and QH_2
b. Blocking of the proton gradient between cytochrome c_1 and cytochrome c
c. Dissociating of cytochrome c from mitochondrial membranes
d. Inhibiting of mitochondrial ATPase (ATP synthase)
e. Uncoupling of electron transfer between NADH and flavoprotein

225. The yield from complete oxidation of glycogen is approximately 4 kcal/g. However, under physiologic conditions, glycogen is highly hydrated, such that the true physiologic yield is only approximately 1.5 kcal/g. Under similar physiologic conditions, what is the approximate yield from the oxidation of triacylglyceride stores?

a. 1 kcal/g
b. 2 kcal/g
c. 4 kcal/g
d. 9 kcal/g
e. 24 kcal/g

226. Which reaction in the figure below occurs in both muscle and liver but has substantially different qualities in the two?

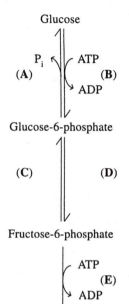

a. Reaction A
b. Reaction B
c. Reaction C
d. Reaction D
e. Reaction E

227. Nervous stimulation of skeletal muscle causes the release of calcium from sarcoplasmic reticulum and leads to muscle contraction. Simultaneously, the increased calcium concentration causes

a. A dramatic rise in cyclic AMP levels
b. Inactivation of glycogen phosphorylase
c. Activation of phosphorylase kinase
d. Activation of cyclic AMP phosphodiesterase
e. Activation of protein phosphatase

228. A teenage girl is brought to the medical center because of her complaints that she gets too tired when asked to participate in gym class. A consulting neurologist finds muscle weakness in the girl's arms and legs. When no obvious diagnosis can be made, biopsies of her muscles are taken for tests. Chemistries reveal greatly elevated amounts of triacylglycerides esterified with primarily long-chain fatty acids. Pathology reports the presence of significant numbers of lipid vacuoles in the muscle biopsy. Which one of the following is the most likely diagnosis?

a. Fatty acid synthase deficiency
b. Tay-Sachs disease
c. Carnitine deficiency
d. Biotin deficiency
e. Lipoprotein lipase deficiency

229. A newborn infant has severe respiratory problems. Over the next few days, it is observed that the baby has severe muscle problems, demonstrates little development, and has neurological problems. A liver biopsy reveals a very low level of acetyl CoA carboxylase, but normal levels of the enzymes of glycolysis, gluconeogenesis, the citric acid cycle, and the pentose phosphate pathway. What is the most likely cause of the infant's respiratory problems?

a. Low levels of phosphatidyl choline
b. Biotin deficiency
c. Ketoacidosis
d. High levels of citrate
e. Glycogen depletion

230. Which of the following statements about mammalian energy metabolism is true?

a. ATP is only formed in the absence of Q_2
b. ATP hydrolysis is an exergonic reaction
c. ATP is only formed in the presence of Q_2
d. Heat produced by ATP hydrolysis specifically drives other reactions
e. NADH cannot be utilized to form ATP

231. Which of the following correctly describes the intermediate 3-hydroxy-3-methylglutaryl CoA?

a. It inhibits the conversion of cholesterol to sex steroids
b. It is formed only in the cytoplasm
c. It inhibits the first step in cholesterol synthesis
d. It is formed by condensation of two molecules of acetyl CoA
e. It is an intermediate in the synthesis of cholesterol

232. Electrons from $FADH_2$ of flavoproteins entering the respiratory chain shown in question 212 first proceed through step

233. Which of the following enzymes is activated by cAMP during fasting?

a. Phospholipase D
b. Lipoprotein lipase
c. Thiokinase
d. Acetyl coenzyme A carboxylase
e. Pancreatic lipase
f. Carnitine acyltransferase I
g. Diacylglycerol lipase
h. Hormone-sensitive lipase
i. Thiolase

234. What enzyme often malfunctions in diseases associated with the symptoms of high blood triacylglyceride levels and steatorrhea?

a. Phospholipase D
b. Lipoprotein lipase
c. Thiokinase
d. Acetyl coenzyme A carboxylase
e. Pancreatic lipase

235. Which enzyme is an allosteric regulator of another enzyme on the list?

a. Acetyl coenzyme A carboxylase
b. Pancreatic lipase
c. Carnitine acyltransferase I
d. Diacylglycerol lipase
e. Hormone-sensitive lipase

236. Which of the descriptions below best fits inositol 1,4,5-triphosphate?

a. A depositor of calcium in endoplasmic reticulum
b. An inhibitor of protein kinase C
c. A second messenger produced by the action of phospholipase C
d. An ionophore
e. A calcium detector

237. Cholera toxin causes massive and often fatal diarrhea by

a. Inactivating G_i protein
b. Irreversibly activating adenylate cyclase
c. Locking G_s protein into an inactive form
d. Rapidly hydrolyzing G protein GTP to GDP
e. Preventing GTP from interacting with G protein

238. A healthy 70-kg man eats a well-balanced diet containing adequate calories and 62.5 g of high-quality protein per day. Measured in grams of nitrogen, his daily nitrogen balance is

a. +10 g
b. +6.25 g
c. 0 g
d. −6.25 g
e. −10 g

239. In patients fed an equal amount (on a molar basis) of carbohydrates and fats, the respiratory quotient is

a. 2.72
b. 1.00
c. 0.86
d. 0.72
e. 0.10

240. The problem of regenerating NAD⁺ from NADH for cytoplasmic processes by using mitochondria is solved in the most energy-efficient manner by which one of the following intercellular shuttle systems?

a. Citrate → pyruvate shuttle
b. Dihydroxyacetone phosphate → α-glycerophosphate shuttle
c. Malate → aspartate shuttle
d. Citrate → citrate shuttle
e. Lactate → pyruvate shuttle

241. Which one of the following tissues can metabolize glucose, fatty acids, and ketone bodies for ATP production?

a. Liver
b. Muscle
c. Hepatocytes
d. Brain
e. Red blood cells

Bioenergetics and Energy Metabolism

Answers

208. The answer is b. (*Murray, pp 123–148. Scriver, pp 2367–2424. Sack, pp 159–175. Wilson, pp 287–317.*) Although metabolic poisons do uncouple oxidation of NADH from production of ATP, the uncoupling of oxidative phosphorylation does occur under certain normal biologic conditions. In brown fat (so called because of the large number of blood vessels), oxidation is uncoupled from phosphorylation so that heat is produced. This phenomenon is observed in newborn mammals, including humans, hibernating animals, and certain mammals that use it as an adaptation to the cold. In brown fat, fatty acids act as uncouplers of mitochondria. The catecholamine norepinephrine controls the release of the fatty acids, thereby regulating the process.

209. The answer is c. (*Murray, pp 123–148. Scriver, pp 2367–2424. Sack, pp 159–175. Wilson, pp 287–317.*) In the citric acid cycle, the conversion of α-ketoglutarate to succinate results in decarboxylation, transfer of an H^+/e^- pair to $NADH + H^+$, and the substrate-level phosphorylation of GDP to GTP. The series of reactions involved is quite complex. First, α-ketoglutarate reacts with $NAD^+ + CoA$ to yield succinyl CoA + CO_2 + NADH + H^+. These reactions occur by the catalysis of the α-ketoglutarate dehydrogenase complex, which contains lipoamide, FAD^+, and thiamine pyrophosphate as prosthetic groups. Under the action of succinyl CoA synthetase, succinyl CoA catalyzes the phosphorylation of GDP with inorganic phosphate coupled to the cleavage of the thioester bond of succinyl CoA. Thus, the production of succinate from α-ketoglutarate yields one substrate-level phosphorylation and the production of three ATP equivalents from NADH via oxidative phosphorylation.

210. The answer is d. (*Murray, pp 123–148. Scriver, pp 2367–2424. Sack, pp 159–175. Wilson, pp 287–317.*) All of the poisons shown affect either electron transport or oxidative phosphorylation. Dinitrophenol is unique in that it disconnects the ordinarily tight coupling of electron transport and phosphorylation. In its presence, electron transport continues normally with no oxidative phosphorylation occurring. Instead, heat energy is generated. The same principle is utilized in a well-controlled way by brown fat to generate heat in newborn humans and cold-adapted mammals. The biological uncoupler in brown fat is a protein called thermogenin. Barbiturates, the antibiotic piericidin A, the fish poison rotenone, dimercaprol, and cyanide all act by inhibiting the electron transport chain at some point.

211. The answer is d. (*Murray, pp 123–148. Scriver, pp 2367–2424. Sack, pp 159–175. Wilson, pp 287–317.*) Some monooxygenases found in liver endoplasmic reticulum require cytochrome P450. This cytochrome acts to transfer electrons between NADPH, O_2, and the substrate. It can be an electron acceptor from a flavoprotein. In the mitochondrial electron transport chain, flavoproteins donate electrons to coenzyme Q, which then transfers them to other cytochromes. Flavoproteins that are oxidases often react directly with molecular oxygen to form hydrogen peroxide. Flavoproteins can be NADH dehydrogenases that oxidize NADH and transfer the electrons to coenzyme Q. The electron transfer centers of flavoproteins in the electron transport chain contain nonheme iron and sulfur.

212. The answer is c. (*Murray, pp 123–148. Scriver, pp 2367–2424. Sack, pp 159–175. Wilson, pp 287–317.*) The electron transport chain shown contains three proton pumps linked by two mobile electron carriers. At each of these three sites (NADH–Q reductase, cytochrome reductase, and cytochrome oxidase) the transfer of electrons down the chain powers the pumping of protons across the inner mitochondrial membrane. The blockage of electron transfers by specific point inhibitors leads to a buildup of highly reduced carriers behind the block because of the inability to transfer electrons across the block. In the scheme shown, rotenone blocks step A, antimycin A blocks step B, and carbon monoxide (as well as cyanide and azide) blocks step E. Therefore a carbon monoxide inhibition leads to a highly reduced state of all of the carriers of the chain. Puromycin and chloramphenicol are inhibitors of protein synthesis and have no direct effect upon the electron transport chain.

213. The answer is f. (*Murray, pp 182–189. Scriver, pp 2367–2424. Sack, pp 159–175. Wilson, pp 287–317.*) In contrast to the case with glycolysis, the only site of substrate-level phosphorylation in the tricarboxylic acid cycle is the step catalyzed by succinyl CoA synthetase. In this step, the cleavage of CoA from succinyl CoA to produce succinate is the utilization of a high-energy bond of CoA to phosphorylate GDP with organic phosphate to produce GTP. Since NADH generated by glycolysis in the cytoplasm cannot pass across the mitochondrial membrane, shuttles are used to bring the electrons into the mitochondria for oxidative phosphorylation. In the glycerol phosphate shuttle, NADH + H$^+$ in the cytoplasm reduces dihydroxyacetone phosphate to glycerol phosphate, which is capable of entering the mitochondria. In the mitochondria, the glycerol phosphate is oxidized back to dihydroxyacetone phosphate, which can then diffuse back out into the cytoplasm. During this process, flavin (FADH$_2$) is reduced and is capable of generating 2 ATP via oxidation by the respiratory chain. In contrast, the malate-aspartate shuttle allows the formation of 3 ATP equivalents for each mole of cytoplasmic NADH + H$^+$ generated. The malate-aspartate shuttle is found mainly in the heart and liver. The process of oxidative phosphorylation that is coupled to electron transport occurs because of the proton gradient maintained across the mitochondrial membrane. ATP is formed by mitochondrial ATPase by the movements of protons across this gradient. In the presence of substances like 2,4-dinitrophenol (DNP), oxidation of oxidative phosphorylation is uncoupled. This occurs because DNP carries the protons across the mitochondrial membrane, short-circuiting the phosphorylations that normally occur. While this reaction is not biologically useful, it does mimic the normal uncoupling of phosphorylation that can occur under certain biologic conditions and is used to generate heat to maintain body temperature. This occurs in certain mammals adapted to cold, newborn mammals, and hibernating animals. In these animals, this process of thermogenesis occurs in specialized brown adipose tissue. The uncoupling protein is called thermogenin. Since electron transport is tightly coupled to phosphorylation, under physiologic conditions electrons do not flow through the electron transport chain to O$_2$ unless ADP is simultaneously phosphorylated to ATP. If the level of ADP is low, oxidative phosphorylation does not occur at as high a rate and the rate of oxygen consumption in tissue decreases. Respiratory control is the regulation of the rate of oxidative phosphorylation by ADP levels.

214. The answer is c. (*Murray, pp 123–148. Scriver, pp 2367–2424. Sack, pp 159–175. Wilson, pp 287–317.*) NADH is generated by many biochemical reactions and used as a reducing agent for biosynthesis. In addition, it is part of the transport chain that conveys electrons to oxygen in the mitochondria. Carnitine binds to fatty acids such as octanoic (C8) or palmitoic (C16) acid, forming acylcarnitines that can be transported into the mitochondria for oxidation. A patient with systemic deficiency of carnitine cannot utilize fatty acids for production of energy. All tissues become glucose-dependent, resulting in hypoglycemia and potential death during overnight fasting.

215. The answer is c. *(Murray, pp 123–148. Scriver, pp 2367–2424. Sack, pp 159–175. Wilson, pp 287–317.)* Glucokinase in the liver or hexokinase in other tissues catalyzes the phosphorylation of glucose as the first step of glycolysis. The equilibrium lies far to the right for the reaction as written:

$$\text{glucose} + \text{ATP} \rightarrow \text{glucose-6-phosphate} + \text{ADP} + P_i$$

The $\Delta G^{\circ\prime}$ for the hydrolysis of glucose-6-phosphate is −3.3 kcal/mol. Thus, the $\Delta G^{\circ\prime}$ of the reverse reaction is +3.3 kcal/mol. Since the $\Delta G^{\circ\prime}$ for the hydrolysis of ATP is −7.3 kcal/mol, the $\Delta G^{\circ\prime}$ for the reaction is:

$$(-7.3 \text{ kcal/mol}) + (+3.3 \text{ kcal/mol}) = -4.0 \text{ kcal/mol}$$

The phosphorylation of glucose is a thermodynamically favorable reaction.

216. The answer is c. *(Murray, pp 123–148. Scriver, pp 2367–2424. Sack, pp 159–175. Wilson, pp 287–317.)* Cyclic AMP is synthesized by adenylate cyclase in response to hormonal stimulation of specific receptors in cells. In all eukaryotic cells studied to date, increased cyclic AMP levels activate a cyclic AMP–dependent protein kinase. The protein kinase, in turn, phosphorylates other enzymes, activating or inactivating them. The kinase is made up of two regulatory and two catalytic subunits. Binding of cyclic AMP to the regulatory subunits allows dissociation of the catalytic subunits. The catalytic subunits are active in the dissociated state. Decrease in cellular cyclic AMP levels by phosphodiesterase breakdown of the nucleotide frees the regulatory subunits from cyclic AMP binding. This allows reassociation of regulatory and catalytic subunits and subsequent inactivation.

217. The answer is b. (*Murray, pp 123–148. Scriver, pp 2367–2424. Sack, pp 159–175. Wilson, pp 287–317.*) The chemiosmotic hypothesis of Mitchell describes the coupling of oxidative phosphorylation and electron transport. The movement of electrons along the electron transport chain allows protons to be pumped from the matrix of the mitochondria to the cytoplasmic side. The protons are pumped at three sites in the electron transport chain to produce a proton gradient. When protons flow back through proton channels of the asymmetrically oriented ATPase of the inner mitochondrial membrane, ATP is synthesized.

218. The answer is b. (*Murray, pp 123–148. Scriver, pp 2367–2424. Sack, pp 159–175. Wilson, pp 287–317.*) Aerobic glycolysis can be defined as the oxidative conversion of glucose to two molecules of pyruvate. In the process, two molecules of ATP and two molecules of NADH are produced. Since reducing equivalents from the two molecules of NADH produced in the cytoplasm must be transported into the mitochondrion for oxidation, it is not known how many ATP molecules are produced. On the assumption that two ATP molecules are formed per molecule of NADH oxidized via the glycerol phosphate shuttle, the ATP yield in aerobic glycolysis can be calculated as six ATP molecules per mole of glucose utilized.

219. The answer is a. (*Murray, pp 190–198. Scriver, pp 2367–2424. Sack, pp 159–175. Wilson, pp 287–317.*) Glucose is immediately phosphorylated to form glucose 6-phosphate (G6P) after being transported into all extrahepatic cells by the enzyme hexokinase. Hexokinase has a very low K_m and thus extremely high affinity for glucose, virtually trapping glucose into entering the metabolic pathways of most tissues. G6P is the starting point for glycolysis, glycogenesis, and the pentose phosphate pathway. In contrast, the liver's hexokinase is called glucokinase and it is only active following a meal, when blood glucose levels are above about 5 mM. It has a relatively low affinity and high K_m. In this manner, the liver sequesters and stores glucose as glycogen for later distribution to tissues only when it is in excess.

220. The answer is d. (*Murray, pp 123–148. Scriver, pp 2367–2424. Sack, pp 159–175. Wilson, pp 287–317.*) ATP is synthesized by two reactions in glycolysis. The first molecule of ATP is generated by phosphoglycerate kinase, converting 1,3-diphosphoglycerate to 3-phosphoglycerate. The second molecule of ATP is generated by pyruvate kinase, converting phosphoenolpyruvate to pyruvate.

221. The answer is e. *(Murray, pp 190–198. Scriver, pp 2367–2424. Sack, pp 159–175. Wilson, pp 287–317.)* High-energy phosphate bonds are added to the substrates of glycolysis at three steps in the pathway. Hexokinase— or, in the case of the liver, glucokinase—adds phosphate from ATP to glucose to form glucose-6-phosphate. Strictly speaking, this is not always considered a step of the glycolytic pathway. Phosphofructokinase uses ATP to convert fructose-6-phosphate to fructose-1,6-phosphate. Using NAD⁺ in an oxidation-reduction reaction, inorganic phosphate is added to glyceraldehyde-3-phosphate by the enzyme glyceraldehyde-3-phosphate dehydrogenase to form 1,3-diphosphoglycerate. The enzymes phosphoglycerate kinase and pyruvate kinase transfer substrate high-energy phosphate groups to ADP to form ATP.

222. The answer is a. *(Murray, pp 259–267. Scriver, pp 2367–2424. Sack, pp 159–175. Wilson, pp 287–317.)* Lipolysis of triacylglycerols yields fatty acids and glycerol. The free glycerol is transported to the liver, where it can be phosphorylated to glycerol phosphate and enter the glycolysis or the gluconeogenesis pathways at the level of dihydroxyacetone phosphate. Acetyl CoA and propionyl CoA are produced in the final round of degradation of an odd-chain fatty acid. Acetyl CoA cannot be converted to glucose, but propionyl CoA can. The three carbons of propionyl CoA enter the citric acid cycle after being converted into succinyl CoA. Succinyl CoA can then be converted to oxaloacetate and enter the glycolytic scheme. Ketone bodies, including β-hydroxybutyrate, are produced from acetyl CoA units derived from fatty acid β-oxidation. They may not be converted to glucose. Amino acids are not a product of triacylglycerol breakdown.

223. The answer is b. *(Murray, pp 259–267. Scriver, pp 2367–2424. Sack, pp 159–175. Wilson, pp 287–317.)* Lipolysis is directly regulated by hormones in adipocytes. Epinephrine stimulates adenylate cyclase to produce cyclic AMP, which in turn stimulates a protein kinase. The kinase activates triglyceride lipase by phosphorylating it. Lipolysis then proceeds and results in the release of free fatty acids and glycerol. A futile reesterification of free fatty acids is prevented, since adipocytes contain little glycerol kinase to phosphorylate the liberated glycerol, which must be processed in the liver. Inhibition of lipolysis occurs in the presence of insulin, which lowers cyclic AMP levels. Lipoprotein lipase is not an adipocyte enzyme.

224. The answer is d. (*Murray, pp 123–148. Scriver, pp 2367–2424. Sack, pp 159–175. Wilson, pp 287–317.*) Oligomycin inhibits mitochondrial ATPase and thus prevents phosphorylation of ADP to ATP. It prevents utilization of energy derived from electron transport for the synthesis of ATP. Oligomycin has no effect on coupling but blocks mitochondrial phosphorylation so that both oxidation and phosphorylation cease in its presence.

225. The answer is d. (*Murray, pp 199–207. Scriver, pp 2367–2424. Sack, pp 159–175. Wilson, pp 287–317.*) Fats (triacylglycerols) are the most highly concentrated and efficient stores of metabolic energy in the body. This is because they are anhydrous and reduced. On a dry-weight basis, the yield from the complete oxidation of the fatty acids produced from triacylglycerols is approximately 9 kcal/g, compared with 4 kcal/g for glycogen and proteins. However, under physiologic conditions, glycogen and proteins become highly hydrated, whereas triacylglyceride stores remain relatively free of water. Therefore, while the energy yield from fat stores remains at approximately 9 kcal/g, the actual yields from the oxidation of glycogen and proteins are diluted considerably. Under anhydrous physiologic conditions, fats yield about six times the energy of glycogen stores.

226. The answer is b. (*Murray, pp 123–148. Scriver, pp 2367–2424. Sack, pp 159–175. Wilson, pp 287–317.*) The conversion of glucose to glucose-6-phosphate is different in liver and muscle. In muscle and most other tissues, hexokinase regulates the conversion of glucose to glucose-6-phosphate. When the major regulatory enzyme of glycolysis, phosphofructose kinase, is turned off, the level of fructose-6-phosphate increases and in turn the level of glucose-6-phosphate rises because it is in equilibrium with fructose-6-phosphate. Hexokinase is inhibited by glucose-6-phosphate. However, in the liver, glucose is phosphorylated even when glucose-6-phosphate levels are high because the enzyme regulating transformation of glucose into glucose-6-phosphate is glucokinase. Glucokinase is not inhibited by glucose-6-phosphate in the liver. While hexokinase has a low K_m for glucose and is capable of acting upon low levels of blood glucose, glucokinase has a high K_m for glucose and is effective only when glucose is abundant. Therefore, when blood glucose levels are low, muscle, brain, and other tissues are capable of taking up and phosphorylating glucose, while the liver is not. When blood glucose is abundant, glucokinase in the liver phosphorylates glucose and provides glucose-6-phosphate for the synthesis and storage of glucose as glycogen.

227. The answer is c. *(Murray, pp 123–148. Scriver, pp 2367–2424. Sack, pp 159–175. Wilson, pp 287–317.)* Muscle contraction is caused by the release of calcium from the sarcoplasmic reticulum following nervous stimulation. In addition to stimulating contraction, the calcium released from the sarcoplasmic reticulum binds to a calmodulin subunit on phosphorylase kinase. This activates phosphorylase kinase, converting it from the D form to the A form. The activated phosphorylase then breaks down glycogen and provides glucose for energy metabolism during exercise. In this way, muscle contraction and glucose production from glycogen are coordinated by the transient increase of cytoplasmic calcium levels during muscle contraction.

228. The answer is c. *(Murray, pp 123–148. Scriver, pp 2367–2424. Sack, pp 159–175. Wilson, pp 287–317.)* The most likely cause of the symptoms observed is carnitine deficiency. Under normal circumstances, long-chain fatty acids coming into muscle cells are activated as acyl coenzyme A and transported as acyl carnitine across the inner mitochondrial membrane into the matrix. A deficiency in carnitine, which is normally synthesized in the liver, can be genetic; but it is also observed in preterm babies with liver problems and dialysis patients. Blockage of the transport of long-chain fatty acids into mitochondria not only deprives the patient of energy production, but also disrupts the structure of the muscle cell with the accumulation of lipid droplets. Oral dietary supplementation usually can effect a cure. Deficiencies in the carnitine acyltransferase enzymes I and II can cause similar symptoms.

229. The answer is a. *(Murray, pp 123–148. Scriver, pp 2367–2424. Sack, pp 159–175. Wilson, pp 287–317.)* Acetyl CoA carboxylase deficiency drastically alters the ability of the patient to synthesize fatty acids. The fact that the infant was born at all is due to the body's ability to utilize fatty acids provided to it. However, all processes dependent upon de novo fatty acid biosynthesis are affected. The lungs, in particular, require surfactant, a lipoprotein substance secreted by alveolar type II cells, to function properly. Surfactant lowers alveolar surface tension, facilitating gas exchange. It contains significant amounts of dipalmitoyl phosphatidylcholine. Palmitate is the major end product of de novo fatty acid synthesis. Acetyl CoA carboxylase formation of malonyl CoA is the first step of fatty acid synthesis. Biotin deficiency cannot be the problem because pyruvate carboxylase in gluconeogenesis is not affected. None of the other answers listed would result in all of the symptoms given.

230. The answer is b. *(Murray, pp 123–148. Scriver, pp 2367–2424. Sack, pp 159–175. Wilson, pp 287–317.)* In mammalian systems ATP may be formed in the presence or the absence of molecular oxygen. In glycolysis, ATP is formed by substrate-level phosphorylation. In mitochondria, ATP is formed by the oxidation of NADH. ATP hydrolysis is an exergonic reaction that releases energy. When this released energy is chemically linked to an energy-requiring or endergonic reaction, that reaction is driven. Heat does not drive biologic reactions.

231. The answer is e. *(Murray, pp 230–237. Scriver, pp 2367–2424. Sack, pp 159–175. Wilson, pp 287–317.)* 3-hydroxy-3-methylglutaryl CoA is not an inhibitor of cholesterol synthesis. The compound 3-hydroxy-3-methylglutaryl CoA is formed by the condensation of acetoacetyl CoA and acetyl CoA in the synthetic pathways for both cholesterol and ketone bodies. However, the similar enzymes involved in each pathway are separated in space. 3-hydroxy-3-methylglutaryl CoA produced in mitochondria is cleaved to yield the ketone body acetoacetate, whereas that produced in the cytosol is reduced to form mevalonic acid, which goes on to form cholesterol. The two series of reactions are also separated in time. Synthesis of cholesterol occurs when excess acetyl CoA produced from carbohydrates is available. During fasting, synthesis of cholesterol is inhibited. In contrast, synthesis of ketone bodies is most rapid during fasting, when acetyl CoA is produced by the β-oxidation of mobilized fatty acids.

232. The answer is b. *(Murray, pp 123–148. Scriver, pp 2367–2424. Sack, pp 159–175. Wilson, pp 287–317.)* The entry point into the electron transport chain for electrons from $FADH_2$ flavoproteins is ubiquinone, which is referred to as Q or QH_2 in the reduced state. Ubiquinone carries these electrons to cytochrome oxidase, the next step in the respiratory chain. This late entry into the transport scheme bypasses the first two steps and thus the first of the three proton pumps of oxidative phosphorylation. $FADH_2$ electrons are derived from the dehydrogenase-based enzymatic reactions of (1) succinate oxidation to fumarate in the citric acid cycle; (2) glycerol phosphate oxidation to dihydroxyacetone phosphate in the mitochondrial portion of the glycerol phosphate shuttle; and (3) fatty acyl CoA oxidation to an enoyl CoA during desaturation of fatty acids.

233. The answer is h. *(Murray, pp 123–148. Scriver, pp 2367–2424. Sack, pp 159–175. Wilson, pp 287–317.)* The regulatory enzyme of lipolysis is hormone-sensitive lipase. It is a triacylglyceride lipase of adipose cells regulated by hormones. The hormones that stimulate release of fatty acids into the blood are glucagon, epinephrine, and norepinephrine, all of which activate adipocyte membrane adenylate cyclase. This produces an increased level of cyclic AMP, which activates a protein lipase that, in turn, phosphorylates and activates the sensitive lipase. In contrast, insulin causes dephosphorylation and inhibition, thereby shutting down lipolysis and the release of fatty acids into the bloodstream.

234. The answer is b. *(Murray, pp 238–249. Scriver, pp 2367–2424. Sack, pp 159–175. Wilson, pp 287–317.)* High blood levels of triacylglycerides and fatty stools (steatorrhea) are symptoms often observed following a meal in patients with lipoprotein lipase deficiency (type I lipidemia). Normally, lipoprotein lipase delipidate the triacylglyceride-rich dietary blood lipoproteins known as chylomicrons by cleaving off fatty acids, thereby allowing their absorption into tissues. When absent or malfunctioning, blood chylomicron levels build up and back up, preventing absorption of fats from the lumen of the gut. This leads to steatorrhea. The pancreatic enzyme secreted into the gut to hydrolyze triacylglycerides is unique in that it only cleaves off the 1' and 3' fatty acids. Thus, 2' monoacylglycerides are produced and absorbed into intestinal epithelial cells, where they are reesterified with fatty acids back into triacylglycerides. The triacylglycerides are packaged into chylomicrons for transport through the lymphatic and vascular system.

235. The answer is a. *(Murray, pp 123–148. Scriver, pp 2367–2424. Sack, pp 159–175. Wilson, pp 287–317.)* Of the enzymes on the list shown, only acetyl coenzyme A carboxylase directly produces a product, malonyl CoA, that is an allosteric regulator of another enzyme on the list. Malonyl CoA is the product of the first step in fatty acid synthesis, which occurs during a time of excess acetyl CoA due to satisfied energy and caloric needs of tissues. Malonyl CoA allosterically inhibits carnitine acyl transferase I, which is the major regulatory enzyme of fatty acid oxidation. Fatty acid oxidation occurs during a time of energy need. Thus, when fatty acids are being synthesized during a time of "plenty," the breakdown of fatty acids is shut off.

236. The answer is c. (*Murray, pp 238–249. Scriver, pp 2367–2424. Sack, pp 159–175. Wilson, pp 287–317.*) A variety of agonists activate the plasma membrane–bound enzyme phospholipase C, which hydrolyzes the phosphodiester bond of phosphatidyl inositol 4,5-bisphosphate and consequently releases diacylglycerol (DAG) and inositol 1,4,5-triphosphate (IP$_3$). Phospholipase C is also known as phosphoinositidase and as polyphosphoinositide phosphodiesterase. Both DAG and IP$_3$ are second messengers. DAG activates protein kinase C, which is important in controlling cell division and cell proliferation. IP$_3$ opens calcium channels and allows the rapid release of the calcium stores in endoplasmic reticulum (in smooth muscle, sarcoplasmic reticulum). The elevated levels of calcium ion stimulate smooth-muscle contraction, exocytosis, and glycogen breakdown.

237. The answer is b. (*Murray, pp 123–148. Scriver, pp 2367–2424. Sack, pp 159–175. Wilson, pp 287–317.*) Cholera toxin is an 87-kD protein produced by *Vibrio cholerae*, a gram-negative bacterium. The toxin enters intestinal mucosal cells by binding to G$_{M1}$ ganglioside. It interacts with G$_s$ protein, which stimulates adenylate cyclase. By ADP-ribosylation of G$_s$, the toxin blocks its capacity to hydrolyze bound GTP to GDP. Thus, the G protein is locked in an active form and adenylate cyclase stays irreversibly activated. Under normal conditions, inactivated G protein contains GDP, which is produced by a phosphatase catalyzing the hydrolysis of GTP to GDP. When GDP is so bound to the G protein, the adenylate cyclase is inactive. Upon hormone binding to the receptor, GTP is exchanged for GDP and the G protein is in an active state, allowing adenylate cyclase to produce cyclic AMP. Because cholera toxin prevents the hydrolysis of GTP to GDP, the adenylate cyclase remains in an irreversibly active state, continuously producing cyclic AMP in the intestinal mucosal cells. This leads to a massive loss of body fluid into the intestine within a few hours.

238. The answer is c. *(Murray, pp 123–148. Scriver, pp 2367–2424. Sack, pp 159–175. Wilson, pp 287–317.)* The daily intake of 62.5 g of high-quality protein is above the minimum daily requirement for a 70-kg adult (45 g protein per day). As the obligatory nitrogen losses are covered by the dietary intake, this man will be in nitrogen balance (i.e., 0) and nitrogen loss will equal nitrogen intake.

239. The answer is c. *(Murray, pp 123–148. Scriver, pp 2367–2424. Sack, pp 159–175. Wilson, pp 287–317.)* The respiratory quotient (RQ) can be studied noninvasively by measuring the CO_2 produced and the O_2 consumed following a meal:

$$RQ = \text{moles of } CO_2 \text{ produced/moles of } O_2 \text{ consumed}$$

The RQ varies for each major food group; values are 0.8 for proteins, 0.72 for fats, and 1.0 for carbohydrates. Thus, if more or less equal amounts of fats and carbohydrates are ingested and burned for energy, the RQ is about halfway between the values of either foodstuff alone, i.e., 0.86.

240. The answer is c. *(Murray, pp 123–148. Scriver, pp 2367–2424. Sack, pp 159–175. Wilson, pp 287–317.)* NADH generated from glycolysis must be relieved of an electron to form nicotinamide adenine dinucleotide (NAD_+) so that glycolysis may continue. However, mitochondrial membranes are impermeable to both NADH and NAD^+. The solution to this problem is the transfer of electrons from NADH to molecules that traverse the membrane. In the glycerophosphate shuttle, dihydroxyacetone phosphate (DHAP) is reduced to glycerol-3-phosphate and thereby regenerates NAD^+. The glycerol-3-phosphate diffuses into mitochondria and is oxidized by flavin adenine dinucleotide (FAD) back to DHAP, which can diffuse back into the cytosol. The mitochondrial reduced form of flavin adenine dinucleotide ($FADH_2$) produced yields 2 ATP in the electron transport chain. In the heart and liver, the more energy-efficient malate-aspartate shuttle moves electrons into mitochondria. Cytoplasmic oxaloacetate is reduced to malate, which diffuses into the mitochondria and is oxidized by NAD_+ back to oxaloacetate. The mitochondrial NADH produced yields 3 ATP on electron transport. The mitochondrial oxaloacetate is converted to aspartate, which diffuses into the cytosol, where it is converted back into cytoplasmic oxaloacetate.

241. The answer is b. (*Murray, pp 123–148. Scriver, pp 2367–2424. Sack, pp 159–175. Wilson, pp 287–317.*) Muscle cells are the only cells listed that are capable of utilizing all the energy sources available—glucose, fatty acids, and, during fasting, ketone bodies. Mitochondria are required for metabolism of fatty acids and ketone bodies. Since red blood cells (erythrocytes) do not contain mitochondria, no utilization of these energy sources is possible. Although the brain may utilize glucose and ketone bodies, fatty acids cannot cross the blood-brain barrier. Hepatocytes (liver cells) are the sites of ketone body production, but the mitochondrial enzyme necessary for utilization of ketone bodies is not present in hepatocytes.

Amino Acid, Lipid, and Nucleotide Metabolism

Questions

DIRECTIONS: Each item below contains a question or incomplete statement followed by suggested responses. Select the **one best** response to each question.

242. A child with a large head, multiple fractures, and blue scleras (whites of the eyes) is evaluated for osteogenesis imperfecta (166200). One study involves labeling of collagen chains in tissue culture to assess their mobility by gel electrophoresis. Amino acids labeled with radioactive carbon 14 are added to the culture dishes in order to label the collagen. Which of the following amino acids would not result in labeled collagen?

a.   Serine
b.   Glycine
c.   Aspartate
d.   Glutamate
e.   Hydroxylserine

243. Liver aminotransferases, which are also called transaminases, catalyze the transfer of α-amino groups from many different amino acids to α-ketoglutarate. The intermediate produced is deaminated back to α-ketoglutarate with the formation of ammonium ion. The structure of α-ketoglutarate is shown below. What is the intermediate produced?

a.   Aspartate
b.   Alanine
c.   Oxaloacetate
d.   Glutamate
e.   Pyruvate

$$^-OOC - CH_2 - CH_2 - \overset{\overset{O}{\|}}{C} - COO^-$$

244. In the urea cycle diagram below, which compound is derived from a condensation of CO_2 and NH_4^+?

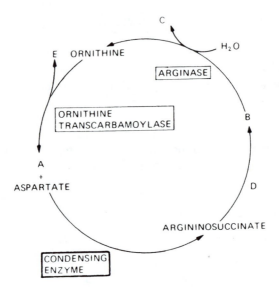

a. Compound A
b. Compound B
c. Compound C
d. Compound D
e. Compound E

245. In the schematic urea cycle diagram in question 244, which compound is considered the end product?

246. The reactions of the urea cycle occur

a. In the cytosol
b. In the mitochondrial matrix
c. In the mitochondrial matrix and the cytosol
d. Only in lysosomes
e. In peroxisomes

247. A newborn becomes progressively lethargic after feeding and increases his respiratory rate. He becomes virtually comatose, responding only to painful stimuli, and exhibits mild respiratory alkalosis. Suspicion of a urea cycle disorder is aroused and evaluation of serum amino acid levels is initiated. In the presence of hyperammonemia, production of which of the following amino acids is always increased?

a. Glycine
b. Arginine
c. Proline
d. Histidine
e. Glutamine

248. The thyroid hormone thyroxine (T_4) is derived from

a. Threonine
b. Tyrosine
c. Thiamine
d. Tryptophan
e. Tyramine

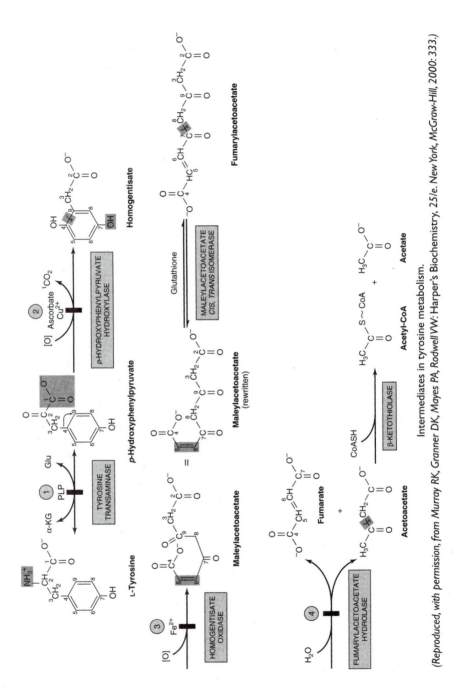

Intermediates in tyrosine metabolism.

(Reproduced, with permission, from Murray RK, Granner DK, Mayes PA, Rodwell VW: Harper's Biochemistry, 25/e. New York, McGraw-Hill, 2000: 333.)

249. Which of the metabolites below is a precursor of tyrosine?

a. L-dihydroxyphenylalanine (dopa)
b. Dopamine
c. Norepinephrine
d. Epinephrine
e. Phenylalanine

250. Which of the following amino acids is a precursor to cysteine?

a. Threonine
b. Methionine
c. Glutamine
d. Lysine
e. Alanine

251. The second and final enzymatic step in the reaction pathway shown is most correctly described as

a. Amination
b. Aminotransferase
c. Transamination
d. Amidation
e. Oxidative deamination

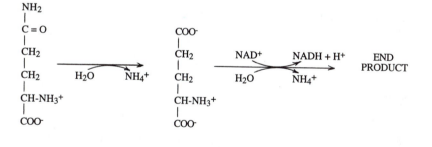

252. An adolescent female develops hemiballismus (repetitive throwing motions of the arms) after anesthesia for a routine operation. She is tall and lanky, and it is noted that she and her sister both had previous operations for dislocated lenses of the eyes. The symptoms are suspicious for the disease homocystinuria (236300). Which of the statements below is descriptive of this disease?

a. Patients may be treated with dietary supplements of vitamin B_{12}
b. Patients may be treated with dietary supplements of vitamin C
c. There is deficient excretion of homocysteine
d. There is increased excretion of cysteine
e. There is a defect in the ability to form homocysteine from methionine by methylation

253. Which clinical laboratory observation below is suggestive of Hartnup disease (neutral amino acid transport deficiency)?

a. Burnt-sugar smell in urine
b. High plasma phenylalanine levels
c. Extremely high levels of citrulline in urine
d. Elevation of glutamine in blood and urine
e. Elevated plasma tyrosine and methionine levels
f. Dark urine
g. High fecal levels of tryptophan and indole derivatives

254. The important reactive group of glutathione in its role as an antioxidant is

a. Serine
b. Sulfhydryl
c. Tyrosine
d. Acetyl coenzyme A (CoA)
e. Carboxyl

255. Which one of the following hormones is derived most completely from tyrosine?

a. Glucagon
b. Thyroxine
c. Insulin
d. Prostaglandins
e. Endorphins

256. A newborn develops jaundice (yellow skin and yellow scleras) that requires laboratory evaluation. Which of the following porphyrin derivatives is conjugated, reacts directly, and is a major component of bile?

a. Bilirubin diglucuronide
b. Stercobilin
c. Biliverdin
d. Urobilinogen
e. Heme
f. Bilirubin
g. Urobilin

257. Which of the following porphyrins gives stools their characteristic brown color?

a. Biliverdin
b. Urobilinogen
c. Heme
d. Stercobilin
e. Urobilin

258. Chylomicrons, intermediate-density lipoproteins (IDLs), low-density lipoproteins (LDLs), and very-low-density lipoproteins (VLDLs) are all serum lipoproteins. What is the correct ordering of these particles from the lowest to the highest density?

a. LDLs, IDLs, VLDLs, chylomicrons
b. Chylomicrons, VLDLs, IDLs, LDLs
c. VLDLs, IDLs, LDLs, chylomicrons
d. Chylomicrons, IDLs, VLDLs, LDLs
e. LDLs, VLDLs, IDLs, chylomicrons

259. A 3-year-old child is brought into the ER while you are on duty. She is cold and clammy and is breathing rapidly. She is obviously confused and lethargic. Her mother indicates she has accidentally ingested automobile antifreeze while playing in the garage. Following gastrointestinal lavage and activated charcoal administration, one of the treatments you immediately initiate involves

a. Intravenous infusion of oxalic acid
b. Nasogastric tube for ethanol administration
c. Flushing out the bladder via a catheter
d. Intramuscular injection of epinephrine
e. Simply waiting and measuring vital signs

260. Ceramide is a precursor to which of the following compounds?

a. Phosphatidyl serine
b. Sphingomyelin
c. Phosphatidyl glycerol
d. Phosphatidyl choline
e. Phosphatidyl ethanolamine

261. Which of the following steps in the biosynthesis of cholesterol is thought to be rate-controlling and the locus of metabolic regulation?

a. Geranyl pyrophosphate → farnesyl pyrophosphate
b. Squalene → lanosterol
c. Lanosterol → cholesterol
d. 3-hydroxy-3-methylglutaryl CoA → mevalonic acid
e. Mevalonic acid → geranyl pyrophosphate

262. Multiple sclerosis is a disease characterized by chronic inflammation. There are significant data to indicate that susceptibility to multiple sclerosis is inherited and causes a primary change in

a. Membrane lipids
b. Anti-inflammatory steroids
c. Blood proteins
d. Stored carbohydrates
e. Nucleotide metabolism

263. Which of the following is most characteristic of a sphingolipidosis?

a. Multifactorial inheritance
b. Variable activities of abnormal enzyme in different patient tissues
c. Deficiency of a hydrolytic enzyme
d. Abnormalities of sphingolipid synthesis
e. Accumulation of ceramide-containing lipids

264. The end product of cytosol fatty acid synthetase in humans is

a. Oleic acid
b. Arachidonic acid
c. Linoleic acid
d. Palmitic acid
e. Palmitoleic acid

265. It has been noted that infants placed on extremely low-fat diets for a variety of reasons often develop skin problems and other symptoms. This is most often due to

a. Lactose intolerance
b. Glycogen storage diseases
c. Antibody abnormalities
d. Deficiency of fatty acid desaturase greater than Δ^9
e. Deficiency of chylomicron and VLDL production

266. The fatty acid synthase complex of mammals

a. Is a dimer of unsimilar subunits
b. Is composed of seven different proteins
c. Dissociates into eight different proteins
d. Catalyzes eight different enzymatic steps
e. Is composed of covalently linked enzymes

267. The primary biochemical lesion in homozygotes with familial hypercholesterolemia (type IIa) is

a. The loss of feedback inhibition of liver hydroxymethylglutaryl CoA reductase
b. The increased production of low-density lipoproteins from very-low-density lipoproteins
c. The loss of apolipoprotein B
d. The malfunctioning of acyl CoA–cholesterol acyl transferase (ACAT)
e. The functional deficiency of plasma membrane receptors for low-density lipoproteins

268. Which one of the following steps results in the formation of a phospholipid?

a. Step A
b. Step B
c. Step C
d. Step D
e. Step E

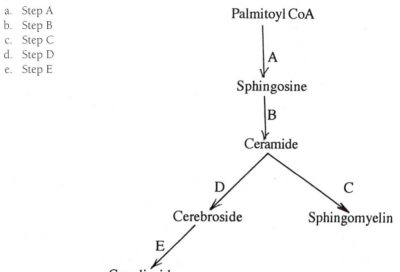

269. Which one of the following apolipoproteins is synthesized in the liver as part of the coat of very-low-density lipoproteins (VLDLs)?

a. AI
b. B48
c. CII
d. B100
e. E

270. Which of the following lipoproteins would contribute to a measurement of plasma cholesterol in a normal person following a 12-h fast?

a. Very-low-density lipoproteins
b. High-density lipoproteins
c. Chylomicrons
d. Chylomicron remnants
e. Adipocyte lipid droplets

271. Which of the following statements correctly describes the enzyme thiokinase?

a. It yields acetyl CoA as a product
b. It yields ADP as a product
c. It yields CoA as a product
d. It forms CoA thioesters as a product
e. It requires β-ketoacyl CoA as a substrate

272. A 15-year-old boy has a long history of school problems and is labeled as hyperactive. His tissues are puffy, giving his face a "coarse" appearance. His IQ tests have declined recently and are now markedly below normal. Laboratory studies demonstrate normal amounts of sphingolipids in fibroblast cultures with increased amounts of glycosaminoglycans in urine. Which of the following enzyme deficiencies might explain the boy's phenotype?

a. Hexosaminidase A
b. Glucocerebrosidase
c. α-L-iduronidase
d. α-galactocerebrosidase
e. β-gangliosidase A

273. Leukocyte samples isolated from the blood of a newborn infant are homogenized and incubated with ganglioside GM$_2$. Approximately 47% of the expected normal amount of N-acetylgalactosamine is liberated during the incubation period. These results indicate that the infant

a. Is a heterozygote (carrier) for Tay-Sachs disease
b. Is homozygous for Tay-Sachs disease
c. Has Tay-Sachs syndrome
d. Will most likely have mental deficiency
e. Has relatively normal β-N-acetylhexosaminidase activity

274. Most of the reducing equivalents utilized for synthesis of fatty acids can be generated from

a. The pentose phosphate pathway
b. Glycolysis
c. The citric acid cycle
d. Mitochondrial malate dehydrogenase
e. Citrate lyase

275. During fatty acid metabolism in humans, coenzyme A (CoA) is different from acyl carrier protein (ACP) in which one of the following ways?

a. Binding of malonic acid with a phosphopantetheine
b. Binding of fatty acids
c. Function in fatty acid oxidation
d. Function in the cytosol
e. Function in fatty acid synthesis

276. For every 2 mol of free glycerol released by lipolysis of triacylglycerides in adipose tissue

a. 2 mol of triacylglycerides is released
b. 2 mol of free fatty acids is released
c. 1 mol of glucose can be synthesized in gluconeogenesis
d. 1 mol of triacylglyceride is released
e. 3 mol of acyl CoA is produced

277. In humans, the formation of the fatty acid $C\text{-}18\text{-}\Delta^9,\Delta^{12}$ can be derived from which of the following?

a. $C\text{-}18$ cis-Δ^9
b. $C\text{-}18$ cis-Δ^6
c. $C\text{-}18$
d. $C\text{-}16$ cis-Δ^6,Δ^9
e. $C\text{-}18$ cis-Δ^9,Δ^{12}

278. Which one of the following compounds is a key intermediate in the synthesis of both triacylglycerols and phospholipids?

a. CDP-choline
b. Phosphatidate
c. Triacylglyceride
d. Phosphatidylserine
e. CDP-diacylglycerol

279. Which of the following is not used in the synthesis of fatty acids?

a. Cobalamin (vitamin B_{12})
b. NADPH
c. AMP
d. $FADH_2$
e. HCO_3^-

280. Which of the diagrammatic structures shown below represents the model of biologic membranes that most successfully accounts for membrane asymmetry?

a. Structure A
b. Structure B
c. Structure C
d. Structure D
e. Structure E

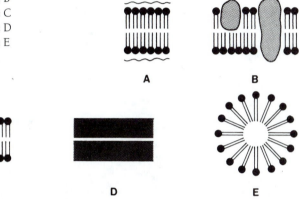

281. Which of the diagrammatic structures shown in question 280 most clearly represents a model of the configuration of lipids obtained during the emulsification process that precedes hydrolysis during digestion?

a. Structure A
b. Structure B
c. Structure C
d. Structure D
e. Structure E

282. A 45-year-old man has a mild heart attack and is placed on diet and mevastatin therapy. Which of the following will be a result of this therapy?

a. Low blood glucose
b. Low blood LDLs
c. High blood cholesterol
d. High blood glucose
e. Low oxidation of fatty acids
f. Ketosis
g. Lipolysis

283. The elongation of fatty acids occurs in which of the diagrammatic structures shown below?

a. Structure A
b. Structure B
c. Structure C
d. Structure D
e. Structure E

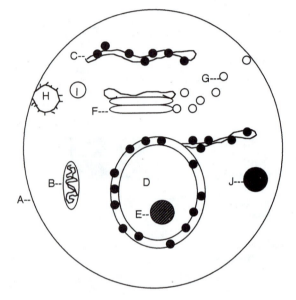

284. The formation of β-hydroxybutyrate occurs in which of the diagrammatic structures shown in question 283?

a. Structure A
b. Structure B
c. Structure C
d. Structure D
e. Structure E

285. Gangliosides and receptors for hormones such as glucagon can be found in which of the diagrammatic structures shown in question 283?

a. Structure A
b. Structure B
c. Structure C
d. Structure D
e. Structure E

286. A control and two patients with hyperlipidemia are studied after an overnight fast. Their plasma lipoprotein electrophoresis patterns are shown below, the control being in the middle lane. One of the patients has a pattern typical of type I lipoprotein lipase deficiency, and the other of type IIa familial hypercholesterolemia. Which of the bands observed in the electrophoretic gel patterns represents a lipoprotein fraction that is abnormally abundant after fasting and that is most enriched in triacylglycerides?

a. Band A
b. Band B
c. Band C
d. Band D
e. Band E
f. Band F
g. Band G
h. Band H
i. Band I

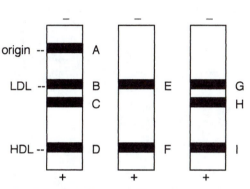

Agarose Gel Electrophoresis Separation Patterns of Plasma Lipoproteins in Three Selected Patients Following a Fast

287. The major source of extracellular cholesterol for human tissues is

a. Very-low-density lipoproteins (VLDLs)
b. Low-density lipoproteins (LDLs)
c. High-density lipoproteins (HDLs)
d. Albumin
e. γ-globulin

288. The synthesis of 3-hydroxy-3-methylglutaryl CoA can occur

a. Only in mitochondria of all mammalian tissues
b. Only in the cytosol of all mammalian tissues
c. Only in the endoplasmic reticulum of all mammalian tissues
d. In both the cytosol and mitochondria
e. In lysosomes

289. When the liver is actively synthesizing fatty acids, a concomitant decrease in β oxidation of fatty acids is due to

a. Inhibition of a translocation between cellular compartments
b. Inhibition by an end product
c. Activation of an enzyme
d. Detergent effects
e. Decreases in adipocyte lipolysis

290. A 4-year-old girl presents in the clinic with megaloblastic anemia and failure to thrive. Blood chemistries reveal orotic aciduria. Enzyme measurements of white blood cells reveal a deficiency of the pyrimidine biosynthesis enzyme orotate phosphoribosyltransferase and abnormally high activity of the enzyme aspartate transcarbamoylase. Which one of the following treatments will reverse all symptoms if carried out chronically?

a. Blood transfusion
b. White blood cell transfusion
c. Dietary supplements of phosphoribosylpyrophosphate (PRPP)
d. Oral thymidine
e. Oral uridine

291. In most patients with gout as well as those with Lesch-Nyhan syndrome, purines are overproduced and overexcreted. Yet the hypoxanthine analogue allopurinol, which effectively treats gout, has no effect on the severe neurological symptoms of Lesch-Nyhan patients because it does not

a. Decrease de novo purine synthesis
b. Decrease de novo pyrimidine synthesis
c. Diminish urate synthesis
d. Increase phosphoribosylpyrophosphate (PRPP) levels
e. Inhibit xanthine oxidase

292. Which of the following would rule out hyperuricemia in a patient?

a. Lesch-Nyhan syndrome
b. Gout
c. Xanthine oxidase hyperactivity
d. Carbamoyl phosphate synthase deficiency
e. Purine overproduction secondary to Von Gierke's disease

293. Which one of the following contributes nitrogen atoms to both purine and pyrimidine rings?

a. Aspartate
b. Carbamoyl phosphate
c. Carbon dioxide
d. Glutamine
e. Tetrahydrofolate

294. Which statement best describes xanthine?

a. It is a direct precursor of guanine
b. It covalently binds to allopurinol
c. It is a substrate rather than a product of the enzyme xanthine oxidase
d. It is oxidized to form uric acid
e. It is oxidized to form hypoxanthine

295. Feedback inhibition of pyrimidine nucleotide synthesis can occur by which of the following means?

a. Increased activity of carbamoyl phosphate synthetase
b. Increased activity of aspartate transcarbamoylase
c. CTP allosteric effects
d. UMP competitive inhibition
e. TTP allosteric effects

296. Purine nucleotide biosynthesis can be inhibited by which of the following?

a. Guanosine triphosphate (GTP)
b. Uridine monophosphate (UMP)
c. Adenosine monophosphate (AMP)
d. Adenosine triphosphate (ATP)
e. Inosine diphosphate (IDP)

297. Which base derivative can serve as a precursor for the synthesis of two of the other base derivatives shown?

a. Cytidine triphosphate (CTP)
b. Uridine monophosphate (UMP)
c. Deoxythymidine monophosphate (dTMP)
d. Adenosine triphosphate (ATP)
e. Deoxyadenosine monophosphate (dAMP)

298. Which is the rate-controlling step of pyrimidine synthesis that exhibits allosteric inhibition by cytidine triphosphate (CTP)?

a. Aspartate transcarbamoylase
b. Hypoxanthine-guanine phosphoribosyl transferase (HGPRT) 5-fluorouracil
c. Thymidylate synthase
d. Ribose-phosphate pyrophosphokinase
e. Xanthine oxidase

299. Which of the following compounds is a required substrate for purine biosynthesis?

a. 5-methyl thymidine
b. Ara C
c. Ribose phosphate
d. 5-phosphoribosylpyrophosphate (PRPP)
e. 5-fluorouracil

300. Which of the following compounds is an analogue of hypoxanthine?

a. Ara C
b. Allopurinol
c. Ribose phosphate
d. 5-phosphoribosylpyrophosphate (PRPP)
e. 5-FU

301. A pentose with a 5′-phosphate group, a 2′-hydroxyl group, and a 1′-pyrimidine group describes which of the following structures?

a. Cytosine
b. Guanosine
c. Thymidine
d. Thymidylate
e. Cytidylate

302. Which of the activated groups or units is most closely associated with uridine diphosphate (UDP)?

a. Electrons
b. Phosphoryl
c. Acyl
d. Aldehyde
e. Glucose

Amino Acid, Lipid, and Nucleotide Metabolism

Answers

242. The answer is e. (*Murray, pp 307–346. Scriver, pp 1667–1724. Sack, pp 121–138. Wilson, pp 287–317.*) Collagen has an unusual amino acid composition in that approximately one-third of collagen molecules are glycine. The amino acid proline is also present in a much greater amount than in other proteins. In addition, two somewhat unusual amino acids, 4-hydroxyproline and 5-hydroxylysine, are found in collagen. Hydroxy-proline and hydroxylysine per se are not incorporated during the synthesis of collagen. Proline and lysine are hydroxylated by specific hydroxylases after collagen is synthesized. A reducing agent such as ascorbate (vitamin C) is needed for the hydroxylation reaction to occur. In its absence, the disease known as scurvy occurs. Only proline or lysine residues located on the amino side of glycine residues are hydroxylated. The hydroxylysine residues of collagen are important sites of glycosylation of disaccharides of glucose and galactose.

243. The answer is d. (*Murray, pp 307–346. Scriver, pp 1667–1724. Sack, pp 121–138. Wilson, pp 287–317.*) Amino acid degradation ultimately leads to the formation of ammonium ion (NH_4^+), which is toxic in significant amounts. In the liver of humans, as in most terrestrial vertebrates, NH_4^+ is produced and converted into urea for excretion. For many amino acids, the conversion of α-amino groups into ammonium ion and then into urea is carried out by two groups of enzymes. Transaminases (aminotransferases) transfer α-amino groups to α-ketoglutarate to form glutamate, which is then oxidatively deaminated by glutamate dehydrogenase to release free ammonium ion that can be converted to urea.

244. The answer is e. (*Murray, pp 307–346. Scriver, pp 1909–1964. Sack, pp 121–138. Wilson, pp 287–317.*) In the liver, the urea cycle converts excess NH_4^+ to a form amenable to excretion by the kidneys. Free NH_4^+ condenses with CO_2 to form carbamoyl phosphate in a reaction catalyzed by carbamoyl phosphate synthetase. This is an energy-expensive, essentially irreversible reaction requiring two molecules of ATP. Carbamoyl phosphate (compound E in the urea cycle diagram) then combines with ornithine to produce citrulline in the first step of the urea cycle proper. The second nitrogen of urea is derived from the amino acid aspartate, which condenses with citrulline to form arginosuccinase in the second step of the cycle. This step is catalyzed by arginosuccinase synthetase and also requires a molecule of ATP.

245. The answer is c. *(Murray, pp 307–346. Scriver, pp 1909–1964. Sack, pp 121–138. Wilson, pp 287–317.)* In humans and other land mammals, excess NH_4^+ is converted into urea (compound C in the urea cycle diagram in question 244) in the liver for excretion by the kidneys. Malfunctions of the urea cycle can lead to hyperammonemia and result in brain damage. Urea is composed of two nitrogen groups and a carbonyl group. One nitrogen and the carbon are derived from free NH_4^+ and CO_2 condensed to form carbamoyl phosphate (compound E). The other nitrogen is derived from the amino group of aspartate.

246. The answer is c. *(Murray, pp 307–346. Scriver, pp 1909–1964. Sack, pp 121–138. Wilson, pp 287–317.)* The steps of the urea cycle are divided between the mitochondrial matrix and cytosol of liver cells in mammals. The formation of ammonia, its reaction with carbon dioxide to produce carbamoyl phosphate, and the conversion to citrulline occur in the matrix of mitochondria. Citrulline diffuses out of the mitochondria, and the next three steps of the cycle, which result in the formation of urea, all take place in the cytosol. Peroxisomes have single membranes, in contrast to the double membranes of mitochondria. They house catalase and enzymes for medium- to long-chain fatty acid oxidation.

247. The answer is e. *(Murray, pp 307–346. Scriver, pp 1909–1964. Sack, pp 121–138. Wilson, pp 287–317.)* Partial blockage of the urea cycle leads to conditions ranging from lethargy and episodic vomiting to mental retardation. A complete block is incompatible with life. A major reason for the toxicity is the severe depletion of ATP levels caused by the siphoning off of α-ketoglutarate from the citric acid cycle in an attempt to consume ammonia. Glutamate dehydrogenase and glutamine synthetase, respectively, catalyze the following reaction:

$$\alpha\text{-ketoglutarate} + NH_4^+ \rightarrow \text{glutamate} + NH_4^+ \rightarrow \text{glutamine}$$

As can be seen, this is the reverse order of steps whereby glutamine is successively deaminated first to glutamate and then to α-ketoglutarate by the enzymes glutaminase and glutamate dehydrogenase, respectively. It is thought that the high level of ammonia ions shifts the equilibrium of the dehydrogenase in favor of the formation of glutamate. Depending on the step in the urea cycle that is blocked, levels of arginine may be decreased.

248. The answer is b. (*Murray, pp 307–346. Scriver, pp 4029–4076. Sack, pp 121–138. Wilson, pp 287–317.*) Thyroxine is a derivative of tyrosine. It is formed by the iodination and joining of peptide-linked tyrosyl residues of thyroglobulin. Proteolysis of thyroglobulin yields thyroxine. Thyroxine is also called tetraiodothyronine, or T_4, because of the four iodine atoms of the thyroid hormone.

249. The answer is e. (*Murray, pp 307–346. Scriver, pp 1667–1724. Sack, pp 121–138. Wilson, pp 287–317.*) In humans, tyrosine can be formed by the hydroxylation of phenylalanine. This reaction is catalyzed by the enzyme phenylalanine hydroxylase. A deficiency of phenylalanine hydroxylase results in the disease called phenylketonuria [PKU(261600)]. In this disease it is usually the accumulation of phenylalanine and its metabolites rather than the lack of tyrosine that is the cause of the severe mental retardation ultimately seen. Once formed, tyrosine is the precursor of many important signal molecules. Catalyzed by tyrosine hydroxylase, tyrosine is hydroxylated to form L-dihydroxyphenylalanine (dopa), which in turn is decarboxylated to form dopamine in the presence of dopa decarboxylase. Then, norepinephrine and finally epinephrine are formed from dopamine. All of these are signal molecules to some degree. Dopa and inhibitors of dopa decarboxylase are used in the treatment of Parkinson's disease, a neurologic disorder. Norepinephrine is a transmitter at smooth-muscle junctions innervated by sympathetic nerve fibers. Epinephrine and dopamine are catecholamine transmitters synthesized in sympathetic nerve terminals and in the adrenal gland. Tyrosine is also the precursor of thyroxine, the major thyroid hormone, and melanin, a skin pigment.

250. The answer is b. (*Murray, pp 307–346. Scriver, pp 1667–1724. Sack, pp 121–138. Wilson, pp 287–317.*) Methionine is the only sulfur-containing amino acid of the group, and is a precursor for the sulfur-containing amino acid cysteine. Threonine has an aliphatic side chain with a hydroxyl group, glutamine and lysine have amino group side chains, and alanine has a methyl side chain. Homocysteine is a sulfur-containing amino acid that is not found in proteins, being an intermediate in the formation of cysteine from the sulfur-containing amino acid methionine. Homocysteine and methionine are also components of the activated methyl cycle in which S-adenosylmethionine is regenerated. S-adenosylmethionine is one of the major donors of methyl groups. Methionine is an essential amino acid and must be derived from the diet.

251. The answer is e. *(Murray, pp 307–346. Scriver, pp 1667–1724. Sack, pp 121–138. Wilson, pp 287–317.)* In the kidney double deamination of glutamine reaction, two ammonia molecules are produced for excretion. In the first step, glutamine is deaminated to glutamate in a monoxidative reaction catalyzed by glutaminase. Then, glutamate dehydrogenase oxidatively deaminates glutamate to α-ketoglutarate. Glutamate dehydrogenase can use either NAD^+, as shown, or $NADP^+$ in the reactions. This second reaction is also found in the liver, where α-amino groups originally transaminated from many amino acids are funneled to glutamate to free ammonium ion for ultimate conversion to urea.

252. The answer is e. *(Murray, pp 307–346. Scriver, pp 2007–2056. Sack, pp 121–138. Wilson, pp 287–317.)* In the synthesis of cysteine, the following sequence of steps occurs, where SAM is S-adenosylmethionine, CS is cystathionine synthase, cys is cysteine, and α-KG is α-ketoglutarate:

$$\text{methionine} \rightarrow \text{SAM} \rightarrow \text{homocysteine} + \text{adenosine}$$
$$\text{homocysteine} + \text{serine} \rightarrow \text{cystathionine} \rightarrow \text{cys} + \alpha\text{-KG} + NH_4^+$$
$$(CS, B_6)$$

Cystathionine synthetase, a pyridoxal phosphate (vitamin B_6) enzyme, catalyzes the condensation of serine and homocysteine to form cystathionine. A deficiency of this enzyme leads to a buildup of homocysteine, which oxidizes to form homocystine. This may result in mental retardation, but sometimes causes dislocated lenses and a tall, asthenic build reminiscent of Marfan's syndrome. Patients with homocystinuria also have a clotting diathesis, requiring care to avoid dehydration during anesthesia. Their cysteine deficiency must be made up from dietary sources. In some cases, dietary intake of vitamin B_6 (pyrixodal phosphate) may alleviate symptoms because of its requirement by the crucial enzymes.

253. The answer is g. *(Murray, pp 307–346. Scriver, pp 2079–2108. Sack, pp 121–138. Wilson, pp 287–317.)* In Hartnup disease, a defect in the transport process for neutral amino acids is most pronounced in intestinal and renal transport. Neutral aminoaciduria is observed as well as increased fecal excretion of indole derivations due to bacterial conversion of unabsorbed dietary tryptophan. Pellagra-like symptoms can be seen due to the lack of tryptophan for niacin biosynthesis. Hyperammonia can be caused by a variety of urea cycle defects including carbamoyl phosphate synthase I deficiency (237300). The high levels of NH_4^+ in the blood lead to very high levels of glutamine synthesis that may well be responsible for the subsequent brain damage. Deficiency of liver phenylalanine hydroxylase causes phenylketonuria [PKU(261600)]. Consequently, high levels of phenylalanine are not converted to tyrosine. Phenylalanine and its metabolites accumulate in blood, leading to mental retardation if infants are not placed on a phenylalanine-restricted diet. Urine darkens upon standing due to the high levels of homogentisate that result from of a deficiency in homogentisate oxidase in the disease alkaptonuria (203500). This is a deficiency in the pathway of tyrosine breakdown.

254. The answer is b. *(Murray, pp 307–346. Scriver, pp 2007–2056. Sack, pp 121–138. Wilson, pp 287–317.)* The antioxidant activity of glutathione is dependent upon maintenance of its reduced state. The enzyme glutathione reductase transfers electrons from NADPH via FAD to oxidized glutathione. Oxidized glutathione is composed of two glutathione molecules held together by a disulfide bridge. Reduced glutathione is a tripeptide with a free sulfhydryl group. It is the presence of the free sulfhydryl group that is of importance to the antioxidant activity of glutathione. In red blood cells, the function of cysteine residues of hemoglobin and other proteins is maintained by the reducing power of glutathione.

255. The answer is b. *(Murray, pp 307–346. Scriver, pp 1667–1724. Sack, pp 121–138. Wilson, pp 287–317.)* Two of the major hormones are derived from the amino acid tyrosine: the adrenal hormone epinephrine and the thyroid hormone thyroxine (tetraiodothyronine). Epinephrine is the catabolic antagonist of insulin, a polypeptide hormone, and is similar in action to glucagon, a liver-specific polypeptide hormone. Thyroxine is important in governing the basal metabolic rate.

256. The answer is a. *(Murray, pp 359–374. Scriver, pp 2961–3104. Sack, pp 121–138. Wilson, pp 287–317.)* Jaundice refers to the yellow color of the skin and eyes caused by increased levels of bilirubin in the blood. It has many causes, including increased production of bilirubin due to hemolytic anemia or malaria, blockage in the excretion of bilirubin due to liver damage, or obstruction of the bile duct. In newborns, jaundice is normal (physiologic) due to liver immaturity. Only excess jaundice is evaluated, based on the age of the infant. High levels of bilirubin in serum (indirect bilirubin) points toward hemolysis from maternofetal blood group incompatibility, while high levels of bilirubin diglucuronide (one of several conjugated bilirubins tested as direct bilirubin) suggest liver/gastrointestinal disease.

Reticuloendothelial cells degrade red blood cells following approximately 120 days in the circulation. The steps in the degradation of heme include (1) formation of the green pigment biliverdin by the cleavage of the porphyrin ring of heme; (2) formation of the red-orange pigment bilirubin by the reduction of biliverdin; (3) uptake of bilirubin by the liver and the formation of bilirubin diglucuronide; and (4) active excretion of bilirubin into bile and eventually into the stool. The change in color of a bruise from bluish-green to reddish-orange reflects the heme degradation and the change in color of the bile pigments biliverdin and bilirubin. Bilirubin, which is quite insoluble, is transported to the liver attached to albumin. In the liver, bilirubin is conjugated to two glucuronic acid molecules to form bilirubin diglucuronide. Bilirubin diglucuronide is transported against a concentration gradient into the bile. If bilirubin is not conjugated, it is not excreted.

257. The answer is d. *(Murray, pp 359–374. Scriver, pp 2961–3104. Sack, pp 121–138. Wilson, pp 287–317.)* Once bile is excreted into the gut, bilirubin diglucuronide is hydrolyzed and reduced by bacteria to form urobilinogen, which is colorless. Much of the urobilinogen of the stools is further oxidized by intestinal bacteria to stercobilin, which gives stools their characteristic brown color. Some urobilinogen is reabsorbed by the gut into the portal blood, transported to the kidney, and converted and excreted as urobilin, which gives urine its characteristic yellow color.

258. The answer is b. *(Murray, pp 258–297. Scriver, pp 2705–2716. Sack, pp 121–138. Wilson, pp 362–367.)* Chylomicrons are triglyceride-rich transport particles containing dietary lipids. Very-low-density lipoproteins (VLDLs) are triglyceride- and cholesterol-containing particles from the liver that contain endogenously packaged lipids. Delipidation of triglycerides from VLDLs leads to formation of intermediate forms (IDLs), and finally to a cholesterol-enriched small particle, the low-density lipoprotein (LDL). Thus, VLDL → IDL → LDL. The following table summarizes the characteristics of these plasma lipoproteins.

Type	Average Density (g/cm³)	% Triglyceride	% Cholesterol (and Esters)
Chylomicrons	0.92	85	7
VLDLs	0.97	55	20
IDLs	——————Intermediate——————		
LDLs	1.03	10	45

259. The answer is b. *(Murray, pp 230–267. Scriver, pp 2297–2326. Sack, pp 121–138. Wilson, pp 287–320.)* Untreated ethylene glycol of antifreeze can be converted to the kidney toxin oxalate crystals. This occurs by oxidation of ethylene glycol. The first committed step in this process is the oxidation of ethylene glycol to an aldehyde by alcohol dehydrogenase. This is normally the route for converting ethanol (drinking alcohol) to acetate. Patients who have ingested ethylene glycol or wood alcohol (methanol) are placed on a nearly intoxicating dose of ethanol by a nasogastric tube together with intravenous saline and sodium bicarbonate. This treatment is carried out intermittently along with hemodialysis until no traces of ethylene glycol are seen in the blood. Ethanol acts as a competitive inhibitor of alcohol dehydrogenase with respect to ethylene glycol or methanol metabolism.

260. The answer is b. *(Murray, pp 230–267. Scriver, pp 2297–2326. Sack, pp 121–138. Wilson, pp 287–320.)* The most common sphingolipid in mammals is sphingomyelin. Ceramide, the basic structure from which all sphingolipids are derived, is composed of the 18-carbon sphingosine connected via its

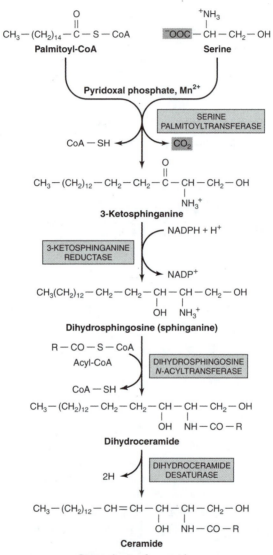

Biosynthesis of ceramide.

(Reproduced, with permission, from Murray RK, Granner DK, Mayes PA, Rodwell VW: Harper's Biochemistry, 25/e. New York, McGraw-Hill, 2000: 264.)

amino group to a fatty acid by an amide linkage. The fatty acid is usually long-chain (18 to 26 carbons) and is saturated or monosaturated. Except for the lack of the glycerol backbone, sphingolipids are quite similar in structure and physical properties to the phospholipids phosphatidyl choline and phosphatidyl ethanolamine. Either phosphoryl choline or phosphoryl ethanolamine is the head group attached to ceramide. If a neutral sugar residue is the polar head group attached to ceramide, a cerebroside is formed. If oligosaccharide head groups containing sialic acid are used, gangliosides are formed. All sphingolipids are important membrane constituents.

261. The answer is d. (*Murray, pp 258–297. Scriver, pp 2705–2716. Sack, pp 121–138. Wilson, pp 362–367.*) Regulation of cholesterol metabolism is by definition exerted at the "committed" and rate-controlling step. This is the reaction catalyzed by 3-hydroxy-3-methylglutaryl CoA reductase. Reductase activity is reduced by fasting and by cholesterol feeding and thus provides effective feedback control of cholesterol metabolism. The statin class of drugs act at this site.

262. The answer is a. (*Murray, pp 230–267. Scriver, pp 2297–2326. Sack, pp 121–138. Wilson, pp 287–320.*) Multiple sclerosis is a demyelination disease characterized by chronic inflammation. The primary losses are of the phospholipids and sphingolipids composing myelin membrane sheets of nerves in white matter. Consequently, brain white matter eventually looks like gray matter. High levels of sphingolipids and phospholipids are observed in the cerebrospinal fluid.

263. The answer is e. (*Murray, pp 230–267. Scriver, pp 2297–2326. Sack, pp 121–138. Wilson, pp 287–320.*) Sphingolipidoses are lipid storage diseases that exhibit Mendelian (autosomal or X-linked recessive) inheritance. To date, all lipidoses studied demonstrate accumulation of a ceramide-containing sphingolipid due to the genetic deficiency of a specific hydrolytic enzyme involved in the breakdown of the sphingolipid in question. This leads to the accumulation of the sphingolipid because its synthetic rate is normal. Since the decrease in activity of the abnormal hydrolytic enzyme is similar in all tissues, diagnostic tests measuring the enzyme can easily be set up using skin biopsies or blood cell measurements. Heterozygous carriers can be screened and receive genetic counseling. Examples of sphingolipidoses include Tay-Sachs disease (272800), Sandhoff's disease (268800), and Gaucher's disease (230800).

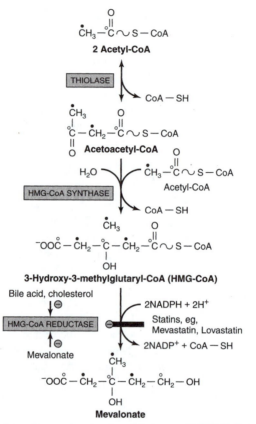

Biosynthesis of mevalonate, showing the critical step of HMG-CoA reductase that is inhibited by statins. The open and solid circles indicate the fates of carbons in acetyl CoA.

(Reproduced, with permission, from Murray RK, Granner DK, Mayes PA, Rodwell VW: Harper's Biochemistry, 25/e. New York, McGraw-Hill, 2000: 286.)

264. The answer is d. (Murray, pp 230–267. Scriver, pp 2297–2326. Sack, pp 121–138. Wilson, pp 287–320.) In humans, the end product of fatty acid synthesis in the cytosol is palmitic acid. The specificity of cytosolic multienzyme, single-protein fatty acid synthetase is such that once the C16 chain length is reached, a thioesterase clips off the fatty acid. Elongation as well as desaturation of de novo palmitate and fatty acids obtained from the diet occur by the action of enzymes in the membranes of the endoplasmic reticulum.

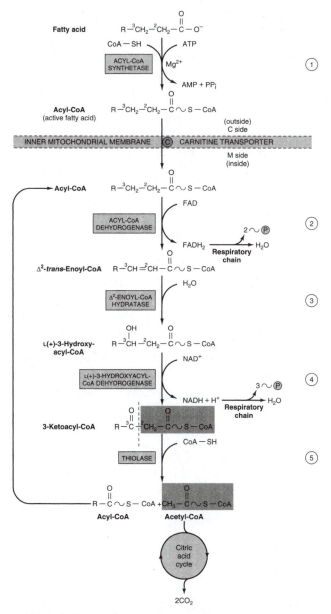

β oxidation of fatty acids. Long-chain acyl CoA is cycled through reactions 2 through 5, and one acetyl CoA moiety is removed with each cycle.

(Reproduced, with permission, from Murray RK, Granner DK, Mayes PA, Rodwell VW: Harper's Biochemistry, 25/e. New York, McGraw-Hill, 2000: 241.)

265. The answer is d. *(Murray, pp 258–297. Scriver, pp 2705–2716. Sack, pp 121–138. Wilson, pp 362–367.)* Infants placed on chronic low-fat formula diets often develop skin problems, impaired lipid transport, and eventually poor growth. This can be overcome by including linoleic acid to make up 1 to 2% of the total caloric requirement. Essential fatty acids are required because humans have only Δ^4, Δ^5, Δ^6, and Δ^9 fatty acid desaturase. Only plants have desaturase greater than Δ^9. Consequently, certain fatty acids such as arachidonic acid cannot be made "from scratch" (de novo) in humans and other mammals. However, linoleic acid, which plants make, can be converted to arachidonic acid. Arachidonate and eicosapentaenoate are 20-carbon prostanoic acids that are the starting point of the synthesis of prostaglandins, thromboxanes, and leukotrienes.

266. The answer is e. *(Murray, pp 230–267. Scriver, pp 2297–2326. Sack, pp 121–138. Wilson, pp 287–320.)* The fatty acid synthase complex of mammals is composed of two identical subunits. Each of the subunits is a multienzyme complex of seven enzymes and the acyl carrier protein component. All the components are covalently linked together; thus, all the components are on a single polypeptide chain, which functions in the presence of another identical polypeptide chain. Each cycle of fatty acid synthesis employs the acyl carrier protein and six enzymes: acetyl transferase, malonyl transferase, β-ketoacyl synthase, β-ketoacyl reductase, dehydratase, and enoyl reductase. When the final fatty acid length is reached (usually C16), thioesterase hydrolyzes the fatty acid off of the synthase complex.

267. The answer is e. *(Murray, pp 258–297. Scriver, pp 2705–2716. Sack, pp 121–138. Wilson, pp 362–367.)* In normal persons, plasma cholesterol levels average about 175 mg/dL. The level is about 300 mg/dL in heterozygotes with the autosomal dominant genotype and about 680 mg/dL in homozygotes. The single mutagenic defect results in a functional loss of low-density lipoprotein (LDL) receptors on the plasma membranes of cells other than those of the liver. This prevents the normal clearing of LDLs from the blood plasma by endocytosis.

268. The answer is c. *(Murray, pp 230–267. Scriver, pp 2297–2326. Sack, pp 121–138. Wilson, pp 287–320.)* Ceramide is the basic unit composing all sphingolipids, which include sphingomyelin and gangliosides. Sphingomyelin, which usually contains phosphocholine as a polar head group, is the only phospholipid that does not have a glycerol backbone. In contrast, gangliosides have complex oligosaccharide head groups.

269. The answer is d. *(Murray, pp 258–297. Scriver, pp 2705–2716. Sack, pp 121–138. Wilson, pp 362–367.)* The shell of apoproteins coating blood transport lipoproteins is important in the physiologic function of the lipoproteins. Some of the apoproteins contain signals that target the movement of the lipoproteins in and out of specific tissues. B48 and E seem to be important in targeting chylomicron remnants to be taken up by liver. B100 is synthesized as the coat protein of VLDLs and marks their end product, LDLs, for uptake by peripheral tissues. Other apoproteins are important for the solubilization and movement of lipids and cholesterol in and out of the particles. C-II is a lipoprotein lipase activator that VLDLs and chylomicrons receive from HDLs. The A apoproteins are found in HDLs and are involved in lecithin–cholesterol acyl transferase (LCAT) regulation.

270. The answer is b. *(Murray, pp 230–267. Scriver, pp 2297–2326. Sack, pp 121–138. Wilson, pp 287–320.)* In the postabsorptional (postprandial) state, plasma contains all the lipoproteins: chylomicrons derived from dietary lipids packaged in the intestinal epithelial cells and their remnants; very-low-density lipoproteins (VLDLs), which contain endogenous lipids and cholesterol packaged in the liver; low-density lipoproteins (LDLs), which are end products of delipidation of VLDLs; and high-density lipoprotins (HDLs), which are synthesized in the liver. HDLs are in part catalytic, since transfer of their CII apolipoprotein to VLDLs or chylomicrons activates lipoprotein lipase. In normal patients, only LDLs and HDLs remain in plasma following a 12-h fast, since both chylomicrons and VLDLs have been delipidated. Most of the cholesterol measured in blood plasma at this time is present in the cholesterol-rich LDLs. However, HDL cholesterol also contributes to the measurement.

271. The answer is d. *(Murray, pp 230–267. Scriver, pp 2297–2326. Sack, pp 121–138. Wilson, pp 287–320.)* Fatty acids must be activated before being oxidized. In this process, they are linked to CoA in a reaction catalyzed by thiokinase (also known as acyl CoA synthetase). ATP is hydrolyzed to AMP plus pyrophosphate in this reaction. In contrast, the enzyme thiolase cleaves off acetyl CoA units from β-ketoacyl CoA, while it forms thioesters during β oxidation.

272. The answer is c. *(Murray, pp 230–267. Scriver, pp 3421–3452. Sack, pp 121–138. Wilson, pp 287–320).* The two major groups of lysosomal storage disease are sphingolipidoses and mucopolysaccharidoses. An absence of α-L-iduronidase, as in Hurler's syndrome (252800) and Scheie's syndrome (252800), leads to accumulations of dermatan sulfate and heparan sulfate. Scheie's syndrome is less severe, with corneal clouding, joint degeneration, and increased heart disease. Hurler's syndrome has the same symptoms plus mental and physical retardation leading to early death. The later onset in this child is compatible with a diagnosis of Scheie's syndrome. Note that Hurler's and Scheie's syndromes result from mutations at the same locus—hence their identical McKusick numbers. The reasons for the differences in disease severity are unknown. All of the other enzyme deficiencies listed lead to the lack of proper breakdown of sphingolipids and their accumulation as gangliosides, glucocerebrosides, and sphingomyelins. Symptoms of lipidoses may include organ enlargement, mental retardation, and early death.

273. The answer is a. *(Murray, pp 230–267. Scriver, pp 3827–3876. Sack, pp 121–138. Wilson, pp 287–320.)* Gangliosides are continually synthesized and broken down. The specific hydrolases that degrade gangliosides by sequentially removing terminal sugars are found in lysosomes. In the lipid storage disease known as Tay-Sachs disease (272800), ganglioside GM_2 accumulates because of a deficiency of β-N-acetylhexosaminidase, a lysosomal enzyme that removes the terminal N-acetylgalactosamine residue. Homozygotes produce virtually no functional enzyme and suffer weakness, retardation, and blindness. Death usually occurs before infants are 3 years old. Carriers (heterozygotes) of the autosomal recessive disease produce approximately 50% of the normal levels of enzyme but show no ill effects. In high-risk populations, such as Ashkenazi Jews, screening for carrier status may be performed.

274. The answer is a. *(Murray, pp 230–267. Scriver, pp 2297–2326. Sack, pp 121–138. Wilson, pp 287–320.)* The sources of NADPH for synthesis of fatty acids are the pentose phosphate pathway and cytosolic malate formed during the transfer of acetyl groups to the cytosol as citrate. The enzyme citrate lyase splits citrate into acetyl CoA and oxaloacetate. The oxaloacetate is reduced to malate by NADH. NADP-linked malate enzyme catalyzes the oxidative decarboxylation of malate to pyruvate and carbon dioxide. Thus, the diffusion of excess citrate from the mitochondria to the cytoplasm of cells not only provides acetyl CoA for synthesis of fatty acids but NADPH as well. One NADPH is produced for each acetyl CoA produced. However, most of the NADPHs needed for synthesis of fatty acids are derived from the pentose phosphate pathway. For this reason, adipose tissue has an extremely active pentose phosphate pathway.

275. The answer is c. (*Murray, pp 230–267. Scriver, pp 2297–2326. Sack, pp 121–138. Wilson, pp 287–320.*) During oxidation of fatty acids in the mitochondrial matrix, fatty acids are processed while being attached to the phosphopantetheine group of coenzyme A (CoA). Acyl carrier protein (ACP) is only involved as part of the fatty acid synthase multienzyme complex in the cytosol. The phosphopantetheine group of ACP binds malonic acid, releasing the CoA group of malonyl CoA. It then condenses malonic acid with an acetyl group derived from acetyl CoA in the first round of synthesis. In subsequent rounds, the growing acyl chain is condensed with malonyl CoA.

276. The answer is c. (*Murray, pp 230–267. Scriver, pp 2297–2326. Sack, pp 121–138. Wilson, pp 287–320.*) During lipolysis, triglycerides are split into three free fatty acids and glycerol. The free fatty acids, as well as the free glycerol, diffuse into the bloodstream, where they are circulated throughout the body. The free fatty acids are used as an energy source for many tissues, primarily muscle. The free glycerol that is released cannot be phosphorylated back to glycerol-3-phosphate in the adipose tissue because it lacks glycerol kinase. However, the free glycerol released in lipolysis is taken up by the liver, where it can be phosphorylated to glycerol-3-phosphate. The phosphorylated glycerol can enter glycolysis or gluconeogensesis at the level of triose phosphates. If gluconeogenesis occurs, for every 2 mol of glycerol-3-phosphate, 1 mol of glucose can be synthesized.

277. The answer is e. (*Murray, pp 230–267. Scriver, pp 2297–2326. Sack, pp 121–138. Wilson, pp 287–320.*) In mammals, a variety of fatty acids are considered essential and cannot be synthesized. These include linoleate (C-18 *cis*-Δ^9, Δ^{12}) and linolenate (C-18 *cis*-Δ^9, Δ^{12}, Δ^{15}). Either these fatty acids or fatty acids for which they are precursors must be supplied in the diet as starting points for synthesis of a variety of other unsaturated fatty acids that lead to the synthesis of prostaglandins, thromboxanes, and leukotrienes. For example, arachidonate, a 20-carbon fatty acid with four double bonds, is derived from linolenate. Arachidonate gives rise to some prostaglandins, thromboxanes, and leukotrienes. Some fatty acids must be obtained in the diet because of the limitations governing enzymes of fatty acid synthesis in humans; that is, double bonds cannot be introduced beyond the 9–10 bond position of carbons in the fatty acid chain, and subsequent double bonds after the first must be separated by two single bonds. Thus, linolenate and linoleate cannot be synthesized in humans.

278. The answer is b. (*Murray, pp 230–267. Scriver, pp 2297–2326. Sack, pp 121–138. Wilson, pp 287–320.*) Diacylglycerol-3-phosphate, more commonly known as phosphatidate, is an intermediate common to the synthesis of both triacylglycerol and phospholipids. In a two-step process, glycerol phosphate is successively acylated by two acyl CoAs to lysophosphatidate, which contains a fatty acid group in the 1′ position, and then phosphatidate, which contains fatty acid groups in the 1′ and 2′ positions with a phosphate group in the 3′ position. From that point, pathways for synthesis of phospholipids and triacylglycerol diverge. If storage lipid is to be produced, phosphatidate is dephosphorylated by a phosphatase and then acylated by acyl CoA to form triacylglycerol. In contrast, if phospholipids are to be produced, phosphatidate is activated by CTP in a reaction that produces CDP-diacylglycerol and pyrophosphate. Phosphatidylserine, phosphatidylinositol, phosphatidylethanolamine, and phosphatidylcholine can all be derived from CDP-diacylglycerol.

279. The answer is d. (*Murray, pp 230–267. Scriver, pp 2297–2326. Sack, pp 121–138. Wilson, pp 287–320.*) Two major enzyme complexes are involved in the synthesis of fatty acids. The first is acetyl CoA carboxylase, which synthesizes malonyl CoA by the steps shown below for the synthesis of palmitate:

$$7 \text{ acetyl CoA} + 7 \text{ HCO}_3^- + 7 \text{ ATP} \rightarrow 7 \text{ malonyl CoA} + 7 \text{ ADP} + 7 \text{ P}_i$$

Using the malonyl CoA, palmitate is then synthesized by seven cycles of the fatty acid synthetase complex, whose stoichiometry is summarized below:

$$\text{acetyl CoA} + 7 \text{ malonyl CoA} + 14 \text{ NADPH} \rightarrow$$
$$\text{palmitate} + 7 \text{ CO}_2 + 14 \text{ NAD}^+ + 8 \text{ CoA} + 6 \text{ H}_2\text{O}$$

As can be seen from the equations above, the necessary amount of malonyl CoA is synthesized. Palmitate is subsequently synthesized from malonyl CoA and one initial acetyl CoA. Thus, acetyl CoA, NADPH, ATP, and HCO_3^- are all necessary in this process. In contrast, $FADH_2$ is not utilized in fatty acid synthesis, but is one of the products of fatty acid oxidation. Vitamin B_{12} is required for conversion of propionic acid to methylmalonic acid, a step in the β oxidation of odd-numbered fatty acid chains.

280. The answer is b. (*Murray, pp 230–267. Scriver, pp 2297–2326. Sack, pp 121–138. Wilson, pp 287–320.*) The fluid mosaic model of membrane structure shown in the question describes plasma membranes as a mosaic of globular proteins in a phospholipid bilayer. The lipids as well as the proteins are in a fluid and dynamic state capable of translational (side-to-side) movement, but not "flip-flop"-type movements. Hence, both the phospholipid and protein components are amphipathic, with a highly polar end in contact with the aqueous phase and hydrophobic residues buried within the membrane. Integral proteins may be embedded in the membrane or exposed on only one side, or they may extend completely through the membrane with different portions of the proteins exposed to opposite sides of the membrane. In contrast to the fluid mosaic model, the models of protein-coated bimolecular layer of lipid diagrammed in A and the unit membrane "railroad track" shown in D (which is based on osmium tetroxide fixed membranes) suggest that membranes are simply bimolecular layers of lipid coated with protein that does not penetrate the lipid. A simple bimolecular layer of lipid is shown in C, and a micelle of lipids is diagrammatically illustrated in E.

281. The answer is e. (*Murray, pp 230–267. Scriver, pp 2297–2326. Sack, pp 121–138. Wilson, pp 287–320.*) The process of emulsification of hydrophobic fat globules by the detergent action of phospholipids and bile acids in the gut breaks the globules down to mixed micelles. The formation of small micelles from large fat globules greatly increases the surface area available for the action of hydrolytic lipases in the gut. Mixed micelle formation is dependent upon the amphipathic properties of bile acids and phospholipids that allow them to act as detergents. Simply put, the hydrophobic moieties (fatty acid chains) of phospholipids are inserted into the hydrophobic fat globules and the hydrophilic polar head groups interact with and face the water, in essence forming a monomolecular layer around the fat (triacylglycerides). This successful strategy of mixed micelles is used to solve many potential problems, including the transport of blood lipoproteins.

282. The answer is b. (*Murray, pp 258–297. Scriver, pp 2705–2716. Sack, pp 121–138. Wilson, pp 362–367.*) Mevastatin, an analogue of mevalonic acid, acts as a feedback inhibitor of 3′-hydroxy-3′-methylglutaryl CoA (HMG-CoA) reductase, the regulated enzyme of cholesterol synthesis. Effective treatment with mevastatin, along with a low-fat diet, decreases levels of blood cholesterol. The lowering of cholesterol also lowers the amounts of the lipoprotein that transports cholesterol to the peripheral tissues, low-density lipoprotein (LDL). Since lipids like cholesterol and triglycerides are insoluble in water, they must be associated with lipoproteins for transport and salvage between their major site of synthesis (liver) and the peripheral tissues. Those lipoproteins associated with more insoluble lipids thus have lower density during centrifugation (see the table in answer 258), a technique that separates the lowest-density chylomicrons from very-low-density lipoproteins (VLDLs with pre-β lipoproteins), low-density lipoproteins (LDLs with β-lipoproteins), intermediate-density lipoproteins (IDLs), and high-density lipoproteins (HDLs with α-lipoproteins). Each type of lipoprotein has typical apolipoproteins such as the apo B100 and apo B48 (translated from the same messenger RNA) in LDL. LDL is involved in transporting cholesterol from the liver to peripheral tissues, while HDL is a scavenger of cholesterol. The ratio of HDL to LDL is thus a predictor of cholesterol deposition in blood vessels, the cause of myocardial infarctions (heart attacks). The higher the HDL/LDL ratio, the lower the rate of heart attacks.

283. The answer is c. (*Murray, pp 230–267. Scriver, pp 2297–2326. Sack, pp 121–138. Wilson, pp 287–320.*) Fatty acid synthesis in the cytosol terminates at palmitate, a C16 saturated fatty acid. Elongation of acyl groups can occur from palmitate as well as from other dietary saturated and unsaturated fatty acids of lengths C10 and greater. Longer-chain elongation of fatty acids occurs in the endoplasmic reticulum (structure C) using malonyl CoA as the acetyl donor and NADPH as the reductant. Very-long-chain and long-chain fatty acids are preferentially catabolized in peroxisomes (structure J). Other structures diagrammed in the figure are the plasma membrane (A), mitochondrion (B), nucleoplasm (D), nucleolus (E), Golgi apparatus (F), secretory vesicles (G), caveolae such as those taking up low-density lipoprotein from its receptor (H), and lysosomes (I).

284. The answer is b. *(Murray, pp 230–267. Scriver, pp 2297–2326. Sack, pp 121–138. Wilson, pp 287–320.)* The ketone bodies, β-hydroxybutyrate and acetoacetate, are synthesized in liver mitochondria from acetyl CoA. The liver produces ketone bodies under conditions of fasting associated with high rates of fatty acid oxidation. Higher amounts of β-hydroxybutyrate than acetoacetate are produced, since high liver levels of NADH lead to the dehydrogenation of acetoacetate.

285. The answer is a. *(Murray, pp 230–267. Scriver, pp 2297–2326. Sack, pp 121–138. Wilson, pp 287–320.)* Plasma membranes are unique as compared to intracellular membranes in that their composition contains cholesterol, glycoproteins, and glycolipids known as gangliosides. Plasma membranes of the cells of different tissues are distinguished from each other due to the properties that make them unique. Hormone receptors allow each cell type to respond to systemic stimulation appropriately. All chronic hormone receptors are localized to plasma membranes and upon stimulation release a second messenger into the interior of the cell. Glucagon, like epinephrine and norepinephrine, stimulates adenylate cyclase to produce cyclic AMP. Glucagon is found on the plasma membranes of liver and adipose tissue cells.

286. The answer is a. *(Murray, pp 258–297. Scriver, pp 2705–2716. Sack, pp 121–138. Wilson, pp 362–367.)* Patients with type I lipoprotein lipase deficiency are not able to rapidly delipidate chylomicrons, which carry dietary triacylglycerides, or VLDLs, which carry lipids packaged by the liver. The electrophoretic pattern (left lane in the figure) after fasting is thus similar to that of a normal patient after a meal—the chylomicrons (band A), LDLs with β-lipoproteins (band B), VLDLs with pre-β-lipoproteins (band C), and HDLs with α-lipoproteins (band D) are all present because chylomicrons and VLDLs are not degraded normally. Hepatic lipase, ordinarily released by the liver to deal with chylomicron remnant and HDL metabolism, must slowly deal with the lipemia (lipoprotein buildup in blood) caused by the lack of lipoprotein lipase. In addition to the lipemia, steatorrhea (fatty stools) and stomach cramps are symptoms of lipoprotein lipase deficiency. A well-controlled low-fat diet is part of the therapy. In contrast, the electrophoretic pattern of patients with type IIa familial hypercholesterolemia [143890 (right lane)] can appear, at first glance, to be normal, since only the LDL and HDL bands are expected following an overnight fast. However, closer inspection reveals an abnormally high accumulation of LDLs (band G), which cause the hypercholesterolemia. Since LDLs are a final stage in the catabolism of VLDLs, the high load of cholesterol being transported from the liver may cause some VLDLs to be present after fasting (band H) along with HDL scavenger lipoproteins (band I). In patients heterozygous for the disease, approximately one-half the normal amount of B100 LDL receptors are present. In homozygous patients, no B100 LDL receptors are present and most (~70%) of the LDL must be cleared by the liver. In such patients, blood cholesterol levels are extraordinarily high and lead to profound early atherosclerosis and death.

287. The answer is b. (*Murray, pp 258–297. Scriver, pp 2705–2716. Sack, pp 121–138. Wilson, pp 362–367.*) The uptake of exogenous cholesterol by cells results in a marked suppression of endogenous cholesterol synthesis. Low-density human lipoprotein not only contains the greatest ratio of bound cholesterol to protein but also has the greatest potency in suppressing endogenous cholesterogenesis. LDLs normally suppress cholesterol synthesis by binding to a specific membrane receptor that mediates inhibition of hydroxymethylglutaryl (HMG) coenzyme A reductase. In familial hypercholesterolemia (143890), the LDL receptor is dysfunctional, with the result that cholesterol synthesis is less responsive to plasma cholesterol levels. Suppression of HMG CoA reductase is attained using inhibitors (statins) that mimic the structure of mevalonic acid, the natural feedback inhibitor of the enzyme.

288. The answer is d. (*Murray, pp 258–297. Scriver, pp 2705–2716. Sack, pp 121–138. Wilson, pp 362–367.*) The synthesis of 3-hydroxy-3-methylglutaryl CoA requires the condensation of three acetyl CoA groups. The two enzymatic steps involved are the first two steps of cholesterol synthesis and ketone body synthesis. While cholesterol synthesis occurs in the cytosol of most mammalian tissues, ketone body synthesis can only occur in the mitochondria of liver cells. Not only are cholesterol synthesis and ketone body synthesis separated by compartmentalization, they are separated by metabolic needs. Cholesterol synthesis is an anabolic pathway that takes place when acetyl CoA production from excess dietary precursors is possible. In contrast, ketone body production by the liver occurs when acetyl CoA levels from β oxidation are high. This catabolic situation exists during fasting, starvation, and uncontrolled diabetes.

289. The answer is a. *(Murray, pp 258–297. Scriver, pp 2705–2716. Sack, pp 121–138. Wilson, pp 362–367.)* Under conditions of active synthesis of fatty acids in the cytosol of hepatocytes, levels of malonyl CoA are high. Malonyl CoA is the activated source of two carbon units for fatty acid synthesis. Malonyl CoA inhibits carnitine acyltransferase I, which is located on the cytosolic face of the inner mitochondrial membrane. Thus, long-chain fatty acyl CoA units cannot be transported into mitochondria where β oxidation occurs, and translocation from cytosol to mitochondrial matrix is prevented. In this situation compartmentalization of membranes as well as inhibition of enzymes comes into play.

290. The answer is e. *(Murray, pp 375–401. Scriver, pp 2663–2704. Sack, pp 121–138. Wilson, pp 287–320.)* Orotic aciduria is the buildup of orotic acid due to a deficiency in one or both of the enzymes that convert it to UMP. Either orotate phosphoribosyltransferase and orotidylate decarboxylase are both defective, or the decarboxylase alone is defective. UMP is the precursor of UTP, CTP, and TMP. All of these end products normally act in some way to feedback-inhibit the initial reactions of pyrimidine synthesis. Specifically, the lack of CTP inhibition allows aspartate transcarbamoylase to remain highly active and ultimately results in a buildup of orotic acid and the resultant orotic aciduria. The lack of CTP, TMP, and UTP leads to a decreased erythrocyte formation and megaloblastic anemia. Uridine treatment is effective because uridine can easily be converted to UMP by omnipresent tissue kinases, thus allowing UTP, CTP, and TMP to be synthesized and feedback-inhibit further orotic acid production.

291. The answer is a. (*Murray, pp 375–401. Scriver, pp 2513–2570. Sack, pp 121–138. Wilson, pp 287–320.*) Most forms of gout are probably X-linked recessive with deficiencies in phosphoribosyl pyrophosphate (PRPP) synthase, the first step of purine synthesis. Some patients may have a partial deficiency of hypoxanthine-guanine phosphoribosyl transferase (HGPRTase), which salvages hypoxanthine and guanine by transferring the purine ribonucleotide of PRPP to the bases and forming iosinate and guanylate, respectively. In all of these patients, the hypoxanthine analogue allopurinol has two actions: (1) it inhibits xanthine oxidase, which catalyzes the oxidation of hypoxanthine to xanthine and then to uric acid stones and tissue deposits; and (2) it forms an inactive allopurinol ribonucleotide from PRPP in a reaction catalyzed by HGPRTase, thereby decreasing the rate of purine synthesis. In contrast, because of the total loss of HGPRTase activity in Lesch-Nyhan patients, the allopurinol ribonucleotide cannot be formed. Thus, PRPP levels are not decreased and de novo purine synthesis continues unabated. The gouty arthritis caused by urate crystal formation is relieved in Lesch-Nyhan patients, but their neurological symptoms are not.

292. The answer is d. (*Murray, pp 375–401. Scriver, pp 2513–2570. Sack, pp 121–138. Wilson, pp 287–320.*) Carbamoyl phosphate (CAP) synthase I is found in mitochondrial matrix and is the first step in urea synthesis, condensing CO_2 and NH_4^+. Hyperammonemia occurs when CAP is deficient. CAP synthase II forms CAP as the first step in pyrimidine synthesis. Its complete deficiency would probably be a lethal mutation. When its activity is decreased, purine catabolism to uric acid is decreased, decreasing the possibility of hyperuricemia. In contrast, gout, Lesch-Nyhan syndrome, high xanthine oxidase activity, and von Gierke's disease [glycogen storage disease type Ia (232200)] all lead to increased urate production and excretion.

293. The answer is a. (*Murray, pp 375–401. Scriver, pp 2513–2570. Sack, pp 121–138. Wilson, pp 287–320.*) During purine ring biosynthesis, the amino acid glycine is completely incorporated to provide C4, C5, and N7. Glutamine contributes N3 and N9, aspartate provides N1, and derivatives of tetrahydrofolate furnish C2 and C8. Carbon dioxide is the source of C6. In pyrimidine ring synthesis, C2 and N3 are derived from carbamoyl phosphate, while N1, C4, C5, and C6 come from aspartate.

Ribose 5-phosphate + ATP

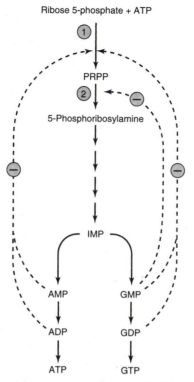

a. Control of the rate of de novo purine synthesis. Solid lines represent metabolite flow and dashed lines feedback inhibition (⊖) by end products of the pathway. *(Reproduced, with permission, from Murray RK, Granner DK, Mayes PA, Rodwell VW: Harper's Biochemistry, 25/e. New York, McGraw-Hill, 2000: 391.)* *(See following page for panel b.)*

294. The answer is d. *(Murray, pp 375–401. Scriver, pp 2513–2570. Sack, pp 121–138. Wilson, pp 287–320.)* Xanthine oxidase catalyzes the last two steps in the degradation of purines. Hypoxanthine is oxidized to xanthine, and xanthine is further oxidized to uric acid. Thus, xanthine is both product and substrate in this two-step reaction. In humans, uric acid is excreted via the urine. Allopurinol, an analogue of xanthine, is used in gout to block uric acid production and deposition of uric acid crystals in the kidneys and joints. It acts as a suicide inhibitor of xanthine oxidase after it is converted to alloxanthine. Guanine can also be a precursor of xanthine.

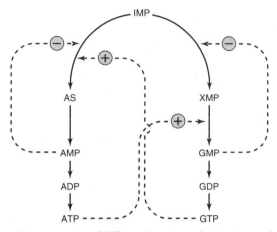

b. Regulation of the conversion of IMP to adenosine and guanosine nucleotides. Solid lines represent metabolite flow and dashed lines represent positive ($\oplus$) or negative ($\ominus$) feedback inhibition.

(Reproduced, with permission, from Murray RK, Granner DK, Mayes PA, Rodwell VW: Harper's Biochemistry, 25/e. New York, McGraw-Hill, 2000: 391.)

295. The answer is c. *(Murray, pp 375–401. Scriver, pp 2513–2570. Sack, pp 121–138. Wilson, pp 287–320.)* The steps of pyrimidine nucleotide biosynthesis are summarized in the figure below. The first step in pyrimidine synthesis is the formation of carbamoyl phosphate. The enzyme catalyzing this step, carbamoyl phosphate synthetase (1), is feedback-inhibited by UMP through allosteric effects on enzyme structure (not by competitive inhibition with its substrates). The enzyme of the second step, aspartate transcarbamoylase, is composed of catalytic and regulatory subunits. The regulatory subunit binds CTP or ATP. TTP has no role in the feedback inhibition of pyrimidine synthesis. Decreased rather than increased activity of enzymes 1 and 2 would be produced by allosteric feedback inhibition.

$$\text{Glutamine} + CO_2 + ATP \overset{1}{-\!\!\!-\!\!\!\longrightarrow} \text{Carbamoyl phosphate}$$
$$\Big|$$
$$2 \leftarrow \text{Aspartate}$$
$$\downarrow$$
$$\text{CTP} \leftarrow 5\!-\!\text{UTP} \leftarrow 4\!-\!\text{UMP} \leftarrow 3\!-\!\text{Carbamoyl aspartate}$$

296. The answer is c. *(Murray, pp 375–401. Scriver, pp 2513–2570. Sack, pp 121–138. Wilson, pp 287–320.)* Several control sites exist in the path of purine synthesis where feedback inhibition occurs. AMP, GMP, or IMP may inhibit the first step of the pathway, which is the synthesis of 5-phosphoribosyl-1-pyrophosphate (PRPP). PRPP synthetase is specifically inhibited. All three nucleotides can inhibit glutamine PRPP aminotransferase, which catalyzes the second step of the pathway. AMP blocks the conversion of IMP to adenylosuccinate. GMP inhibits the formation of xanthylate from IMP. Thus, blockage rather than enhancement of IMP metabolism to AMP and GMP effectively inhibits purine biosynthesis.

297. The answer is b. *(Murray, pp 375–401. Scriver, pp 2513–2570. Sack, pp 121–138. Wilson, pp 287–320.)* The nitrogenous bases are aromatic compounds. The pyrimidines—uracil, thymine, and cytosine—contain one heterocyclic ring each. The purines—adenine and guanine—are derivatives of pyrimidines and consist of a pyrimidine ring joined with an imidazole ring. All the bases except for uracil are found in DNA; uracil replaces thymine in RNA. The ribose monophosphate form of uracil (UMP) serves as a precursor for cytidine triphosphate (UMP → UDP → UTP → CTP). In these series of reactions, the uracil moiety is aminated with an amine contributed by glutamine, to form cytosine. UMP also gives rise to the deoxyribose monophosphate form of uridylate (dUMP), which forms deoxythymidylate in a reaction catalyzed by thymidylate synthase. In this reaction, uracil is methylated with a methylene contributed by N5,N10-methylenetetrahydrofolate (M-THF). The widely used chemotherapy drug methotrexate (amethopterin) blocks the regeneration of THF to M-THF, preventing the thymidylate synthase reaction and blocking rapidly dividing cells from synthesizing DNA. Another chemotherapeutic drug, fluorouracil, is converted to fluorodeoxyuridylate (F-dUMP) by in vivo enzymes. F-dUMP is a suicide inhibitor of thymidylate synthase, which forms an irreversible covalent complex with the enzyme.

299. The answer is c. *(Murray, pp 375–401. Scriver, pp 2513–2570. Sack, pp 121–138. Wilson, pp 287–320.)* 5'-phosphoribosyl-1-pyrophosphate (PRPP) donates the ribose phosphate unit of nucleotides and is absolutely required for the beginning of the synthesis of purines. In fact, the enzymes regulating the synthesis of PRPP and the subsequent synthesis of phosphoribosylamine from PRPP are all end product–inhibited by inosine monophosphate (IMP), adenosine monophosphate (AMP), and guanosine monophosphate (GMP), the products of this reaction pathway. Allopurinol, an analogue of hypoxanthine, is a drug used to correct gout. It accomplishes this by inhibiting the production of urate from hypoxanthine and in doing so undergoes suicide inhibition of xanthine oxidase. 5-fluorouracil is an analogue of thymidine that inhibits thymidylate synthetase and is used in cancer chemotherapy. Cytosine arabinoside (Ara C), an inhibitor of RNA synthesis, also takes advantage of rapid nucleic acid synthesis in cancer cells and is used in chemotherapy.

300. The answer is b. *(Murray, pp 375–401. Scriver, pp 2513–2570. Sack, pp 121–138. Wilson, pp 287–320.)* The degradation of purines to urate can lead to gout when an elevated level of urate is present in serum, causing the precipitation of sodium urate crystals in joints. The excessive production of urate in many patients seems to be connected to a partial deficiency of hypoxanthine-guanine phosphoribosyl transferase (HGPRT). Allopurinol, an analogue of hypoxanthine, is a drug used to correct gout. It accomplishes this by inhibiting the production of urate from hypoxanthine and in doing so undergoes suicide inhibition of xanthine oxidase. Ribose phosphate and PRPP are required for purine synthesis. 5-fluorouracil (5-FU) and cytosine arabinoside (Ara C) are cancer chemotherapy agents, the former being an analogue of thymine that inhibits thymidylate synthetase and the latter an inhibitor of RNA synthesis.

301. The answer is e. *(Murray, pp 375–401. Scriver, pp 2513–2570. Sack, pp 121–138. Wilson, pp 287–320.)* Only cytidylate (CMP) has a 5′-phosphate group, a ribose (pentose) group with a 2′-hydroxyl, and a pyrimidine base. Two purines [adenine (A) and guanine (G)] and two pyrimidines [cytosine (C) and thymine (T)] occur in DNA. In RNA, uracil (U) replaces thymine. Hypoxanthine and inosine are biosynthetic precursors to the bases in nucleic acids. Bases form nucleosides through bonding of a nitrogen with the C1 carbon (1′-carbon) of a pentose sugar. Adenosine, guanosine, and cytidine can form ribonucleotides with ribose (2′- and 3′-hydroxyl groups) or deoxyribonucleotides with deoxyribose (3′-hydroxyl group only). Uridine occurs only as the ribonucleoside, thymidine as the deoxyribonucleotide (actually as thymidylate deoxyribonucleotide synthesized from uridylate by thymidylate synthetase). Ribonucleotides (adenylate, guanidylate, cytidylate, uridylate) have a phosphate ester on the 5′-hydroxyl of ribose (note that the *ribo-*

prefix is usually omitted). Deoxyribonucleotides have a phosphate ester on the 5'-hydroxyl of deoxyribose (deoxyadenylate, deoxyguanidylate, deoxycytidylate, and thymidylate). Thymidylate does not need the *deoxy-* prefix since it only forms as a deoxyribonucleotide. The phosphate ester may be formed of one, two, or three phosphate groups (e.g., AMP, ADP, or ATP).

302. The answer is e. *(Murray, pp 375–401. Scriver, pp 2513–2570. Sack, pp 121–138. Wilson, pp 287–320.)* The activated form of glucose utilized for the synthesis of glycogen and galactose is UDP-glucose, which is formed from the reaction of glucose-1-phosphate and UTP. The vitamin lipoic acid is covalently bound to the ε-amino group of a lysine residue of the enzyme dihydrolipoyl transacetylase. The amide-linked lipolysine residue is known as lipoamide and is an activated carrier of acyl groups derived from the hydroxyethyl derivative of thiamine pyrophosphate. In this manner, lipoamide functions as one of the coenzymes in oxidative decarboxylation reactions. In reductive synthesis such as fatty acid synthesis, NADPH is the major electron donor. This may be contrasted to NADH, which is utilized for the generation of ATP via electron transport.

Nutrition

Vitamins and Minerals

Questions

DIRECTIONS: Each item below contains a question or incomplete statement followed by suggested responses. Select the **one best** response to each question.

303. A middle-aged man presents with congestive heart failure with elevated liver enzymes. His skin has a grayish pigmentation. The levels of liver enzymes are higher than those usually seen in congestive heart failure, suggesting an inflammatory process (hepatitis) with scarring (cirrhosis) of the liver. A liver biopsy discloses a marked increase in iron storage. In humans, molecular iron (Fe) is

a. Stored primarily in the spleen
b. Stored in combination with ferritin
c. Excreted in the urine as Fe^{++}
d. Absorbed in the intestine by albumin
e. Absorbed in the ferric (Fe^{+++}) form

304. Humans most easily tolerate a lack of which of the following nutrients?

a. Protein
b. Iodine
c. Carbohydrate
d. Lipid
e. Calcium

305. A deficiency of vitamin B_{12} causes

a. Cheilosis
b. Beriberi
c. Pernicious anemia
d. Scurvy
e. Rickets

306. In adults, a severe deficiency of vitamin D causes

a. Night blindness
b. Osteomalacia
c. Rickets
d. Osteogenesis imperfecta
e. Osteopetrosis

307. Which of the following vitamins would most likely become deficient in a person who develops a completely carnivorous lifestyle?

a. Thiamine
b. Niacin
c. Cobalamin
d. Pantothenic acid
e. Vitamin C

308. Which of the following statements regarding vitamin A is true?

a. It is not an essential vitamin
b. It is related to tocopherol
c. It is a component of rhodopsin
d. It is derived from ethanol
e. It is also known as opsin

309. Fully activated pyruvate carboxylase depends upon the presence of

a. Malate and niacin
b. Acetyl CoA and biotin
c. Acetyl CoA and thiamine pyrophosphate
d. Oxaloacetate and biotin
e. Oxaloacetate and niacin

310. Pantothenic acid is a constituent of the coenzyme involved in

a. Decarboxylation
b. Acetylation
c. Dehydrogenation
d. Reduction
e. Oxidation

311. Studies of the actions of two anticoagulants—dicumarol and war-farin (the latter also a hemorrhagic rat poison)—have revealed that

a. Vitamin C is necessary for the synthesis of fibrinogen
b. Vitamin C activates fibrinogen
c. Vitamin K is a clotting factor
d. Vitamin K is essential for γ-carboxylation of glutamate
e. The action of vitamin E is antagonized by these compounds

312. Biotin is involved in which of the following types of reactions?

a. Hydroxylations
b. Carboxylations
c. Decarboxylations
d. Dehydrations
e. Deaminations

313. Which of the following vitamins is the precursor of CoA?

a. Riboflavin
b. Pantothenate
c. Thiamine
d. Cobamide
e. Pyridoxamine

314. In the Far East, beriberi is a serious health problem. It is character-ized by neurologic and cardiac symptoms. Beriberi is caused by a defi-ciency of

a. Choline
b. Ethanolamine
c. Thiamine
d. Serine
e. Glycine

315. Both acyl carrier protein (ACP) of fatty acid synthetase and coenzyme A (CoA)

a. Contain reactive phosphorylated tyrosine groups
b. Contain thymidine
c. Contain phosphopantetheine-reactive groups
d. Contain cystine-reactive groups
e. Carry folate groups

316. Which one of the following transfers acyl groups?

a. Thiamine pyrophosphate
b. Lipoamide
c. ATP
d. NADH
e. FADH

317. Which one of the following cofactors must be utilized during the conversion of acetyl CoA to malonyl CoA?

a. Thiamine pyrophosphate
b. Acyl carrier protein (ACP)
c. NAD_1
d. Biotin
e. FAD

318. Which one of the following enzymes requires a coenzyme derived from the vitamin whose structure is shown below?

a. Enoyl CoA hydratase
b. Phosphofructokinase
c. Glucose-6-phosphatase
d. Glucose-6-phosphate dehydrogenase
e. Glycogen phosphorylase

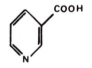

319. Coenzymes derived from the vitamin shown below are required by enzymes involved in the synthesis of which of the following?

a. ATP
b. UTP
c. CTP
d. NADH
e. NADPH

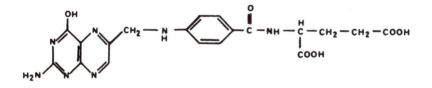

320. Coenzymes derived from the vitamin shown below are required by which one of the following enzymes?

a. Lactate dehydrogenase
b. Glutamate dehydrogenase
c. Pyruvate dehydrogenase
d. Malate dehydrogenase
e. Glyceraldehyde-3-phosphate dehydrogenase

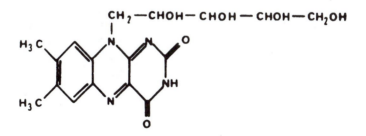

321. Which of the structures in the figure below is involved in amino transferase (transamination and deamination) and decarboxylation reactions of amino acids?

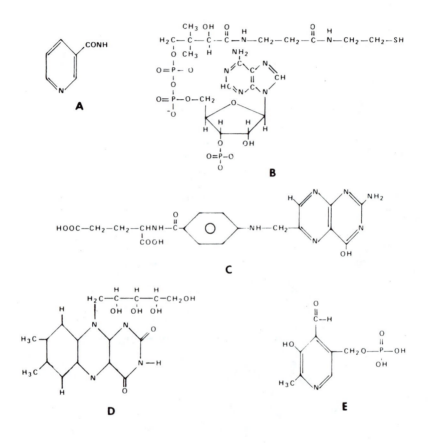

a. Structure A
b. Structure B
c. Structure C
d. Structure D
e. Structure E

322. Which of the compounds in the figure in question 321 is the precursor of the electron donor used in reductive biosynthesis?

a. Structure A
b. Structure B
c. Structure C
d. Structure D
e. Structure E

323. Which of the following is a coenzyme?

a. Glucose-6-phosphate
b. Glucose-1-phosphate
c. Calcium ion
d. Lipoic acid
e. UDP-glucose

324. Which one of the following is a cofactor and not a coenzyme?

a. Biotin
b. Tetrahydrofolic acid
c. Copper
d. Methylcobalamin
e. Pyridoxal phosphate

325. Which of the following statements describing vitamin K is true?

a. Vitamin K is broken down by intestinal bacteria
b. Vitamin K is obtained by eating citrus fruits, spinach, and cabbage
c. Vitamin K is not found in dairy or meat products; it is obtained by eating egg yolk and liver
d. Vitamin K is required for liver synthesis of prothrombin
e. Vitamin K prevents thrombosis

326. A term infant is born at home and does well with breast-feeding. Two days later, the mother calls frantically because the baby is bleeding from the umbilical cord and nostrils. The most likely cause is

a. Deficiency of vitamin C due to a citrus-poor diet during pregnancy
b. Hypervitaminosis A due to ingestion of beef liver during pregnancy
c. Deficiency of vitamin K because infant intestines are sterile
d. Deficiency of vitamin K because of disseminated intravascular coagulation (disseminated clotting due to infantile sepsis)
e. Deficiency of vitamin E due to maternal malabsorption during pregnancy

327. Which of the following statements regarding vitamin A is true?

a. Vitamin A promotes maintenance of epithelial tissue
b. Vitamin A is necessary for hearing but not for vision
c. Vitamin A is synthesized in skin
d. All vitamin A derivatives are safe to use during pregnancy
e. Vitamin A is a form of calciferol

328. Which of the following conditions most rapidly produces a functional deficiency of vitamin K?

a. Coumadin therapy to prevent thrombosis in patients prone to clot formation
b. Broad-spectrum antibiotic therapy
c. Lack of red meat in the diet
d. Lack of citrus fruits in the diet
e. Premature birth

329. A 3-month-old boy presents with poor feeding and growth, low muscle tone (hypotonia), elevation of blood lactic acid (lactic acidemia), and mild acidosis (blood pH 7.3 to 7.35). The ratio of pyruvate to lactate in serum is elevated, and there is decreased conversion of pyruvate to acetyl coenzyme A in fibroblasts. Which of the following compounds might be considered for therapy?

a. Pyridoxine
b. Thiamine
c. Free fatty acids
d. Biotin
e. Ascorbic acid

330. A homeless person is brought into the emergency room with psychotic imagery and alcohol on his breath. Which of the following compounds is most important to administer?

a. Glucose
b. Niacin
c. Nicotinic acid
d. Thiamine
e. Riboflavin

331. Which of the following vitamins becomes a major electron acceptor, aiding in the oxidation of numerous substrates?

a. Vitamin B_6
b. Niacin
c. Riboflavin
d. Thiamine
e. Vitamin B_1

332. Which of the following vitamins can act without phosphorylation?

a. Pyridoxine
b. Lipoamide
c. Niacin
d. Thiamine
e. Riboflavin

333. A 2-year-old child presents with chronic cough and bronchitis, growth failure, and chronic diarrhea with light-colored, foul-smelling stools. A deficiency of which of the following vitamins should be considered?

a. Vitamin A
b. Vitamin C
c. Vitamin B_1
d. Vitamin B_2
e. Vitamin B_6

334. Pantothenic acid is important for which of the following steps or pathways?

a. Pyruvate carboxylase
b. Fatty acid synthesis
c. Pyruvate carboxykinase
d. Gluconeogenesis
e. Glycolysis

335. Which of the following enzymes requires a phosphorylated derivative of the vitamin shown below?
a. Pyruvate carboxylase
b. Pyruvate dehydrogenase
c. Phosphoenolpyruvate carboxykinase
d. Glucokinase
e. Fructokinase

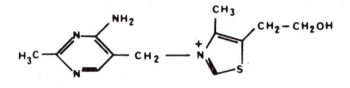

336. A deficiency of which of the following vitamins is associated with the occurrence of neural tube defects (anencephaly and spina bifida)?
a. Ascorbic acid (vitamin C)
b. Thiamine (vitamin B_1)
c. Riboflavin (vitamin B_2)
d. Niacin (vitamin B_3)
e. Biotin
f. Pantothenic acid
g. Folic acid
h. Cobalamin (vitamin B_{12})

337. An African American infant presents with prominent forehead, bowing of the limbs, broad and tender wrists, swellings at the costochondral junctions of the ribs, and irritability. Which of the following treatments are recommended?
a. Lotions containing retinoic acid
b. Diet of baby food containing leafy vegetables
c. Diet of baby food containing liver and ground beef
d. Milk and sunlight exposure
e. Removal of eggs from diet

Vitamins and Minerals

Answers

303. The answer is b. (*Murray, pp 627–661. Scriver, pp 3127–3164. Sack, pp 121–138. Wilson, pp 287–320.*) Ferrous iron (Fe^{++}) is the form absorbed in the intestine by ferritin, transported in plasma by transferrin, and stored in the liver in combination with ferritin or as hemosiderin. There is no known excretory pathway for iron, either in the ferric or ferrous form. For this reason, excessive iron uptake over a period of many years may cause hemochromatosis (235200), the likely diagnosis for this man. This is a condition of extensive hemosiderin deposition in the liver, myocardium, pancreas, and adrenals. The resulting symptoms include liver cirrhosis, congestive heart failure, diabetes mellitus, and changes in skin pigmentation.

304. The answer is c. (*Murray, pp 627–661. Scriver, pp 3897–3964. Sack, pp 121–138. Wilson, pp 287–320.*) Certain amino acids and lipids are dietary necessities because humans cannot synthesize them. The energy usually obtained from carbohydrates can be obtained from lipids and the conversion of some amino acids to intermediates of the citric acid cycle. These alternative substrates can thus provide fuel for oxidation and energy plus reducing equivalents for biosynthesis. Iodine is important for thyroid hormone synthesis, while calcium is essential for muscle contraction and bone metabolism.

305. The answer is c. (*Murray, pp 627–661. Scriver, pp 3897–3964. Sack, pp 121–138. Wilson, pp 287–320.*) Pernicious anemia results from an inability to absorb vitamin B_{12} from the gastrointestinal tract. This may be due to a deficiency of intrinsic factor, surgical gastrectomy, or small bowel disease. The earliest clinical signs of pernicious anemia do not appear until 3 to 5 years following the onset of vitamin B_{12} deficiency. The term *pernicious* indicates a potential fatal outcome. Cheilosis is dryness and scaling of the lips that is characteristic of riboflavin (vitamin B_2) deficiency. Scurvy is caused by vitamin C deficiency and is characterized by bleeding gums and bone disease. Rickets is softening and deformation of the bones due to vitamin D deficiency or defects in vitamin D processing. The word *beriberi* is Singhalese for "I cannot," referring to muscular atrophy and paralysis caused by the inflammation of multiple nerves (polyneuritis). Beriberi is caused by thiamine (vitamin B_1) deficiency and is common in Asians who subsist on a diet of polished white rice.

306. The answer is b. *(Murray, pp 627–661. Scriver, pp 3897–3964. Sack, pp 121–138. Wilson, pp 287–320.)* Osteomalacia is the name given to the disease of bone seen in adults with vitamin D deficiency. It is analogous to rickets, which is seen in children with the same deficiency. Both disorders are manifestations of defective bone formation. The osteogenesis imperfectas are a group of genetic bone disorders caused by collagen gene mutations. Osteopetrosis is a hardening of the bones that occurs in certain hereditary conditions. Night blindness is associated with vitamin A deficiency.

307. The answer is e. *(Murray, pp 627–661. Scriver, pp 3897–3964. Sack, pp 121–138. Wilson, pp 287–320.)* Ascorbic acid (vitamin C) is found in fresh fruits and vegetables. Deficiency of ascorbic acid produces scurvy, the "sailor's disease." Ascorbic acid is necessary for the hydroxylation of proline to hydroxyproline in collagen, a process required in the formation and maintenance of connective tissue. The failure of mesenchymal cells to form collagen causes the skeletal, dental, and connective tissue deterioration seen in scurvy. Thiamine, niacin, cobalamin, and pantothenic acid can all be obtained from fish or meat products. The nomenclature of vitamins began by classifying fat-soluble vitamins as A (followed by subsequent letters of the alphabet such as D, E, and K) and water-soluble vitamins as B. Components of the B vitamin fraction were then given subscripts, e.g., thiamine (B_1), riboflavin (B_2), niacin [nicotinic acid (B_3)], panthothenic acid (B_5), pyridoxine (B_6), and cobalamin (B_{12}). The water-soluble vitamins C, biotin, and folic acid do not follow the B nomenclature.

308. The answer is c. *(Murray, pp 627–661. Scriver, pp 3897–3964. Sack, pp 121–138. Wilson, pp 287–320.)* The retinal pigment rhodopsin is composed of the 11-*cis*-retinal form of vitamin A coupled to opsin. Light isomerizes 11-*cis*-retinal to all-*trans*-retinal, which is hydrolyzed to free all-*trans*-retinal and opsin. In order for regeneration of rhodopsin to occur, 11-*cis*-retinal must be regenerated. This dark reaction involves the isomerization of all-*trans*-retinal to 11-*cis*-retinal, which combines with opsin to reform rhodopsin. A deficiency of vitamin A, which is often derived from the β-carotene of plants, results in night blindness.

309. The answer is b. (*Murray, pp 627–661. Scriver, pp 3897–3964. Sack, pp 121–138. Wilson, pp 287–320.*) Pyruvate carboxylase catalyzes the conversion of pyruvate to oxaloacetate in gluconeogenesis:

$$\text{pyruvate} + HCO_3^- + ATP \rightarrow \text{oxaloacetate} + ADP + P_i$$

In order for pyruvate carboxylase to be ready to function, it requires biotin, Mg^{++}, and Mn^{++}. It is allosterically activated by acetyl CoA. The biotin is not carboxylated until acetyl CoA binds the enzyme. By this means, high levels of acetyl CoA signal the need for more oxaloacetate. When ATP levels are high, the oxaloacetate is consumed in gluconeogenesis. When ATP levels are low, the oxaloacetate enters the citric acid cycle. Gluconeogenesis only occurs in the liver and kidneys.

310. The answer is b. (*Murray, pp 627–661. Scriver, pp 3897–3964. Sack, pp 121–138. Wilson, pp 287–320.*) Pantothenic acid, also called coacetylase, is a component of coenzyme A (CoA). Acetyl CoA is the activated form of acetate employed in acetylation reactions, including the citric acid cycle and lipid and cholesterol metabolism. A deficiency of pantothenic acid would limit CoA and have deadly consequences in mammals. However, since it is common in foodstuffs, there is little evidence of pantothenic acid deficiency in humans.

311. The answer is d. (*Murray, pp 627–661. Scriver, pp 3897–3964. Sack, pp 121–138. Wilson, pp 287–320.*) In order to be converted to thrombin during clot formation, prothrombin must bind Ca^{++}, which allows it to anchor to platelet membranes produced by injury. Prothrombin's affinity for Ca^{++} is dependent on the presence of 10 γ-carboxyglutamate residues found in the first 35 amino acid residues of its amino terminal region. The vitamin K–dependent γ-carboxylation of prothrombin is a posttranslational modification that occurs as nascent prothrombin is synthesized on liver rough endoplasmic reticulum and passes into the lumen of the reticulum. The anticoagulants warfarin and dicumarol are structural analogues that block the γ-carboxylation of prothrombin by substituting for vitamin K. Hence, the prothrombin produced has a weak affinity for Ca^{++} and cannot properly bind to platelet membranes in order to be converted to thrombin. A simplified diagram of the final steps of fibrin clot formation is given below.

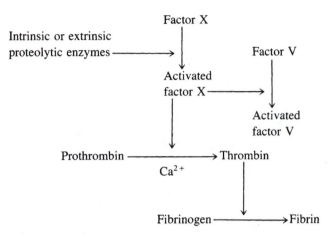

312. The answer is b. *(Murray, pp 627–661. Scriver, pp 3897–3964. Sack, pp 121–138. Wilson, pp 287–320.)* The vitamin biotin is the cofactor required by carboxylating enzymes such as acetyl CoA, pyruvate, and propionyl CoA carboxylases. The fixation of CO_2 by these biotin-dependent enzymes occurs in two stages. In the first, bicarbonate ion reacts with adenosine triphosphate (ATP) and the biotin carrier protein moiety of the enzyme; in the second, the "active CO_2" reacts with the substrate—e.g., acetyl CoA.

313. The answer is b. *(Murray, pp 627–661. Scriver, pp 3897–3964. Sack, pp 121–138. Wilson, pp 287–320.)* Pantothenate is the precursor of CoA, which participates in numerous reactions throughout the metabolic scheme. CoA is a central molecule of metabolism involved in acetylation reactions. Thus a deficiency of pantothenic acid would have severe consequences. There is no documented deficiency state for pantothenate, however, since this vitamin is common in foodstuffs.

314. The answer is c. *(Murray, pp 627–661. Scriver, pp 3897–3964. Sack, pp 121–138. Wilson, pp 287–320.)* In the Far East, rice is a staple of the diet. When rice is unsupplemented, beriberi can be manifest, since rice is low in vitamin B_1 (thiamine). Thiamine pyrophosphate is the necessary prosthetic group of enzymes that transfers activated aldehyde units. Such enzymes include transketolase, pyruvate dehydrogenase, and α-ketoglutarate dehydrogenase. Beriberi is a wasting disease whose symptoms include pain in the limbs induced by peripheral neuropathy, weak musculature, and heart enlargement. Yeast products, whole grains, nuts, and pork are rich in thiamine. Choline, ethanolamine, and serine are polar head groups of phospholipids. Glycine is a common amino acid.

315. The answer is c. *(Murray, pp 627–661. Scriver, pp 3897–3964. Sack, pp 121–138. Wilson, pp 287–320.)* The almost universal carrier of acyl groups is coenzyme A (CoA). However, acyl carrier protein (ACP) also functions as a carrier of acyl groups. In fatty acid synthesis, ACP carries the acyl intermediates. The reactive prosthetic group of both ACP and CoA is a phosphopantetheine sulfhydryl. In ACP, the phosphopantetheine group is attached to the 77-residue polypeptide chain via a serine hydroxyl. In CoA, the phosphopantetheine is linked to the 5'-phosphate of adenosine that is phosphorylated in its 3'-hydroxyl.

316. The answer is b. *(Murray, pp 627–661. Scriver, pp 3897–3964. Sack, pp 121–138. Wilson, pp 287–320.)* Lipoamide, like CoA, transfers acetyl groups, but it is a catalytic cofactor in an enzyme complex rather than a stoichiometric cofactor like CoA. A reactive disulfide of lipoamide links the acetyl group to be transferred. Lipoamide becomes acetyllipoamide and then dihydrolipoamide as it first accepts and then transfers an acyl group. This reaction and the regeneration of lipoamide are catalyzed by different parts of the dehydrogenase enzyme complexes of pyruvate dehydrogenase and isocitrate dehydrogenase. ATP transfers phosphoryl groups and thiamine pyrophosphate transfers aldehyde groups. NADH and FADH transfer protons.

317. The answer is d. *(Murray, pp 627–661. Scriver, pp 3897–3964. Sack, pp 121–138. Wilson, pp 287–320.)* The key enzymatic step of fatty acid synthesis is the carboxylation of acetyl CoA to form malonyl CoA. The carboxyl of biotin is covalently attached to an ε-amino acid group of a lysine residue of acetyl CoA carboxylase. The reaction occurs in two stages. In the first step, a carboxybiotin is formed:

$$HCO_3^- + \text{biotin-enzyme} + ATP \rightarrow CO_2\text{-biotin-enzyme} + ADP + P_i$$

In the second step, the CO_2 is transferred to acetyl CoA to produce malonyl CoA:

$$CO_2\text{-biotin-enzyme} + \text{acetyl CoA} \rightarrow \text{malonyl CoA} + \text{biotin-enzyme}$$

None of the other cofactors listed are involved in this reaction.

318. The answer is d. *(Murray, pp 627–661. Scriver, pp 3897–3964. Sack, pp 121–138. Wilson, pp 287–320.)* The vitamin whose structure appears in the question is nicotinic acid (niacin), which gives rise to the nicotinamide adenine dinucleotide coenzymes NAD^+ and $NADP^+$. NAD^+ is a cofactor required by all dehydrogenases. NADPH is a cofactor produced by the pentose phosphate shunt. It is utilized in reductive synthesis of compounds such as fatty acids.

319. The answer is a. *(Murray, pp 627–661. Scriver, pp 3897–3964. Sack, pp 121–138. Wilson, pp 287–320.)* The structure shown in the question is the vitamin folic acid. Tetrahydrofolic acid, the active cofactor derived from folic acid, is required in two steps of purine synthesis and thus required in the de novo synthesis of ATP and GTP. CTP and TTP are pyrimidine base derivatives, and although de novo synthesis of the pyrimidine ring does not require tetrahydrofolate, the formation of thymine from uracil does. NADH and NADPH require niacin for their synthesis.

320. The answer is c. *(Murray, pp 627–661. Scriver, pp 3897–3964. Sack, pp 121–138. Wilson, pp 287–320.)* The structure shown in the question is that of the vitamin riboflavin. It is a precursor of two cofactors involved in electron transport systems, riboflavin 5′-phosphate, also known as flavin mononucleotide (FMN), and flavin adenine dinucleotide (FAD). Strictly speaking, these compounds are not nucleotides, as they contain the sugar alcohol ribitol, not ribose. The cofactors are strongly bound to their apoenzymes and function as dehydrogenation catalysts. Pyruvate dehydrogenase is a multienzyme complex and contains the enzyme dihydrolipoyl dehydrogenase, which has as its prosthetic group two molecules of FAD per molecule of enzyme. In the overall reaction, the reduced FAD is reoxidized by NAD^+. Succinate dehydrogenase also contains tightly bound FAD, one molecule per molecule of enzyme. Glutamate, lactate, malate, and glyceraldehyde-3-

phosphate dehydrogenases all use nicotinamide dinucleotide cofactors and do not contain FAD as a prosthetic group.

321. The answer is e. *(Murray, pp 627–661. Scriver, pp 3897–3964. Sack, pp 121–138. Wilson, pp 287–320.)* The coenzyme pyridoxal phosphate is a versatile compound that aids in the catalysis of many reactions involving amino acids. This includes amino transferase reactions such as transamination (e.g., glutamic-oxaloacetic transaminase), deamination (e.g., serine dehydratase), decarboxylation (glutamate decarboxylase), and transulfuration (e.g., cystathionine synthetase and cystathionase). Using the same type of mechanism, pyridoxal phosphate is important for the operation of glycogen phosphorylase. All of these reactions using pyridoxal phosphate catalysis have a number of features in common. First, a Schiff-base intermediate is formed with a specific lysine group at the active site of the appropriate enzymes. Then, in the reactions involving amino acids, the amino acid substrate is exchanged to form the Schiff-base with the amino acid substrate. Finally, the proteinated form of pyridoxal phosphate acts as an electron sink to stabilize the catalytic intermediates that are negatively charged. In other words, the ring nitrogen of pyridoxal phosphate attracts electrons from the amino acid substrate, which allows the product Schiff-base to be hydrolyzed. Pyridoxine (vitamin B_6) is found in many different foods. Therefore, deficiency usually only results from the administration of a number of commonly used drugs that act as pyridoxine antagonists (e.g., isoniazid and penicillamine).

322. The answer is a. *(Murray, pp 627–661. Scriver, pp 3897–3964. Sack, pp 121–138. Wilson, pp 287–320.)* The major contributor of electrons in reductive biosynthetic reactions is nicotinamide adenine dinucleotide phosphate ($NADPH + H^+$), which is derived by reduction of NAD^+. NAD^+ is formed from the vitamin niacin (also called nicotinate). Niacin can be formed from tryptophan in humans. In the synthesis of NAD^+, niacin reacts with 5-phosphoribosyl-1-pyrophosphate to form nicotinate ribonucleotide. Then, AMP is transferred from ATP to nicotinate ribonucleotide. Finally, the amide group of glutamate is transferred to the niacin carboxyl group to form the final product, NAD^+. $NADP^+$ is derived from NAD^+ by phosphorylation of the 2′-hydroxyl group of the adenine ribose moiety. The reduction of $NADP^+$ to $NADPH + H^+$ occurs primarily through the hexose monophosphate shunt.

323. The answer is d. *(Murray, pp 627–661. Scriver, pp 3897–3964. Sack, pp 121–138. Wilson, pp 287–320.)* A coenzyme is a nonprotein organic molecule that binds to an enzyme to aid in its catalytic function. Usually it is involved in the transfer of a specific functional group. A coenzyme usually binds loosely and can be separated from the enzyme. When a coenzyme binds tightly to an enzyme, it is spoken of as a prosthetic group of the enzyme. Coenzymes can be viewed as a second substrate for the enzyme, often undergoing chemical changes that counterbalance those of the substrate. Lipoic acid is a short-chain fatty acid with two sulfhydryl groups. Lipoic acid is a coenzyme involved in pyruvate dehydrogenase and α-ketoglutarate dehydrogenase reactions, taking part in the reactions. Each of these reactions also uses thiamine pyrophosphate, CoA, FAD^+, and NAD^+. Glucose-1-phosphate, glucose-6-phosphate, or UDP-glucose function as primary substrates of enzymatic reactions and/or induce structural changes in the enzyme (allosteric regulators) to influence enzyme activity. Calcium and other metal ions do not undergo chemical changes during the enzyme reaction and are classified as cofactors. While many coenzymes are derived by modification of vitamins such as CoA from pantothenic acid or FAD from riboflavin, some coenzymes do not contain vitamins. For example, ubiquinone (oxidized) or ubiquinol (reduced) is in fact coenzyme Q, which is involved in transferring hydrogen ion atoms and electrons in the oxidative phosphorylation system. Since humans can synthesize ubiquinones and lipoic acid, these substances are not considered vitamins.

324. The answer is d. *(Murray, pp 627–661. Scriver, pp 3897–3964. Sack, pp 121–138. Wilson, pp 287–320.)* Cofactors are distinguished from coenzymes because cofactors do not function in group transfer and do not undergo chemical reactions (other than changes in valence due to oxidation/reduction). Cofactors are usually metallic ions rather than organic molecules. Examples of cofactors include copper in cytochrome oxidase, iron in all the cytochromes, magnesium for all enzymes utilizing ATP, and zinc in lactate dehydrogenase. Methylcobalamin, biotin, tetrahydrofolic acid, and pyridoxal phosphates all assist with enzyme catalysis by transfer of groups from or to the primary substrate.

325. The answer is d. *(Murray, pp 627–661. Scriver, pp 3897–3964. Sack, pp 121–138. Wilson, pp 287–320.)* The major role of vitamin K is in the synthesis of prothrombin and other clotting factors (e.g., VII, IX, and X). Vitamin K acts on the inactive precursor molecules of these proteins, allowing carboxylation of glutamic acid residues to γ-carboxyglutamate. A true vitamin K deficiency is unusual because vitamin K is found in a variety of foods and can be produced by intestinal bacteria. Liver, egg yolk, spinach, cauliflower, and cabbage are some of the sources of vitamin K. Vitamin K is not involved in the prevention of thrombosis (blood clots that can lead to stroke or heart failure), but is actually required for the formation of blood clots. In fact, a method for preventing thrombosis involves the use of drugs that interfere with vitamin K, such as dicumarol and warfarin, a synthetic analogue of vitamin K. Both of these compounds interfere with the formation of γ-carboxyglutamate.

326. The answer is c. (*Murray, pp 627–661. Scriver, pp 3897–3964. Sack, pp 121–138. Wilson, pp 287–320.*) Hemorrhagic disease of the newborn is caused by poor transfer of maternal vitamin K through the placenta and by lack of intestinal bacteria in the infant for synthesis of vitamin K. The intestine is sterile at birth and becomes colonized over the first few weeks. Because of these factors, vitamin K is routinely administered to newborns. Deficiencies of the fat-soluble vitamins A, E, D, and K can occur with intestinal malabsorption, but avid fetal uptake during pregnancy usually prevents infantile symptoms. Hypervitaminosis A can cause liver toxicity but not bleeding, and deficiencies of E (neonatal anemia) or C (extremely rare in neonates) have other symptoms besides bleeding.

327. The answer is a. (*Murray, pp 627–661. Scriver, pp 3897–3964. Sack, pp 121–138. Wilson, pp 287–320.*) Vitamin A is essential for the normal differentiation of epithelial tissue as well as normal reproduction. Yellow and dark green vegetables as well as fruits are good sources of carotenes, which serve as precursors of vitamin A. However, egg yolk, butter, cream, and liver and kidneys are good sources of performed vitamin A. Vitamin A is necessary for vision, not hearing. The visual pigment rhodopsin is formed from the protein opsin and 11-*cis*-retinal. During the photobleaching of rhodopsin, all-*trans*-retinal plus opsin is formed from dissociated rhodopsin, causing an impulse that is transmitted by the optic nerve to the brain. 11-*cis*-retinal is isomerized from *trans*-retinal, which spontaneously combines with opsin to reform rhodopsin, making it ready for another photochemical cycle. all-*trans*-retinoic acid (tretinoin) has been found to be effective for topical treatment of psoriasis. Another form of vitamin A is

13-*cis*-retinoic acid (Accutane), which has been found to be effective in the treatment of severe cases of acne. Accutane causes birth defects of the face and brain if taken during the first trimester of pregnancy. Vitamin A is not synthesized in the skin. Vitamin D (derivatives of calciferol) can be synthesized in the skin under the influence of sunlight from 7-dehydrocholesterol, an intermediate in cholesterol synthesis.

328. The answer is a. (*Murray, pp 627–661. Scriver, pp 3897–3964. Sack, pp 121–138. Wilson, pp 287–320.*) Vitamin K is essential for the posttranscriptional modification of prothrombin by γ-carboxylation of glutamate residues. A functional deficiency exists in patients treated with analogues of vitamin K such as the coumadin derivatives. The analogues act as anticoagulants by competing with vitamin K and preventing the production of functional prothrombin. By administration of vitamin K, hemorrhage can be prevented in such patients. Vitamin K is normally obtained from green, leafy vegetables in the diet (not from citrus fruits or red meat). Intestinal bacteria also synthesize the vitamin, but even broad-spectrum antibiotic therapy does not completely sterilize the intestine. A deficiency of vitamin K can cause hemorrhage disease in newborn infants since their intestines do not have the bacteria that produce vitamin K and since vitamin K does not cross the placenta. The neonatal deficiency occurs in term or premature infants.

329. The answer is b. (*Murray, pp 627–661. Scriver, pp 2275–2296. Sack, pp 121–138. Wilson, pp 287–320.*) An elevation of pyruvate and a deficiency of acetyl CoA suggest a deficiency of pyruvate dehydrogenase (PDH). This multisubunit enzyme assembly contains pyruvate dehydrogenase, dihydrolipoyl transacetylase, dihydrolipoyl dehydrogenase, and two enzymes involved in regulation of the overall enzymatic activity of the complex. PDH requires thiamine pyrophosphate as a coenzyme, dihydrolipoyl transacetylase requires lipoic acid and CoA, and dihydrolipoyl dehydrogenase has an FAD prosthetic group that is reoxidized by NAD^+. Biotin, pyridoxine, and ascorbic acid are not coenzymes for PDH. An ATP-dependent protein kinase can phosphorylate PDH to decrease activity, and a phosphatase can activate PDH. Increases of ATP, acetyl CoA, or NADH (increased energy charge) and of fatty acid oxidation increase phosphorylation of PDH and decrease its activity. PDH is less active during starvation, increasing pyruvate, decreasing glycolysis, and sparing carbohydrates. Free fatty acids decrease PDH activity and would not be appropriate therapy for PDH deficiency. PDH deficiency (246900, 312170) exhibits genetic heterogeneity, as would be expected from its multiple subunits, with autosomal and X-linked recessive forms. The infant also could be classified as having Leigh's disease (266150), a heterogenous group of disorders with hypotonia and lactic acidemia that can include PDH deficiency.

330. The answer is d. *(Murray, pp 627–661. Scriver, pp 3897–3964. Sack, pp 121–138. Wilson, pp 287–320.)* Chronic alcoholics are at risk for thiamine deficiency, which is thought to play a role in the incoordination (ataxia) and psychosis that can become chronic (Wernicke-Korsakoff syndrome). The thiamine deficiency produces relative deficiency of the pyruvate dehydrogenase complex. The administration of glucose without checking glucose levels can therefore be dangerous, since excess glucose is converted to pyruvate by glycolysis. The low rate of pyruvate dehydrogenase conversion of pyruvate to coenzyme A (and entry into the citric acid cycle) causes pyruvate to be converted to lactate (through lactate dehydrogenase). Lactic acidosis can be fatal. Chronic alcoholics can be deficient in the other vitamins mentioned, but thiamine is most likely to help the neurologic symptoms.

331. The answer is b. *(Murray, pp 627–661. Scriver, pp 3897–3964. Sack, pp 121–138. Wilson, pp 287–320.)* Nicotinamide adenine dinucleotide (NAD$^+$) is the functional coenzyme derivative of niacin. It is the major electron acceptor in the oxidation of molecules, generating NADH, which is the major electron donor for reduction reactions. Thiamine (also known as vitamin B$_1$) occurs functionally as thiamine pyrophosphate and is a coenzyme for enzymes such as pyruvate dehydrogenase. Riboflavin (vitamin B$_2$) functions in the coenzyme forms of flavin mononucleotide (FMN) or flavin adenine dinucleotide (FAD). When concentrated, both have a yellow color due to the riboflavin they contain. Both function as prosthetic groups of oxidation-reduction enzymes or flavoproteins. Flavoproteins are active in selected oxidation reactions and in electron transport, but they do not have the ubiquitous role of NAD$^+$.

332. The answer is b. *(Murray, pp 627–661. Scriver, pp 3897–3964. Sack, pp 121–138. Wilson, pp 287–320.)* All the vitamins listed except lipoamide contain at least one phosphate in their cofactor form. Thiamine (vitamin

B$_1$) is converted to thiamine pyrophosphate simply by the addition of pyrophosphate. It is involved in aldehyde group transfer. Niacin (nicotinic acid) is esterified to adenine dinucleotide and its two phosphates to form nicotinamide adenine dinucleotide. Pyridoxine (vitamin B$_6$) is converted to either pyridoxal phosphate or pyridoxamine phosphate before complexing with enzymes. Riboflavin becomes flavin mononucleotide by obtaining one phosphate (riboflavin 5'-phosphate). If it complexes with adenine dinucleotide via a pyrophosphate ester linkage, it becomes flavin adenine dinucleotide.

333. The answer is a. (*Murray, pp 627–661. Scriver, pp 3897–3964. Sack, pp 121–138. Wilson, pp 287–320.*) Vitamins A, D, E, and K are all fat-soluble. The physical characteristics of fat-soluble vitamins derive from the hydrophobic nature of the aliphatic chains composing them. The other vitamins listed are water-soluble, efficiently administered orally, and rapidly absorbed from the intestine. Fat-soluble vitamins must be administered intramuscularly or as oral emulsions (mixtures of oil and water). In intestinal disorders such as chronic diarrhea or malabsorption due to deficient digestive enzymes, fat-soluble vitamins are poorly absorbed and can become deficient. Supplementation of fat-soluble vitamins is thus routine in disorders like cystic fibrosis (219700), a cause of respiratory and intestinal disease that is the likely diagnosis in this child.

334. The answer is b. (*Murray, pp 627–661. Scriver, pp 3897–3964. Sack, pp 121–138. Wilson, pp 287–320.*) Pantothenic acid is phosphorylated and complexed with the amino acid cysteine to form 4-phosphopantetheine, the precursor for coenzyme A (CoA) and the acyl carrier protein (ACP) that participates in fatty acid synthesis. The thiol group of 4-phosphopantetheine is a carrier of acyl groups in CoA (A stands for acetylation or acetyl group) and ACP (fatty acyl groups). CoA is one of the major molecules in metabolism, carrying a pantetheine group bound to adenosine ribonucleotide-3'-phosphate via a 5'-diphosphate (pyrophosphate). Acetyl groups are linked to the reactive terminal sulfhydryl group to produce acetyl CoA, which has a high acetyl transfer potential. CoA carries and transfers acetyl groups in much the same way as ATP transfers activated phosphoryl groups. CoA is involved in fatty acid synthesis, fatty acid β oxidation, and the citric acid cycle; it is not involved in glycolysis or gluconeogenesis, where acetyl transfer does not occur.

Gluconeogenesis generates glucose by converting pyruvate to oxalo-acetate (via pyruvate carboxylase) to phosphoenopyruvate (via phos-phoenopyruvate carboxykinase) to fructose-1,6-bisphosphate (through reversal of glycolytic enzymes) to fructose-6-phosphate (via fructose-1,6-bisphosphatase) to glucose-6-phosphate (through reversal of phospho-hexose isomerase) to glucose (through glucose-6-phosphatase). Special enzymes are required at steps where reversal of glycolysis is not energeti-cally feasible.

335. The answer is b. (*Murray, pp 627–661. Scriver, pp 3897–3964. Sack, pp 121–138. Wilson, pp 287–320.*) The vitamin shown in the question is thi-amine (vitamin B_1), which requires phosphorylation to thiamine pyrophos-phate for activity. Thiamine is required for the reactions catalyzed by pyruvate dehydrogenase, transketolases, and α-ketoglutarate dehydroge-nase. In all these reactions, thiamine is involved with oxidative decarboxy-lation. The five-member thiazole ring of thiamine pyrophosphate forms a carbanion (carbon between the nitrogen and sulfur) that can react with C=O groups, causing elimination of the carbonyl group (COOH) as CO_2. Kinases such as those in glycolysis require ATP as a cofactor, while pyru-vate carboxylase and other carboxylases require biotin to transfer an acti-vated carbonyl group.

336. The answer is g. (*Murray, pp 627–661. Scriver, pp 3897–3964. Sack, pp 121–138. Wilson, pp 287–320.*) Spina bifida, or myelomeningocele, is a defect of the lower neural tube that produces an exposed spinal cord in the thoracic or sacral regions. Exposure of the spinal cord usually causes nerve damage that results in paralysis of the lower limbs and urinary bladder. Anencephaly is a defect of the anterior neural tube that results in lethal brain anomalies and skull defects. Folic acid is necessary for the develop-ment of the neural tube in the first few weeks of embryonic life, and the children of women with nutritional deficiencies have higher rates of neural tube defects. Since neural tube closure occurs at a time when many women are not aware that they are pregnant, it is essential that all women of child-bearing age take a folic acid supplement of approximately 0.4 mg per day. Frank folic acid deficiency can also cause megaloblastic anemia because of a decreased synthesis of the purines and pyrimidines needed for cells to make DNA and divide. Deficiencies of thiamine in chronic alcoholics are related to Wernicke-Korsakoff syndrome, which is characterized by loss of memory, lackadaisical behavior, and a continuous rhythmic movement of the eyeballs. Thiamine dietary deficiency from excess of polished rice can cause beriberi. Niacin deficiency leads to pellagra, a disorder that produces skin rash (dermatitis), weight loss, and neurologic changes including depression and dementia. Riboflavin deficiency leads to mouth ulcers (stomatitis), cheilosis (dry, scaly lips), scaly skin (seborrhea), and photophobia. Since biotin is widely distributed in foods and is synthesized by intestinal bacteria, biotin deficiency is rare. However, the heat-labile molecule avidin, found in raw egg whites, binds biotin tightly and blocks its absorption, causing dermatitis, dehydration, and lethargy. Lactic acidosis results as a buildup of lactate due to the lack of functional pyruvate carboxylase when biotin is missing. Vitamin C deficiency leads to scurvy, which causes bleeding gums and bone disease.

Vitamin B_{12} can be deficient due to a lack of intrinsic factor, which is a glycoprotein secreted by gastric parietal cells. A lack of intrinsic factor or a dietary deficiency of cobalamin can cause pernicious anemia and neuropsychiatric symptoms. The only known treatment for intrinsic factor deficiency (vitamin B_{12} deficiency) is intramuscular injection of cyanocobalamin throughout the patient's life.

337. The answer is d. (*Murray, pp 627–661. Scriver, pp 3897–3964. Sack, pp 121–138. Wilson, pp 287–320.*) People with bowed legs and other bone malformations were quite common in the northeastern United States following the industrial revolution. This was caused by childhood diets lacking foods with vitamin D and by minimal exposure to sunlight due to the dawn-to-dusk working conditions of the textile mills. Vitamin D is essential for the metabolism of calcium and phosphorus. Soft and malformed bones result from its absence. Liver, fish oil, and egg yolks contain vitamin D, and milk is supplemented with vitamin D by law. In adults, lack of sunlight and a diet poor in vitamin D lead to osteomalacia (soft bones). Darkskinned peoples are more susceptible to vitamin D deficiency.

Biotin deficiency can be caused by diets with excess egg white, leading to dehydration and acidosis from accumulation of carboxylic and lactic acids. Retinoic acid is a vitamin A derivative that can be helpful in treating acne but not vitamin D deficiency. Leafy vegetables are a source of B vitamins such as niacin and cobalamin.

Hormones and Integrated Metabolism

Questions

DIRECTIONS: Each item below contains a question or incomplete statement followed by suggested responses. Select the **one best** response to each question.

338. Which of the following statements accurately describes sex hormones?

a. They bind specific membrane receptors
b. They interact with DNA directly
c. They cause release of a proteinaceous second messenger from the cell membrane
d. They enhance transcription when bound to receptors
e. They inhibit translation through specific cytoplasmic proteins

339. Epinephrine stimulation of lipolysis in adipocytes is thought to differ from epinephrine stimulation of glycogenolysis in the liver in which way?

a. Glucagon, not epinephrine, stimulates lipolysis in adipocytes
b. The mechanism of hormone-receptor interaction is thought to be fundamentally different in each tissue
c. Phosphorylase kinase is activated directly by a second messenger in adipocytes, but not in the liver
d. Adenosine 3′,5′-cyclic monophosphate (cyclic AMP) is the second messenger in adipocytes, but not in the liver
e. Only protein kinase is interposed as an amplification factor between the second messenger and the physiologically important enzymes in adipocytes

340. Which of the following is noted in Cushing's syndrome, a disease of the adrenal cortex?

a. Decreased production of epinephrine
b. Excessive production of epinephrine
c. Excessive production of vasopressin
d. Excessive production of cortisol
e. Decreased production of cortisol

341. Increased reabsorption of water from the kidney is the major consequence of which of the following hormones?

a. Cortisol
b. Insulin
c. Vasopressin
d. Glucagon
e. Aldosterone

342. Lack of glucocorticoids and mineralocorticoids might be a consequence of which of the following defects in the adrenal cortex?

a. Androstenedione deficiency
b. 17α-hydroxyprogesterone deficiency
c. Estrone deficiency
d. C-21-hydroxylase deficiency
e. Testosterone deficiency

343. A patient presents with a complaint of muscle weakness following exercise. Neurological examination reveals that the muscles supplied by cranial nerves are most affected. You suspect myasthenia gravis. Your diagnosis is confirmed when lab tests indicate antibodies in the patient's blood against

a. Acetylcholinesterase
b. Muscle endplates
c. Cranial nerve synaptic membranes
d. Cranial nerve presynaptic membranes
e. Acetylcholine receptors

344. Which of the following hormones can cause hyperglycemia without known effects on glycogen or gluconeogenesis?

a. Thyroxine
b. Epinephrine
c. Glucocorticoids
d. Epidermal growth factor
e. Glucagon

345. Which of the following statements correctly describes insulin?

a. It is an anabolic signal to cells that glucose is scarce
b. It is converted from proinsulin to insulin primarily following secretion from β cells
c. It does not have a prohormone form
d. It is a small polypeptide composed of a single chain bridged by disulfide groups
e. Its action is antagonistic to that of glucagon

346. Insulin has many direct effects on various cell types from such tissues as muscle, fat, liver, and skin. Which of the following cellular activities is decreased following exposure to physiologic concentrations of insulin?

a. Plasma membrane transfer of glucose
b. Glucose oxidation
c. Gluconeogenesis
d. Lipogenesis
e. Formation of ATP, DNA, and RNA

347. Following release of norepinephrine by sympathetic nerves and epinephrine by the adrenal medulla, which of the following metabolic processes is decreased?

a. Glycolysis
b. Lipolysis
c. Gluconeogenesis
d. Glycogenolysis
e. Ketogenesis

348. Which of the following statements about prostaglandins is true?

a. They are precursors to arachidonic acid
b. They release arachidonic acid from membranes through the action of phospholipase A
c. They were first observed to cause uterine contraction and lowering of blood pressure
d. Although found in many organs, they are synthesized only in the prostate and seminal vesicles
e. They may be converted to leukotrienes by lipoxygenase

349. Which of the following hormones promotes hypoglycemia?

a. Epinephrine
b. Norepinephrine
c. Insulin
d. Glucagon
e. Glucocorticoids

350. The absorption of glucose from the gut into intestinal mucosal cells is coupled to Na^+,K^+-ATPase. In contrast, the movement of glucose from the intestinal epithelial cells into the submucosal bloodstream occurs through passive transport. Given these facts, which of the following statements can be true at one time or another?

a. Cytosolic levels of glucose in intestinal mucosal cells are regulated by levels of glucose in skeletal muscle cells
b. Free glucose levels in the lumen of the intestine can never be higher than levels in intestinal cells
c. Plasma glucose levels are much higher than intestinal cell cytosolic levels of glucose
d. Levels of glucose in the intestinal lumen are always higher than those in the cytosol of intestinal epithelial cells
e. Levels of plasma glucose are approximately equal to levels in the cytosol of intestinal epithelial cells

351. Which of the following proteins is responsible for secretion of pancreatic juice into the intestine?

a. Cholecystokinin
b. Gastrin
c. Insulin
d. Intrinsic factor
e. Secretin

352. Which step in the diagram below is thought to be responsible for the effect of anti-inflammatory steroids?

a. Step A
b. Step B
c. Step C
d. Step D
e. Step E

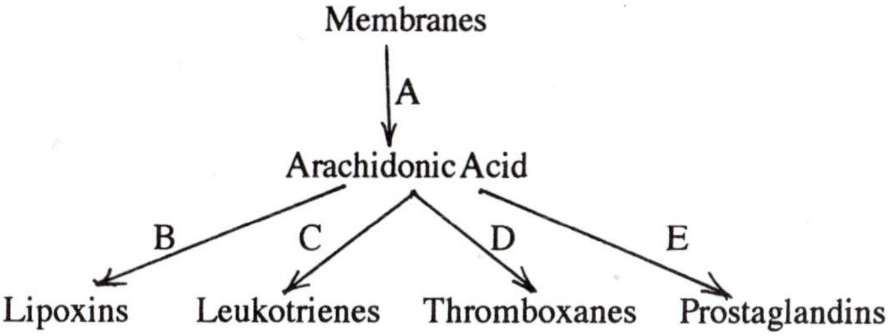

Membranes

|A
↓

Arachidonic Acid

B   C   D   E

Lipoxins   Leukotrienes   Thromboxanes   Prostaglandins

353. A compound normally used to conjugate bile acids is

a. Acetate
b. Glucuronic acid
c. Glutathione
d. Sulfate
e. Glycine

354. The reactions leading to the synthesis of squalene (C30) from dimethylallyl pyrophosphate (C5) are

a. Sequential condensation of five-carbon units
b. Sequential condensation, then cyclization, of five-carbon units
c. Sequential condensation of five-carbon-pyrophosphate units
d. Sequential condensation of 5-carbon units to 15-carbon units, then condensation of 15-carbon units
e. Sequential condensation of 5-carbon units to 10-carbon units, then sequential condensation of 10-carbon units

355. Which of the following effects of the steroid digitalis is observed after treatment of congestive heart failure?

a. Decrease in cytosolic sodium levels
b. Inhibition of Na^+,K^+-ATPase
c. Decrease in the force of heart muscle contraction
d. Stimulation of the plasma membrane ion pump
e. Decrease in cytosolic calcium

356. Which of the following involves isoprenoids?

a. The chromophore of visual pigments
b. Carnitine
c. Vitamin C
d. Thiamine
e. Ketone bodies

357. Aspirin inhibits which of the following enzymes?

a. Lipoprotein lipase
b. Lipoxygenase
c. Cyclooxygenase
d. Phospholipase D
e. Phospholipase A_2

358. Which of the following processes yields arachidonic (5,8,11,14-eicosatetraenoic) acid in mammals?

a. Elongation of stearic acid
b. Chain elongation and one desaturation of linolenic (9,12,15-octadecatrienoic) acid
c. Chain elongation and two desaturations of linoleic (9,12-octadecadienoic) acid
d. Desaturation of oleic acid
e. Elongation of palmitic acid

359. A patient stung by a bee is rushed into the emergency room with a variety of symptoms including increasing difficulty in breathing due to vasal and bronchial construction. While your subsequent treatment is to block the effects of histamine and other acute-phase reactants released by most cells, you must also block the slow-reacting substance of anaphylaxis (SRS-A), which is the most potent constrictor of the muscles enveloping the bronchial passages. What is SRS-A composed of?

a. Thromboxanes
b. Interleukins
c. Complement
d. Leukotrienes
e. Prostaglandins

360. Which of the following is an essential fatty acid?

a. Palmitic acid
b. Linoleic acid
c. Arachidonic acid
d. Oleic acid
e. Eicosatetraenoic acid

361. The central ring structure shown below is found in which of the following compounds?

a. Adrenocorticotropin
b. Aldosterone
c. Geranyl phosphate
d. Prostaglandin
e. Vitamin C

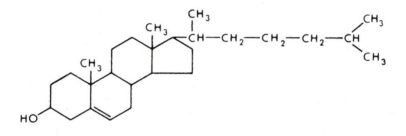

362. Which of the following compounds serves as a primary link between the citric acid cycle and the urea cycle?

a. Malate
b. Succinate
c. Isocitrate
d. Citrate
e. Fumarate

363. Which one of the following can be converted to an intermediate of either the citric acid cycle or the urea cycle?

a. Tyrosine
b. Lysine
c. Leucine
d. Tryptophan
e. Aspartate

364. Most major metabolic pathways are considered to be either mainly anabolic or catabolic. Which of the following pathways is most correctly considered to be amphibolic?

a. Lipolysis
b. Glycolysis
c. β oxidation of fatty acids
d. Citric acid cycle
e. Gluconeogenesis

365. Which one of the following products of protein metabolism is decreased below normal levels during the early stages of starvation?

a. Urea
b. Anabolic enzymes
c. CO_2
d. NH_4^+
e. Glucose

366. Which one of the following is a correct statement about the regulation and sequence of reactions in metabolic pathways?

a. The initial step in many pathways is a major determinant of control
b. The sequence of steps in catabolic pathways is usually the exact reverse of the biosynthetic sequence
c. Enzymes found in an anabolic pathway are rarely found in the corresponding catabolic pathway
d. A small set of large precursors serves as the starting point for most biosynthetic processes in energy metabolism
e. Steps in both anabolic and catabolic pathways are usually irreversible

367. Which one of the following statements is correct regarding the well-fed state?

a. NADPH production by the hexose monophosphate shunt is decreased
b. Acetoacetate is the major fuel for muscle
c. Glucose transport into adipose tissue is decreased
d. The major fuel used by the brain is glucose
e. Amino acids are utilized for glucose production

368. During an overnight fast, the major source of blood glucose is

a. Dietary glucose from the intestine
b. Hepatic glycogenolysis
c. Gluconeogenesis
d. Muscle glycogenolysis
e. Glycerol from lipolysis

369. The jinga bean, found in the jungles of Brazil, is unique in that it is composed almost exclusively of protein. Studies have shown that, immediately following a meal composed exclusively of jinga beans, which one of the following occurs?

a. A decreased release of epinephrine
b. A complete absence of liver glycogen
c. Hypoglycemia
d. An increased release of insulin
e. Ketosis caused by the metabolism of ketogenic amino acids

370. Approximately 3 h following a well-balanced meal, blood levels of which of the following are elevated?

a. Fatty acids
b. Glucagon
c. Glycerol
d. Epinephrine
e. Chylomicrons

371. If a homogenate of liver cells is centrifuged to remove all cell membranes and organelles, which of the following enzyme activities will remain in the homogenate?

a. Glucose-6-phosphate dehydrogenase
b. Glycogen synthetase
c. Aconitase
d. Acyl CoA hydratase
e. Hydroxybutyrate dehydrogenase

372. Which of the following descriptions of calcium is correct?

a. Calcium is abundant in the body as deposits of calcium sulfate
b. Calcium ion is required as a cofactor for many reactions
c. Calcium freely diffuses across the endoplasmic reticulum of muscle cells
d. Calcium is most highly concentrated in muscle
e. Calcium is mostly excreted by the kidney

373. Which of the following enzymes is active in adipocytes following a heavy meal?

a. Glycogen phosphorylase
b. Glycerol kinase
c. Hormone-sensitive triacylglyceride lipase
d. Glucose-6-phosphatase
e. Phosphatidate phosphatase

374. Which of the following tissues is capable of contributing to blood glucose?

a. Skeletal muscle
b. Adipose tissues
c. Cardiac muscle
d. Duodenal epithelium
e. Cartilage

375. Which of the following statements correctly describes metabolism?

a. Fatty acids can be precursors of glucose
b. High energy levels turn on glycolysis
c. Synthesis and degradation of a substance do not occur at the same time
d. Phosphorylation activates enzymes that store fat and glycogen
e. Guanosine triphosphate (GTP) is the major donor for enzyme phosphorylation

376. Which of the following is appropriate for a patient with renal failure?

a. High-carbohydrate diet
b. High-protein diet
c. Low-fat diet
d. High-fiber diet
e. Free water of at least 3 L per day

377. Which of the clinical conditions listed below can be associated with the malabsorption of iron?

a. Anemia
b. Tetany
c. Hyperchylomicronemia
d. Porphyria
e. Hemophilia

378. An adolescent presents with abdominal discomfort, abdominal fullness, excess gas, and weight loss. Blood glucose, cholesterol, and alkaline phosphatase levels are normal. There is no jaundice or elevations. The stool tests positive for reducing substances. Which of the clinical conditions listed below is the most likely diagnosis?

a. Diabetes mellitus
b. Starvation
c. Nontropical sprue
d. Milk intolerance
e. Gallstones

379. Which of the following diseases reflects the loss of ability to move specific molecules between membrane-separated cellular compartments?

a. McArdle's phosphorylase disease
b. Carnitine deficiency
c. Methanol poisoning
d. Ethylene glycol poisoning
e. Diphtheria

380. Which set of blood values most closely correlates with a patient who has conducted a hunger strike for 1 month?

		Concentration of Blood Fuels (mM)		
	Glucose	Free Fatty Acids	Ketone Bodies	Amino Acids
a.	2.00	3.0	10.00	5.0
b.	4.50	1.5	5.00	4.7
c.	12.00	2.0	10.00	4.5
d.	4.50	0.5	0.02	4.5
e.	4.49	2.0	8.00	3.1

Hormones and Integrated Metabolism

Answers

338. The answer is d. (*Murray, pp 505–626. Scriver, pp 4029–4240. Sack, pp 121–138. Wilson, pp 287–320.*) All steroid hormones, including the sex hormones estrogen, testosterone, and progesterone, act by binding specific cytoplasmic receptors, which then stimulate transcription by binding to specific sites on DNA. These hormones may be contrasted with most non-steroidal hormones, for example epinephrine, which interact with the cell membrane, causing a second-messenger effect. The latter hormones, in contrast to steroids, act in a matter of minutes, while steroid hormones take hours to have a biologic effect. Recent studies have indicated that specific cytoplasmic receptors for steroid hormones have an extraordinarily high affinity for the hormones. In addition, the receptors contain a DNA-binding region that is rich in amino acid residues that form metal binding fingers. Likewise, thyroid hormone receptors contain DNA-binding domains with metal binding fingers. Like steroid hormones, thyroid hormones are transcriptional enhancers.

339. The answer is e. (*Murray, pp 505–626. Scriver, pp 4029–4240. Sack, pp 121–138. Wilson, pp 287–320.*) In humans, both glucagon and epinephrine have been demonstrated to be capable of stimulating adenosine 3′,5′-cyclic monophosphate (cyclic AMP) production in liver, whereas only epinephrine and norepinephrine have been unequivocally shown to be agonists of cyclic AMP accumulation in adipocytes. In rat adipose tissue, glucagon and adrenocorticotropic hormone (ACTH), in addition to the catecholamines, also stimulate adenylate cyclase. The mode of hormone receptor stimulation of adenylate cyclase by epinephrine in both adipocytes and hepatocytes is thought to be basically the same. The primary difference between the two tissues lies in the ultimate physiologic response to the accumulation of second messenger and the mode of amplification. In the liver, cyclic AMP activates a protein kinase, which activates a phosphorylase kinase, which finally activates glycogen phosphorylase to turn on glycogenolysis. The cascade pathway is much simpler in adipose tissue, where cyclic AMP activates a protein kinase, which activates triglyceride lipase to turn on lipolysis of stored triacylglycerides.

340. The answer is d. (*Murray, pp 505–626. Scriver, pp 4029–4240. Sack, pp 121–138. Wilson, pp 287–320.*) A tumor of the adrenal cortex would be expected to affect the production of adrenal steroid hormone. Cortisol and aldosterone are synthesized in the cortex. In Cushing's syndrome, hypersecretion of cortisol occurs. Cortisol is a glucocorticoid that has the effect of encouraging metabolism of proteins, lipids, and carbohydrates. In some cases of Cushing's disease, excessive production of cortisol is due to high levels of ACTH produced as a result of pituitary tumors. Diseases affecting the adrenal medulla might be expected to disrupt or potentiate production of epinephrine in some way. Epinephrine (adrenalin) is synthesized in the medulla.

341. The answer is c. (*Murray, pp 505–626. Scriver, pp 4029–4240. Sack, pp 121–138. Wilson, pp 287–320.*) Vasopressin, which is also called antidiuretic hormone, increases the permeability of the collecting ducts and distal convoluted tubules of the kidney and thus allows passage of water. Like the mineralocorticoid aldosterone, vasopressin results in an expansion of blood volume. However, the mode of action of aldosterone is different; it causes sodium reabsorption, not water reabsorption. Sodium reabsorption indirectly leads to increased plasma osmolality and thus water retention in the blood. Cortisol is a glucocorticoid that potentiates catabolic metabolism chronically. Epinephrine stimulates catabolic metabolism acutely. Insulin acutely favors anabolic metabolism, in large part by allowing glucose and amino acid transport into cells.

342. The answer is d. (*Murray, pp 505–626. Scriver, pp 4029–4240. Sack, pp 121–138. Wilson, pp 287–320.*) Both cortisol and aldosterone contain C-21-hydroxyl groups. Both are also derived from progesterone in the adrenal cortex. In contrast, the sex hormones are synthesized in the ovaries and testicular interstitial cells. In the synthesis of sex hormones, progesterone is converted to 17α-hydroxyprogesterone and then androstenedione, which may either become estrone or testosterone. Testosterone gives rise to estradiol in the ovaries. In the corpus luteum, progesterone is produced.

343. The answer is e. (*Murray, pp 505–626. Scriver, pp 4029–4240. Sack, pp 121–138. Wilson, pp 287–320.*) The major problem in myasthenia gravis is a marked reduction of acetylcholine receptors on the motor endplate where cranial nerves form a neuromuscular junction with muscles. In these patients, autoantibodies against the acetylcholine receptors effectively reduce receptor numbers. Normally, acetylcholine molecules released by the nerve terminal bind to receptors on the muscle endplate, resulting in a stimulation of contraction by depolarizing the muscle membrane. The condition is improved with drugs that inhibit acetylcholinesterase.

344. The answer is a. (*Murray, pp 505–626. Scriver, pp 4029–4240. Sack, pp 121–138. Wilson, pp 287–320.*) Thyroid hormones raise serum glucose levels, but the mechanism is unknown. Epinephrine and glucagon lead to acute hyperglycemic effects by activating liver phosphorylase and the release of glucose from glycogen through a cyclic AMP cascade effect. Glucocorticoids stimulate the liver to produce more gluconeogenic enzymes and promote protein breakdown to form amino acids. Glucocorticoid (a steroid hormone) and thyroxine exert chronic effects and act by binding to intracellular binding proteins (receptors) that eventually act as enhancers of transcription. Epidermal growth factor receptor is similar to the insulin receptor in that it has a tyrosine kinase activity that is activated by the binding of growth factor to the extracellular portion of the protein. Epidermal growth factor does not cause hyperglycemia.

345. The answer is e. (*Murray, pp 505–626. Scriver, pp 4029–4240. Sack, pp 121–138. Wilson, pp 287–320.*) The action of insulin is antagonistic to that of glucagon, which is a catabolic hormone secreted by the α cells of the pancreas. The anabolic hormone called insulin is synthesized on the endoplasmic reticulum of pancreatic β cells as a nascent polypeptide chain called preproinsulin. Immediately following synthesis, the amino terminal signal sequence of 16 residues is cleaved off to form proinsulin. Proinsulin is composed of one continuous polypeptide that contains in sequence an A chain of 21 residues, a connecting peptide (C peptide) of about 30 residues, and a B chain of 30 residues. The molecule is folded so that two disulfide bridges span the A and B chains. The proinsulin molecule is transported from the lumen of the endoplasmic reticulum to the Golgi apparatus, where it is packaged into storage granules. In the Golgi apparatus and in the storage granules, proteolysis of the C peptide occurs. Exocytosis of the granules releases insulin as well as C peptides into the bloodstream. Neither proinsulin nor the C peptide is biologically active.

346. The answer is c. *(Murray, pp 505–626. Scriver, pp 4029–4240. Sack, pp 121–138. Wilson, pp 287–320.)* Gluconeogenesis is a catabolic process for the synthesis of glucose, mainly from the amino acids of degraded proteins. Gluconeogenesis is the adaptive response of the organism to low blood levels of glucose and is, therefore, diminished by insulin. Insulin allows the disposition and utilization of glucose, particularly exogenous glucose. High blood glucose signals pancreatic β cells to secrete insulin. Under these conditions, insulin stimulates the entry of glucose and amino acids into a variety of tissues, including muscle and fat cells. The presence of glucose allows the anabolic processes of glucose oxidation, lipogenesis, and the synthesis of macromolecular precursors, such as nucleotides, to be carried out.

347. The answer is a. *(Murray, pp 505–626. Scriver, pp 4029–4240. Sack, pp 121–138. Wilson, pp 287–320.)* The actions of epinephrine (adrenaline) and norepinephrine are catabolic; that is, these catecholamines are antagonistic to the anabolic functions of insulin and, like glucagon, are secreted in response to low blood glucose or during "fight or flight" stress. Glycolysis is an anabolic process that is decreased in the presence of elevated catecholamines. Unlike glucagon, which only acts on the liver, the catecholamines affect most tissues, including liver and muscle. The catabolic processes increased by secretion of epinephrine and norepinephrine include glycogenolysis, gluconeogenesis, lipolysis, and ketogenesis. Thus, products that increase blood sugar or spare it, such as ketone bodies and fatty acids, are increased.

348. The answer is c. *(Murray, pp 505–626. Scriver, pp 4029–4240. Sack, pp 121–138. Wilson, pp 287–320.)* Although prostaglandins were originally isolated from prostate glands, seminal vesicles, and semen, their synthesis in other organs has been amply documented; indeed, few organs have failed to demonstrate prostaglandin release. Prostaglandins cause platelet aggregation, smooth-muscle contraction, vasodilation, and uterine contraction. Prostaglandins are synthesized from arachidonic acid, a 20-carbon fatty acid with interspersed carbon double bonds. Signals such as angiotensin II, bradykinin, epinephrine, and thrombin can activate phospholipase A_2 and release arachidonic acid from membrane lipids. The arachidonic acid is cyclized by cyclooxygenase to form prostaglandins. Arachidonic acid can also be oxidized to leukotrienes by the action of lipoxygenases.

349. The answer is c. *(Murray, pp 505–626. Scriver, pp 4029–4240. Sack, pp 121–138. Wilson, pp 287–320.)* Insulin promotes glucose uptake by cells to lower blood glucose levels and facilitates amino acid entry into cells, which lowers the amino acid supply available for gluconeogenesis. Both glucagon and epinephrine are antagonists of insulin. They raise blood glucose levels by stimulating glycogenolysis via cyclic AMP mediation. Glucagon acts specifically on the liver and kidneys, whereas epinephrine can stimulate these tissues as well as skeletal muscle and adipocytes. The 11-hydroxy,C-21 adrenocortical steroids known as glucocorticoids promote increased blood levels by being permissive to the actions of glucagon and epinephrine; that is, they promote protein and amino acid degradation to oxaloacetate and pyruvate, which are substrates for gluconeogenesis. In addition, glucocorticoids induce liver production of gluconeogenic enzymes. Hence, by acute stimulation as well as by adaptive changes, glycogenolytic hormones and the glucocorticoids promote hyperglycemia.

350. The answer is e. *(Murray, pp 505–626. Scriver, pp 4029–4240. Sack, pp 121–138. Wilson, pp 287–320.)* The plasma membranes of intestinal epithelial cells contain a sodium gradient that drives the active transport of glucose. The rate and amount of glucose transported depend upon the sodium gradient maintained across the plasma membrane. Sodium ions entering the cell in the company of glucose are pumped out again by Na^+,K^+-ATPase. Once in the cytosol of the intestinal cell, the glucose moves across the cell and diffuses out of the cell into the interstitial fluid of the submucosa and then into the plasma of the capillaries underlying the intestinal epithelium. This occurs for the following reason: while glucose is maintained in blood plasma at an approximately constant level, it is always slowly moving out of the plasma into the cells of tissue that use it. Given that the diffusion from the intestinal cells into the plasma is passive, the intestinal cells and the plasma try to maintain an equilibrium. Thus, plasma glucose levels are always approximately equal to or slightly less than levels in the intestinal cells. Due to the passive maintenance of this equilibrium, it is highly unlikely that the concentration of glucose in the plasma can get much higher than that in the intestinal cell cytosol. It is also unlikely that the levels of glucose in other tissues of the body (for example, muscle) will have any bearing on those found in the intestinal cells.

351. The answer is e. *(Murray, pp 505–626. Scriver, pp 4029–4240. Sack, pp 121–138. Wilson, pp 287–320.)* Secretin, a circulatory hormone liberated in response to peptides or acid in the duodenum, stimulates the flow of pancreatic juice. Gastrin governs acid production by the stomach, and cholecystokinin causes the gallbladder to contract. Cholecystokinin stimulates this contraction after it is released by the duodenum into the circulation, with subsequent emptying of bile into the intestine. The C-terminal octapeptide of cholecystokinin is more than five times as potent as the parent hormone, and its C-terminal pentapeptide is identical to gastrin. Gastrin, produced in specialized cells of the antral mucosa of the stomach, stimulates parietal cells to produce HCl (approximately 0.16 M) and KCl (0.007 M); it also stimulates secretion of glucagon and insulin. Production of gastrin is inhibited by secretin.

352. The answer is a. *(Murray, pp 505–626. Scriver, pp 4029–4240. Sack, pp 121–138. Wilson, pp 287–320.)* The evidence indicates that anti-inflammatory steroids inhibit phospholipase A_2, which is responsible for hydrolyzing arachidonate off of membrane phospholipids. Corticosteroids and their manufactured derivatives are thought to cause induction of the phospholipase A_2–inhibitory protein lipocortin. In this manner, production of all of the derivatives of arachidonic acid (lipoxins, leukotrienes, thromboxanes, and prostaglandins) is shut off. In contrast, nonsteroidal anti-inflammatory agents such as aspirin, indomethacin, and ibuprofen act by inhibiting the cyclooxygenase component of prostaglandin synthase. The synthase is responsible for the first step in the production of prostaglandins (step E) and thromboxanes (step D) from arachidonic acid. The lipoxygenase pathway leads to the synthesis of lipoxins (step B) and leukotrienes (step C).

353. The answer is e. *(Murray, pp 505–626. Scriver, pp 4029–4240. Sack, pp 121–138. Wilson, pp 287–320.)* Bile acids often are conjugated with glycine to form glycocholic acid and with taurine to form taurocholic acid. In human bile, glycocholic acid is by far the more common. The presence of the charged carboxyl group of glycine or the charged sulfate of taurine adds to the hydrophilic nature of the bile acids, thereby increasing their ability to emulsify lipids during the digestive process. Glucuronic acid is used to conjugate bilirubin and many xenobiotics (foreign chemicals), such as polychlorinated biphenyls (PCBs) and insecticides. A hydroxyl group is added to the xenobiotic by the cytochrome P450 system, then conjugated with glucuronide, sulfate, acetate, or glutathione to make it water-soluble for excretion in urine.

354. The answer is d. (*Murray, pp 505–626. Scriver, pp 4029–4240. Sack, pp 121–138. Wilson, pp 287–320.*) In the first stage of cholesterol formation, acetyl coenzyme A condenses to form mevalonate, which is then phosphorylated and decarboxylated to form isopentenyl pyrophosphate. Half of the isopentenyl pyrophosphate isomerizes to form dimethylallyl pyrophosphate. These two isomeric C5 pyrophosphate units (isopentenyl pyrophosphate and dimethylallyl pyrophosphate) condense to form a C10 compound called geranyl pyrophosphate. Isopentenyl pyrophosphate then condenses with geranyl pyrophosphate to form the C15 compound farnesyl pyrophosphate. Finally, two farnesyl pyrophosphates condense in the presence of NADPH to form the C30 compound squalene. Squalene is ultimately cyclized through a series of steps to form cholesterol. Thus, the correct sequence of events leading from C5 units to C30 squalene is sequential condensation of 5-carbon units until a 15-carbon unit is formed, then condensation of two 15-carbon units to form squalene.

355. The answer is b. (*Murray, pp 505–626. Scriver, pp 4029–4240. Sack, pp 121–138. Wilson, pp 287–320.*) Treatment of patients with congestive heart failure is often based on the use of cardiotonic steroids such as digitalis. Digitalis is derived from the foxglove plant and has been used as an herbal treatment for heart problems since ancient times. Digitalis and ouabain are cardiotonic steroids that inhibit the Na^+,K^+-ATPase pump located in the plasma membrane of cardiac muscle cells. They specifically inhibit the dephosphorylation reaction of the ATPase when the cardiotonic steroid is bound to the extracellular face of the membrane. Due to inhibition of the pump, higher levels of sodium are left inside the cell, leading to a diminished sodium gradient. This results in a slower exchange of calcium by the sodium-calcium exchanger. Subsequently, intracellular levels of calcium are maintained at a higher level and greatly enhance the force of contraction of cardiac muscle.

356. The answer is a. (*Murray, pp 505–626. Scriver, pp 4029–4240. Sack, pp 121–138. Wilson, pp 287–320.*) In mammals, β-carotene is the precursor of retinal, which is the basic chromophore of all visual pigments. Isopentenyl pyrophosphate and dimethylallyl pyrophosphate are isoprenoid isomers formed from the repeated condensation of acetyl CoA units. By continued condensation in mammalian systems, cholesterol can be formed. In plant systems, carotenoids are formed. In addition to producing the color of tomatoes and carrots, carotenoids serve as the light-absorbing molecules of photosynthesis. Ketone bodies are derived from condensation of acetyl CoA units but not from isoprenoid units. Vitamin C (ascorbic acid), carnitine, and thiamine (vitamin B_1) are not derived from isoprenoid units.

357. The answer is c. (*Murray, pp 505–626. Scriver, pp 4029–4240. Sack, pp 121–138. Wilson, pp 287–320.*) During the synthesis of prostaglandins, a specific fatty acid is released from the $2'$ position of membrane phospholipids by the action of phospholipase A_2. After its release, the fatty acid can enter either the lipoxygenase pathway, which produces acid with an unknown biologic function, or the prostaglandin cyclooxygenase (also called prostaglandin synthetase) pathway. In the formation of prostaglandins from fatty acids, cyclooxygenase catalyzes formation of a cyclopentane ring and the introduction of three oxygen atoms. The type of prostaglandin produced depends on the starting fatty acid, which is always a derivative of an essential fatty acid. Eicosatrienoic acid yields series 1 prostaglandins, eicosatetraenoic (arachidonic) acid yields series 2 prostaglandins, and eicosapentaenoic acid yields series 3 prostaglandins. Aspirin, like indomethacin, decreases prostaglandin synthesis by inhibiting the oxygenase activity of cyclooxygenase.

358. The answer is c. (*Murray, pp 505–626. Scriver, pp 4029–4240. Sack, pp 121–138. Wilson, pp 287–320.*) In mammals, arachidonic (5,8,11,15-eicosatetraenoic) acid can only be synthesized from essential fatty acids derived from the diet. Linoleic (9,12-octadecadienoic) acid produces arachidonic acid following two desaturations and chain elongation. While linolenic (9,12,15-octadecatrienoic) acid also is an essential fatty acid, desaturation and elongation produce 8,11,14,17-eicosatetraenoic acid, which is distinct from arachidonic acid. Oleic, palmitic, and stearic acids are all nonessential fatty acids that cannot give rise to arachidonic acids in mammals.

359. The answer is d. (*Murray, pp 505–626. Scriver, pp 4029–4240. Sack, pp 121–138. Wilson, pp 287–320.*) Leukotrienes C_4, D_4, and E_4 together compose the slow-reacting substance of anaphylaxis (SRS-A), which is thought to be the cause of asphyxiation in individuals not treated rapidly enough following an anaphylactic shock. SRS-A is up to 1000 times more effective than histamines in causing bronchial muscle constriction. Anti-inflammatory steroids are usually given intravenously to end chronic bronchoconstriction and hypotension following a shock. The steroids block phospholipase A_2 action, preventing the synthesis of leukotrienes from arachidonic acid. Acute treatment involves epinephrine injected subcutaneously initially and then intravenously. Antihistamines such as diphenhydramine are administered intravenously or intramuscularly.

360. The answer is b. (*Murray, pp 505–626. Scriver, pp 4029–4240. Sack, pp 121–138. Wilson, pp 287–320.*) The essential fatty acid linoleic acid, with 18 carbons and two double bonds at carbons 9 and 18 (C-18:2-$\Delta^{9,12}$) is desaturated to form α-linolenic acid (C-18:3-$\Delta^{6,9,12}$), which is sequentially elongated and desaturated to form eicosatrienoic acid (C-20:3-$\Delta^{8,11,14}$) and arachidonic acid (C-20:4-$\Delta^{5,8,11,14}$), respectively. Many of the eicosanoids (20-carbon compounds)—prostaglandins, thromboxanes, and leukotrienes—are derived from arachidonic acid. The scientific name of arachidonic acid is eicosatetraenoic acid. Arachidonic acid can only be synthesized from essential fatty acids obtained from the diet. Palmitic acid (C-16:0) and oleic acid (C-18:1-Δ^9) can be synthesized by the tissues.

361. The answer is b. (*Murray, pp 505–626. Scriver, pp 4029–4240. Sack, pp 121–138. Wilson, pp 287–320.*) Steroid hormones such as aldosterone are ultimate derivatives of cholesterol. The compound illustrated in the question is cholesterol, one of a large group of steroids. Cholesterol, which can be derived from the diet as well as synthesized de novo, is the precursor of all steroids involved in mammalian metabolism. These include the bile acids, the steroid hormones, and vitamin D. Cholesterol cannot be metabolized to carbon dioxide and water in humans. It must be excreted as a component of bile. Adrenocorticotropin (ACTH) is a peptide hormone of the adenohypophysis that influences the secretion of corticosteroid hormones. Prostaglandins are eicosanoid derivatives that are also made up of isoprene units. Geranyl phosphate is a 2-isoprenoid unit precursor in cholesterol synthesis.

362. The answer is e. *(Murray, pp 505–626. Scriver, pp 4029–4240. Sack, pp 121–138. Wilson, pp 287–320.)* All the compounds listed are intermediates of the citric acid cycle. However, only fumarate is an intermediate of both the citric acid and urea cycles. It and arginine are produced from argininosuccinate. Once produced by the urea cycle, fumarate enters the citric acid cycle and is converted to malate and then oxidized to oxaloacetate. Depending upon the organism's needs, oxaloacetate can either enter gluconeogenesis or react with acetyl CoA to form citrate.

363. The answer is e. *(Murray, pp 505–626. Scriver, pp 4029–4240. Sack, pp 121–138. Wilson, pp 287–320.)* Aspartate is a glucogenic amino acid that is also used to carry NH_4^+ into the urea cycle. Aspartate aminotransferase catalyzes the direct transamination of aspartate to oxaloacetate:

$$\text{aspartate} + \alpha\text{-ketoglutarate} \rightarrow \text{oxaloacetate} + \text{glutamate}$$

Oxaloacetate may either be utilized in the citric acid cycle or undergo gluconeogenesis. Argininosuccinate synthetase catalyzes the condensation of citrulline and aspartate to form argininosuccinate:

$$\text{citrulline} + \text{asparate} + \text{ATP} \rightarrow \text{argininosuccinate} + \text{AMP} + \text{PP}_i$$

In this manner, one of the two nitrogens of urea is introduced into the urea cycle.

364. The answer is d. *(Murray, pp 505–626. Scriver, pp 4029–4240. Sack, pp 121–138. Wilson, pp 287–320.)* In general, the corresponding pathways of catabolism and anabolism are not identical (glycolysis versus gluconeogenesis, lipolysis and β oxidation of fatty acids versus fatty acid synthesis and lipogenesis, glycogenolysis versus glycogenesis). However, the citric acid cycle is a central pathway from which anabolic precursors of biosynthetic reactions may derive or into which the complete catabolism of small molecules to carbon dioxide and water may occur. For these reasons, the citric acid cycle is often called an amphibolic pathway.

365. The answer is b. *(Murray, pp 505–626. Scriver, pp 4029–4240. Sack, pp 121–138. Wilson, pp 287–320.)* During the early phases of starvation, the catabolism of proteins is at its highest level. Anabolic enzymes, which are not utilized during starvation, are degraded and their synthesis is repressed. The deamination of amino acids for gluconeogenesis and ketogenesis results in a negative nitrogen balance. Hence, ammonia and urea levels in the urine exceed normal values. The glucose formed from gluconeogenic amino acids becomes the major source of blood glucose following depletion of liver glycogen stores. Complete oxidation of this glucose, as well as the ketone bodies formed from ketogenic amino acids, leads to a relative increase in the CO_2 and H_2O formed from amino acid carbon skeletons.

366. The answer is a. *(Murray, pp 505–626. Scriver, pp 4029–4240. Sack, pp 121–138. Wilson, pp 287–320.)* Although the same intermediates may appear in both anabolic and catabolic pathways, one path is not simply the reverse of the other, because irreversible enzymatic steps often occur in the beginning of the reaction sequence. However, many steps in both anabolic and catabolic pathways are reversible. The same enzymes often appear in many metabolic pathways, but regulatory steps are irreversible. A number of small precursors serve as the building blocks of anabolism, while large energy-storage molecules such as glycogen, lipids, and proteins give rise to smaller molecules during catabolic processes.

367. The answer is d. *(Murray, pp 505–626. Scriver, pp 4029–4240. Sack, pp 121–138. Wilson, pp 287–320.)* Glucose is the major fuel for the brain in the well-fed state. The brain requires a continuous supply of glucose at all times. In fact, if glucose drops to a low level, convulsions may follow. However, during starvation or fasting, the brain is capable of obtaining approximately 75% of its energy from circulating ketone bodies. During the absorptive phase, ketone bodies such as acetoacetate and 3-hydroxybutyrate are low. Circulating amino acids are utilized for protein synthesis. Liver production of NADPH is at a high level because it is needed for fatty acid synthesis. Glucose is actively transported into all cells, including adipocytes, which require it to form glucose-3-phosphate for esterifying fatty acids into triacylglyceride.

368. The answer is b. *(Murray, pp 505–626. Scriver, pp 4029–4240. Sack, pp 121–138. Wilson, pp 287–320.)* In the absorptive phase following a meal, the major source of glucose is glucose taken directly from the intestine into the blood system. Much of this glucose is absorbed into cells and, in particular, into the liver via the action of insulin, where it is stored as glycogen. Once the effects of daytime eating have subsided and all the glucose from absorption has been stored, the normal overnight fast begins. During this period, the major source of blood glucose is hepatic glycogen. Through the effects of glycogenolysis, which are mediated by glucagon, hepatic glycogen is slowly parceled out as glucose to the bloodstream, keeping blood glucose levels normal. In contrast, muscle glycogenolysis has no effect on blood glucose levels because no glucose-6-phosphatase exists in muscle and hence phosphorylated glucose cannot be released from muscle into the bloodstream. Following a more prolonged fast or in the early stages of starvation, gluconeogenesis is needed to produce glucose from glucogenic amino acids and the glycerol released by lipolysis of triacylglycerides in adipocytes. This is because the liver glycogen is depleted and the liver is forced to turn to gluconeogenesis to produce the amounts of glucose necessary to maintain blood levels.

369. The answer is a. *(Murray, pp 505–626. Scriver, pp 4029–4240. Sack, pp 121–138. Wilson, pp 287–320.)* High blood levels of amino acids, in addition to glucose, promote the release of insulin through their action on receptors at the surface of the β cells of the pancreas. While insulin alone could lead to a hypoglycemic effect, hypoglycemia should not be observed because glucagon is also released in response to the elevated levels of circulating amino acids. The balance of glucagon and glucose tends to keep blood levels of glucose within normal ranges while amino acid transport into cells is promoted. Due to the normal insulin levels in the fed state, ketosis and depletion of liver glycogen are not observed. Both of these events occur during fasting and starvation due to the abundance of glucagon and epinephrine in the blood as opposed to the low levels of insulin.

370. The answer is a. *(Murray, pp 505–626. Scriver, pp 4029–4240. Sack, pp 121–138. Wilson, pp 287–320.)* Following digestion, the products of digestion enter the bloodstream. These include glucose, amino acids, triacylglycerides packaged into chylomicrons from the intestine, and very-low-density lipoproteins from the liver. The hormone of anabolism, insulin, is also elevated because of the signaling of the glucose and amino acids in the blood, which allows release of insulin from the β cells of the pancreas. Insulin aids the movement of glucose and amino acids into cells. In contrast, all the hormones and energy sources associated with catabolism are decreased in the blood during this time. Long-chain fatty acids and glycerol released by lipolysis from adipocytes are not elevated. Glucagon and epinephrine are not released. The only time glucose levels rise significantly above approximately 80 mM is following a well-balanced meal when glucose is obtained from the diet. The concentration of glucose reaches a peak 30 to 45 min after a meal and returns to normal within 2 h after eating. This response of blood glucose after eating (mimicked by giving 50 g of oral glucose) is the basis for the glucose tolerance test. In the event of insulin deficiency (diabetes mellitus), the peak glucose concentration is abnormally high and its return to normal is delayed.

371. The answer is a. (*Murray, pp 505–626. Scriver, pp 4029–4240. Sack, pp 121–138. Wilson, pp 287–320.*) Centrifugation of a cellular homogenate at a force of 100,000 × g will pellet all cellular organelles and membranes. Only soluble cellular molecules found in the cytosol will remain in the supernatant. Thus, the enzymes of glycolysis and most of those of gluconeogenesis, fatty acid synthesis, and the pentose phosphate pathway will be in the supernatant. Glucose-6-phosphate dehydrogenase, which results in the formation of 6-phosphoglucono-δ-lactone from glucose-6-phosphate, is the committed step in the pentose phosphate pathway. In the pellet will be the enzymes within mitochondria, including those of the citric acid cycle (aconitase), fatty acid β oxidation (acyl CoA hydratase), and ketogenesis (hydroxybutyrate dehydrogenase). Enzymes of glycogen degradation and synthesis (glycogen synthetase) will also be in the pellet associated with glycogen particles.

372. The answer is b. (*Murray, pp 505–626. Scriver, pp 4029–4240. Sack, pp 121–138. Wilson, pp 287–320.*) Calcium ions and calcium deposits are virtually universal in the structure and function of living things. In humans, calcium ions are required for the activity of many enzymes. Calcium is taken up from the gut in the presence of forms of vitamin D, such as cholecalciferol. Calcium is also primarily excreted through the intestine. When soluble, it is present as a divalent cation. When insoluble, it is found as hydroxyapatite (calcium phosphate) in bone. It is required by muscle cells for contraction and is sequestered into the sarcoplasmic reticulum during relaxation. It is actively transported by a calcium-ATPase across the sarcoplasmic reticulum.

373. The answer is e. *(Murray, pp 505–626. Scriver, pp 4029–4240. Sack, pp 121–138. Wilson, pp 287–320.)* The enzyme phosphatidate phosphatase converts phosphatidic acid to diacylglycerol during synthesis of triacylglycerides. The function of adipose tissue is the storage of fatty acids as triacylglycerols in times of plenty and the release of fatty acids during times of fasting or starvation. Fatty acids taken in by adipocytes are stored by esterification to glycerol-3-phosphate. Glycerol-3-phosphate is derived almost entirely from the glycolytic intermediate dihydroxyacetone phosphate through the action of glycerol-3-phosphate dehydrogenase. Glycolytic enzymes are active in adipocytes during triglyceride synthesis, but those of glycogen degradation (low levels in adipocytes) and gluconeogenesis (i.e., glucose-6-phosphatase) are not. Glycerol kinase is not present to any great extent in adipocytes, so that glycerol freed during lipolysis is not used to reesterify the fatty acids being released. The enzyme triacylglyceride lipase is turned on by phosphorylation by a cyclic AMP–dependent protein kinase following epinephrine stimulation.

374. The answer is d. *(Murray, pp 505–626. Scriver, pp 4029–4240. Sack, pp 121–138. Wilson, pp 287–320.)* Although the liver is the major site of the formation of free glucose to maintain blood glucose levels, the kidneys and intestinal epithelium (e.g., duodenum, jejunum, and ileum) may also release glucose. All of these tissues contain the enzyme glucose-6-phosphatase, an endoplasmic reticulum enzyme that dephosphorylates glucose and allows it to be transferred out of the cells. No other tissues in mammals contain this enzyme.

375. The answer is c. *(Murray, pp 505–626. Scriver, pp 4029–4240. Sack, pp 121–138. Wilson, pp 287–320.)* There are certain properties of metabolism that are considered truisms. (1) Futile cycles involving useless synthesis and degradation of a fuel do not occur simultaneously. (2) Acetyl CoA or substances that produce it, such as fatty acids or ketogenic amino acids, cannot be precursors of glucose. (3) ATP is a major phosphate donor and energy source; it must be present in cells at all times in order for them to function. (4) Protein phosphorylation inactivates enzymes that store glycogen and fat and activates enzymes that increase blood glucose and fatty acids. (5) Low blood glucose stimulates gluconeogenesis and glycogenolysis. (6) Low energy levels stimulate glycolysis and lipolysis. (7) High energy levels inhibit glycolysis and β oxidation of fatty acids.

GTP can be a phosphate donor in reactions such as that catalyzed by phosphoenopyruvate carboxykinase during gluconeogenesis. However, ATP is more commonly used. GTP plays important roles as the energy donor for protein synthesis and in allosteric regulation/covalent modification of the G proteins involved in signal transduction.

376. The answer is a. (*Murray, pp 505–626. Scriver, pp 4029–4240. Sack, pp 121–138. Wilson, pp 287–320.*) A diet high in carbohydrate and fats spares glucose use and inhibits gluconeogenesis, thereby preventing protein catabolism and nitrogen production. A major function of the kidneys is to excrete nitrogen catabolized from proteins in the form of urea. Indeed, the major clinical measures of renal function are products of protein catabolism [blood urea nitrogen (BUN) and blood creatinine]. A diet for a patient with renal failure should therefore minimize protein and nitrogen load. Although 3 L/day of fluid is a normal intake for adults with healthy kidneys, glomerular filtration and water excretion are decreased in renal failure. Water and salt intake (particularly potassium) must therefore be limited in renal failure. Excess water or salt intake in patients with renal disease is manifest clinically by edema (swollen eyelids, swollen lower limbs).

377. The answer is a. (*Murray, pp 505–626. Scriver, pp 4029–4240. Sack, pp 121–138. Wilson, pp 287–320.*) Malabsorption of iron, vitamin B_{12}, or folate can be associated with anemia. Iron-deficiency anemia due to poor diet or improper uptake and/or utilization is diagnosed quite frequently. Due to blood losses during menstruation, adult women are more likely than other people to have iron-deficiency anemia. In this condition, transferrin, the iron-binding protein in plasma, is less than one-third saturated. Tetany is caused by calcium deficiency, producing muscle spasms and cramps. In the several types of porphyria, defects in heme synthesis produce excess porphyrins. The symptoms range from abdominal pain to unusual rashes and behavioral abnormalities. The hemophilias are bleeding disorders caused by clotting factor deficiencies, and hyperchylomicronemia occurs in lipoprotein lipase deficiency.

378. The answer is d. (*Murray, pp 505–626. Scriver, pp 4029–4240. Sack, pp 121–138. Wilson, pp 287–320.*) Milk intolerance may be due to milk protein allergies during infancy, but it is commonly caused by lactase deficiency in older individuals. Intestinal lactase hydrolyzes the milk sugar lactose into galactose and glucose, both reducing sugars that can be detected as reducing substances in the stool. The symptoms of lactose intolerance (lactase deficiency) and other conditions involving intestinal malabsorption include diarrhea, cramps, and flatulence due to water retention and bacterial action in the gut. In nontropical sprue, symptoms seem to result from the production of antibodies in the blood against fragments of wheat gluten. It seems likely that a defect in intestinal epithelial cells allows tryptic peptides from the digestion of gluten to be absorbed into the blood, as well as to exert a harmful effect on intestinal epithelia.

Gallbladder inflammation (cholecystitis) usually presents with acute abdominal pain (colic) with radiation to the right shoulder. The normal composition of bile is about 5% cholesterol, 15% phosphatidylcholine, and 80% bile salt in a micellar liquid form. Increased cholesterol from high-fat diets or genetic conditions can upset the delicate micellar balance, leading to supersaturated cholesterol or cholesterol precipitates that cause gallstone formation. Removal of the gallbladder is a common treatment for this painful condition.

Mobilization of fats with the production of ketone bodies occurs during fasting and starvation, but ketone production is well controlled. During uncontrolled diabetes mellitus, ketogenesis proceeds at a rate that exceeds the buffering capacity of the blood to produce ketoacidosis.

379. The answer is b. (*Murray, pp 505–626. Scriver, pp 4029–4240. Sack, pp 121–138. Wilson, pp 287–320.*) A deficiency in carnitine, carnitine acyltransferase I, carnitine acyltransferase II, or acylcarnitine translocase can lead to an inability to oxidize long-chain fatty acids. This occurs because all of these components are needed to translocate activated long-chain (>10 carbons long) fatty acyl CoA across mitochondrial inner membrane into the matrix where β oxidation takes place. Once long-chain fatty acids are coupled to the sulfur atom of CoA on the outer mitochondrial membrane, they can be transferred to carnitine by the enzyme carnitine acyltransferase I, which is located on the cytosolic side of the inner mitochondrial membrane. Acyl carnitine is transferred across the inner membrane to the matrix surface by translocase. At this point the acyl group is reattached to a CoA sulfhydryl by the carnitine acyltransferase II located on the matrix face of the inner mitochondrial membrane.

McArdle's disease (deficiency of muscle glycogen phosphorylase) is one of several glycogen storage diseases. Muscle cramping and fatigue after exercise are characteristics of muscle glycogen storage diseases (types V and VII), while hypoglycemia, hyperuricemia, and liver disease are characteristics of liver glycogen storage diseases (types I, III, IV, VI, and VIII).

Wood alcohol (methanol) is a cause of death or serious illness (including blindness) among patients who ignorantly substitute it for ethanol or mistakenly ingest it. Ingestion of automotive antifreeze (ethylene glycol) can also result in death if not treated. In both cases, death or serious injury can be averted by quickly administering an intoxicating dose of ethanol. The success of this treatment is based upon the fact that methanol and ethylene glycol are not poisons as such. First, they must be converted by the action of the enzyme alcohol dehydrogenase to precursors of potentially toxic substances. Administration of large doses of ethanol inhibits oxidation of both methanol and ethylene glycol by effectively competing as a preferred substrate for the active sites of alcohol dehydrogenase. Over time, methanol and ethylene glycol are excreted.

One of the primary killers of children prior to immunization was upper respiratory tract infections by *Corynebacterium diphtheriae*. Toxin produced by a lysogenic phage that is carried by some strains of this bacteria causes the lethal effects. It is lethal in small amounts because it blocks protein synthesis. The viral toxin is composed of two parts. The B portion binds a cell's surface and injects the A portion into the cytosol of cells. The A portion ADP-ribosylates a histidine-derived residue of the elongation factor 2 (EF-2) known as diphthamide. This action completely blocks the ability of EF-2 to translocate the growing polypeptide chain.

380. The answer is e. *(Murray, pp 505–626. Scriver, pp 4029–4240. Sack, pp 121–138. Wilson, pp 287–320.)* In a normal postabsorptive patient, blood fuel values are 4.5 mM glucose, 0.5 mM free fatty acids, 0.02 mM ketone bodies, and 4.5 mM amino acids (choice d). Levels of ketone bodies are always low in a fed person. Following several days of starvation, a catabolic homeostasis has set in, such that free fatty acids (1.5 mM) have risen and production of ketone bodies (5 mM) by the liver is proceeding (choice b). At this point, glycogen stores have been depleted. Much of the blood glucose, which is maintained at about 4.5 mM throughout starvation, now comes from gluconeogenesis using increased concentrations of amino acids (4.7 mM) derived from protein breakdown. Most of the brain's fuel supply still derives from glucose at this time. Since the brain accounts for at least 20% of the body's total consumption of fuel, this amount can be considerable. Following prolonged starvation, utilization of glucose and hence catabolism of protein are spared by the induction of increased amounts of brain enzymes to utilize ketone bodies. Thus, in prolonged starvation, the blood concentration of amino acids (3.1 mM) decreases, whereas that of free fatty acids (2 mM) and ketone bodies (8 mM) increases (choice e). Of course, blood glucose is maintained at about 4.5 mM. The lack of insulin in diabetics causes a stimulation of lipolysis, glycogenolysis, gluconeogenesis, and ketogenesis. Thus, the blood values of free fatty acids (2 mM), ketone bodies (10 mM), and amino acids (4.5 mM) should resemble those of a fasting or starving person with one major exception—the high level of blood glucose [12 mM (choice c)]. The lack of insulin does not allow the glucose to enter most cells.

Inheritance Mechanisms and Biochemical Genetics

Inheritance Mechanisms/Risk Calculations

Questions

DIRECTIONS: Each item below contains a question or incomplete statement followed by suggested responses. Select the **one best** response to each question.

381. The age of onset of a degenerative neurologic disease is 35. Epidemiologic study of affected persons indicates that most cases occur in the spring, are isolated (i.e., no neighbors or relatives are affected), and occur equally in men and women. However, a subset of cases consists of two affected siblings in a family. The best description of this disease is

a. Inherited
b. Genetic
c. Sporadic
d. Congenital
e. Familial

382. Juvenile diabetes mellitus is a disorder of carbohydrate metabolism caused by insulin deficiency. The disease often follows a viral infection with inflammation of the pancreatic β cells, but also exhibits genetic predisposition with a 40 to 50% concordance rate in monozygous twins and clustering in families. Juvenile diabetes mellitus is best described as a

a. Congenital disorder
b. Multifactorial disorder
c. Mendelian disorder
d. Sporadic disorder
e. Sex-limited disorder

383. Which phrase best defines the genetic disease category of multifactorial inheritance?

a. Mendelian inheritance
b. Mitochondrial inheritance
c. Most common type of human genetic disease
d. Major cause of miscarriages
e. Maternally derived

384. Assuming that all alleles derive from a single locus, match the mating of an Aa father with an aa mother and their probabilities for genotypes in offspring.

a. 1 AA
b. ½ AA, ½ aa
c. ¼ AA, ½ Aa, ¼ aa
d. ½ AA, ½ Aa
e. ½ Aa, ½ aa

385. A couple has three girls, the last of whom is affected with cystic fibrosis. The first-born daughter marries her first cousin—that is, the son of her mother's sister—and they have a son with cystic fibrosis. The father has a female cousin with cystic fibrosis on his mother's side. Select the pedigree that best represents this family history from the diagrams below.

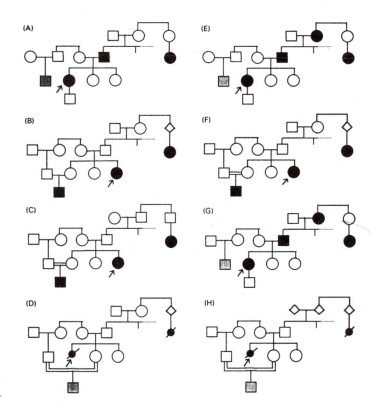

a. Diagram A
b. Diagram B
c. Diagram C
d. Diagram D
e. Diagram E
f. Diagram F
g. Diagram G
h. Diagram H

386. The standard karyotype is performed by photomicroscopy of cells at which mitotic stage?

a. Interphase
b. Prophase
c. Metaphase
d. Anaphase
e. Telophase

387. A couple is referred to the physician because their first three pregnancies have ended in spontaneous abortion. Chromosomal analysis reveals that the wife has two cell lines in her blood, one with a missing X chromosome (45,X) and the other normal (46,XX). Her chromosomal constitution can be described as

a. Chimeric
b. Monoploid
c. Trisomic
d. Mosaic
e. Euploid

388. A child with cleft palate, a heart defect, and extra fifth fingers is found to have 46 chromosomes with extra material on one homologue of the chromosome 5 pair. This chromosomal abnormality is best described by which of the following terms?

a. Polyploidy
b. Balanced rearrangement
c. Ring formation
d. Mosaicism
e. Unbalanced rearrangement

389. A 10-year-old boy is referred to the physician because of learning problems and a lack of motivation in school. His family history is unremarkable. Physical examination is normal except for single palmar creases of the hands and curved fifth fingers (clinodactyly). The physician decides to order a karyotype. Which of the following indications for obtaining a karyotype would best explain the physician's decision in this case?

a. A couple with multiple miscarriages, or a person who is at risk for an inherited chromosome rearrangement
b. A child with ambiguous genitalia who needs genetic sex assignment
c. A child with an appearance suggestive of Down's syndrome or other chromosomal disorder
d. A child with mental retardation and/or multiple congenital anomalies
e. A child who is at risk for cancer

390. Chromosomal analysis reveals a 47,XYY karyotype. Which of the following descriptions best fits this abnormality?

a. Autosomal trisomy
b. A male with Klinefelter's syndrome
c. Sex chromosome aneuploidy
d. A female with Turner's syndrome
e. Sex chromosome triploidy

391. The error in meiosis that produces a 47,XYY karyotype is best described by

a. Meiosis division I of paternal spermatogenesis
b. Meiosis division I of maternal oogenesis
c. Meiosis division II of paternal spermatogenesis
d. Meiosis division II of maternal oogenesis
e. Meiosis division II in either parent

392. A physician makes the diagnosis of 47,XYY in a 16-year old boy. Which of the following options is most appropriate for the physician during the counseling session that follows the chromosome result?

a. Recommend karyotyping of the parents
b. Explain that the recurrence risk for such chromosomal aberrations is about 1%
c. Urge that the school receive a copy of the karyotype since these boys often have behavior problems
d. Recommend testosterone supplementation when the boy reaches puberty
e. Inform the parents that their child will be sterile

393. Which of the following karyotypes is an example of aneuploidy?

a. 46,XX
b. 23,X
c. 69,XXX
d. 92,XXXX
e. 90,XX

394. The proper cytogenetic notation for a female with Down's syndrome mosaicism is

a. 46,XX,+21/46,XY
b. 47,XY,+21
c. 47,XXX/46,XX
d. 47,XX,+21/46,XX
e. 47,XX,+21(46,XX)

395. A female with Turner's syndrome is denoted by which of the following cytogenetic notations?

a. 47,XX,+21
b. 45,X
c. 47,XXX
d. 46,XX,t(14;21)
e. 45,XX,−21

396. Which of the diagrams below depicts a reciprocal translocation?

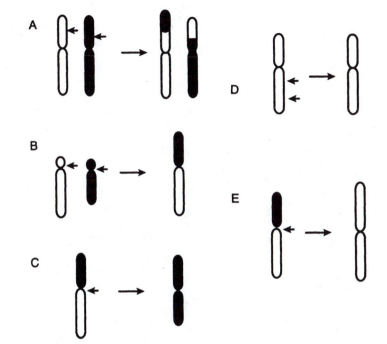

a. Diagram A
b. Diagram B
c. Diagram C
d. Diagram D
e. Diagram E

397. The cytogenetic notation 46,XX,i(6q) refers to which lettered diagram above?

a. Diagram A
b. Diagram B
c. Diagram C
d. Diagram D
e. Diagram E

398. A newborn girl is found to have marked swelling of the dorsal areas of her feet along with a broad (webbed) neck, a broad chest, and a heart murmur that is due to coarctation of the aorta. Her physician suspects a chromosomal disorder and orders a karyotype. Which of the results pictured below is most likely?

a. Result A
b. Result B
c. Result C
d. Result D

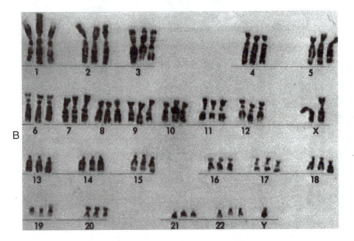

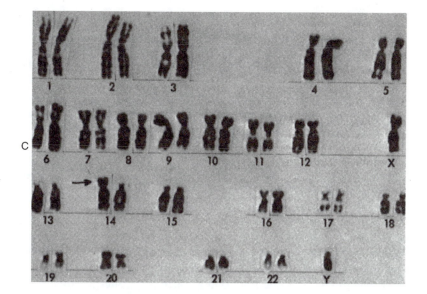

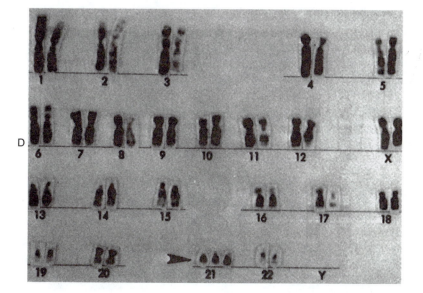

399. A newborn boy feeds poorly, turning blue and choking after breast-feeding. He is also very floppy (hypotonic), has a loud heart murmur, and has some unusual physical findings. These include a flat occiput (brachycephaly), folds over the inner corners of the eyes (epicanthal folds), single creases on the palms (single palmar creases), and a broad space between the first and second toes. Significant in the family history is that one of the parents' three prior children had Down's syndrome. After obtaining a chromosome analysis, which of the results pictured in question 398 is most likely?

a. Result A
b. Result B
c. Result C
d. Result D

400. A 2-week-old baby is hospitalized for inadequate feeding and poor growth. The parents are concerned by the child's weak cry. An experienced grandmother accompanies them, saying she thought the cry sounded like a cat's meow. The grandmother also states that the baby doesn't look much like either parent. The physician orders a karyotype after noting a small head size (microcephaly) and subtle abnormalities of the face. Which of the results pictured below is most likely?

a. Result A
b. Result B
c. Result C
d. Result D
e. Result E

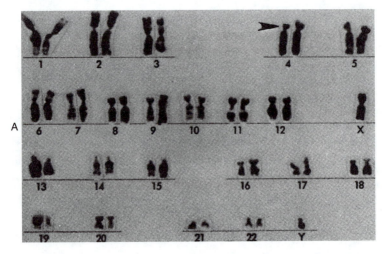

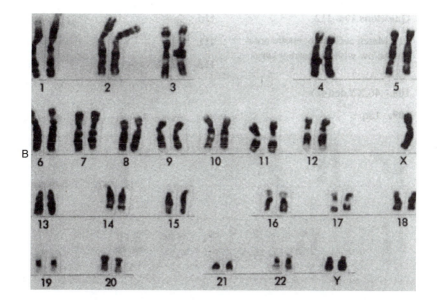

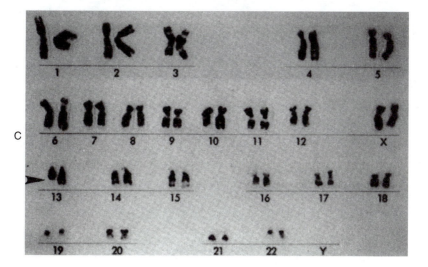

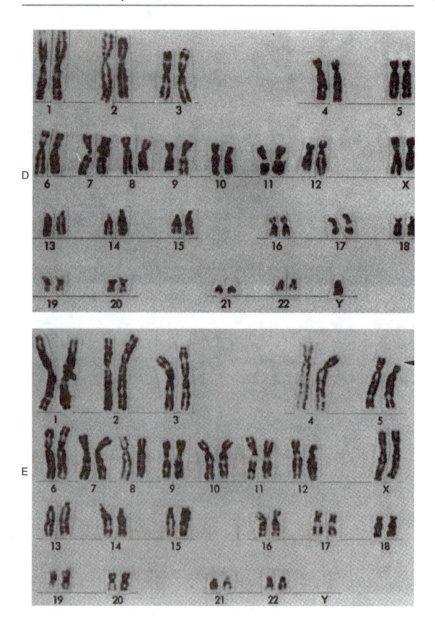

401. Autosomal recessive conditions are correctly characterized by which of the following statements?

a. They are often associated with deficient enzyme activity
b. Both alleles contain the same mutation
c. They are more variable than autosomal dominant conditions
d. Most persons do not carry any abnormal recessive genes
e. Affected individuals are likely to have affected offspring

402. Gardner's syndrome is an autosomal dominant condition characterized by multiple polyps of the intestines, bony tumors, skin cysts, and a high risk of intestinal cancer. A family is encountered in which a great-grandfather, grandmother, and father are affected with Gardner's syndrome and develop intestinal cancer in their thirties. The father brags that none of his four children have inherited Gardner's syndrome because they lack skin cysts and have not had cancer. The chance that at least one child has inherited the Gardner's syndrome allele, and the reason the children have not manifested cancer, are

a. 1/4, ascertainment bias
b. 1/2, variable cancer predisposition
c. 3/4, early-onset disease manifestation
d. 13/16, incomplete medical evaluation
e. 15/16, later-onset disease manifestation

403. Ectrodactyly is an autosomal dominant trait that causes missing middle fingers (lobster claw malformation). A grandfather and grandson both have ectrodactyly, but the intervening father has normal hands by x-ray. Which of the following terms applies to this family?

a. Incomplete penetrance
b. New mutation
c. Variable expressivity
d. Germinal mosaicism
e. Anticipation

404. A 4-year-old boy presents to the physician's office with coarse facies, short stature, stiffening of the joints, and mental retardation. Both parents, a 10-year-old sister, and an 8-year-old brother all appear unaffected. The patient's mother is pregnant. She had a brother who died at 15 years of age with similar findings that seemed to worsen with age. She also has a nephew (her sister's son) who exhibits similar features. Based on the probable mode of inheritance, the risk that her fetus is affected is

a. 100%
b. 67%
c. 50%
d. 25%
e. Virtually 0

405. A couple comes to the physician's office after having had two sons affected with a similar disease. The first-born son is tall and thin and has dislocated lenses and an IQ of 70. He has also experienced several episodes of deep vein thromboses. The chart mentions deficiency of the enzyme cystathionine-β-synthase, but a diagnosis is not given. The second son was treated from an early age with pyridoxine (vitamin B_6) and is less severely affected. No other family members are affected. While taking a family history, the physician discovers that the parents are first cousins. The 38-year-old mother is pregnant, and amniocentesis has demonstrated that the fetus has a 46,XY karyotype. The risk that the fetus will be affected with the same disease is

a. 100%
b. 67%
c. 50%
d. 25%
e. Virtually 0

406. Mr. Smith is affected with Crouzon's syndrome (123500) and has craniosynostosis (i.e., premature closure of the skull sutures) along with unusual facies that includes proptosis secondary to shallow orbits, hypoplasia of the maxilla, and a prominent nose. His son and brother are also affected, although two daughters and his wife are not. Mr. and Mrs. Smith are considering having another child. Their physician counsels them that the risk that the child will be affected with Crouzon's syndrome is

a. 100%
b. 67%
c. 50%
d. 25%
e. Virtually 0

407. A patient presents to the physician's office to ask questions about color blindness. The patient is color-blind, as is one of his brothers. His maternal grandfather was color-blind, but his mother, father, daughter, and another brother are not. His daughter is now pregnant. The risk that her child will be color-blind is

a. 100%
b. 50%
c. 25%
d. 12.5%
e. Virtually 0

408. Little People of America (LPA) is a support group for individuals with short stature that conducts many workshops and social activities. Two individuals with achondroplasia (100800), a common form of dwarfism, meet at an LPA convention and decide to marry and have children. What is their risk of having a child with dwarfism?

a. 100%
b. 75%
c. 50%
d. 25%
e. Virtually 0

409. A woman with cystic fibrosis (219700) marries her first cousin. What is the risk that their first child will have cystic fibrosis?

a. 1/2
b. 1/4
c. 1/8
d. 1/16
e. 1/32

410. A woman with no history of color blindness (304000) marries a color-blind man. What are the risks for this couple of having a son or daughter who is color-blind?

a. 100%
b. 75%
c. 50%
d. 25%
e. Virtually 0

411. A family presents with an unusual type of footdrop and lower leg atrophy that is unfamiliar to their physician. The pedigree below is obtained. Based on the pedigree, what is the risk of individual III-3 having an affected child?

a. 100%
b. 75%
c. 50%
d. 25%
e. Virtually 0

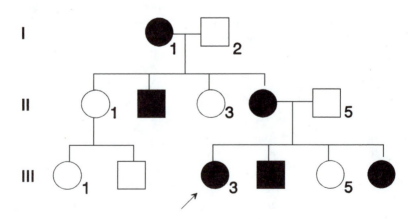

412. A child is evaluated by an ophthalmologist and is found to have retinitis pigmentosa, a disorder characterized by pigmentary granules in the retina and progressive vision loss. The pedigree below is obtained and the family comes in for counseling. What is the risk for individual II-2 of having an affected child if he mates with an unrelated woman?

a. 100%
b. 75%
c. 50%
d. 25%
e. Virtually 0

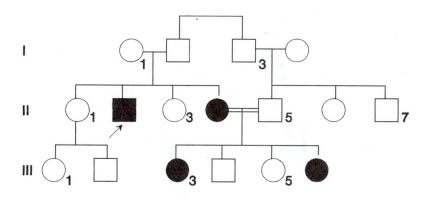

413. A different family with retinitis pigmentosa is encountered, and the pedigree shown below is documented. What is the risk that a son born to individual III-3 would be affected?

a. 100%
b. 75%
c. 50%
d. 25%
e. Virtually 0

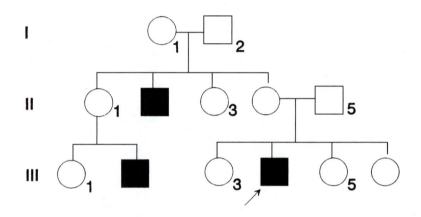

414. Osteogenesis imperfecta (166200) is an autosomal dominant disorder that causes thin, bluish scleras (whites of the eyes), deafness, and multiple bone fractures. Parents have two children with osteogenesis imperfecta, but themselves exhibit no signs of the disease. Which of the following genetic mechanisms is the most likely explanation for two offspring of normal parents to have an autosomal dominant disease?

a. Variable expressivity
b. Uniparental disomy
c. New mutations
d. Germinal mosaicism in one parent
e. Incomplete penetrance

415. Females occasionally have symptoms of X-linked recessive diseases such as Duchenne's muscular dystrophy, hemophilia, or color blindness. The most common explanation is

a. Nonrandom lyonization
b. X chromosome trisomy (47,XXX)
c. X autosome–balanced translocation that disrupts the particular X chromosome locus
d. Turner's syndrome (45,X)
e. 46,XY karyotype in a female

416. Incontinentia pigmenti is an X-linked disorder that is lethal in utero for affected males. The findings vary in females and include pigmented skin lesions, dental abnormalities, patchy areas of alopecia, and mental retardation. Approximately 45% of cases are the result of new mutations. Which of the following descriptions of incontinentia pigmenti is most accurate?

a. X-linked recessive inheritance with spontaneous abortions and few isolated cases
b. X-linked dominant inheritance; 3:1 ratio of females to males in affected sibships
c. X-linked recessive inheritance with spontaneous abortions and many isolated cases
d. X-linked dominant inheritance, 1.5:1 ratio of females to males in affected sibships
e. X-linked dominant inheritance with spontaneous abortions and many isolated cases

417. If parents with three affected children have a higher recurrence risk than parents with two affected children, the disease in question is likely to exhibit

a. Autosomal dominant inheritance
b. Autosomal recessive inheritance
c. X-linked recessive inheritance
d. X-linked dominant inheritance
e. Multifactorial determination inheritance

418. Two parents are both affected with albinism (203100, 203200), but have a normal child. Which of the following terms best applies to this situation?

a. Allelic heterogeneity
b. Locus heterogeneity
c. Variable expressivity
d. Incomplete penetrance
e. New mutation

419. Waardenburg syndrome (193500) is an autosomal dominant condition that accounts for 1.4% of cases of congenital deafness. In addition to deafness, patients with this condition have atypical facies, including lateral displacement of the inner canthi and partial albinism. A mother has Waardenburg syndrome, her husband is unaffected, and they plan to have a family with three children. What is the probability that one of the three children will be affected?

a. 1/8
b. 1/4
c. 3/8
d. 1/3
e. 1/2

420. The major blood group locus in humans produces types A (genotypes AA or AO), B (genotypes BB or BO), AB (genotype AB), or O (genotype OO). For parents who are type AB and type O, what are the possible blood types of their offspring?

a. Type AB child
b. Type B child
c. Type O child
d. Type A or B child
e. Type B or AB child

421. Phenylketonuria [PKU (261600)] is an autosomal recessive disease that causes severe mental retardation if it is undetected. Two normal parents are told by their state neonatal screening program that their third child has PKU. Assuming that the initial screening is accurate, what is the risk that their first child is a carrier for PKU?

a. 100%
b. 67%
c. 50%
d. 25%
e. Virtually 0

422. A couple presents for genetic counseling after their first child is born with achondroplasia (100800), a dwarfing syndrome. The physician obtains the following family history: the husband (George) is the first-born of four male children, and George's next-oldest brother has cystic fibrosis (219700). The wife is an only child, but she had DNA screening because a second cousin had cystic fibrosis and she knows that she is a carrier. There are no other medical problems in the couple or their families. The physician should now draw the pedigree with the female member of any couple on the left. The generations are numbered with Roman numerals and individuals with Arabic numerals; individuals affected with achondroplasia or cystic fibrosis are indicated. Which of the following risk figures applies to the next child born to George and his wife?

a. Achondroplasia 1/2, cystic fibrosis 1/4
b. Achondroplasia 1/2, cystic fibrosis 1/8
c. Achondroplasia virtually 0, cystic fibrosis 1/4
d. Achondroplasia virtually 0, cystic fibrosis 1/6
e. Achondroplasia virtually 0, cystic fibrosis 1/8

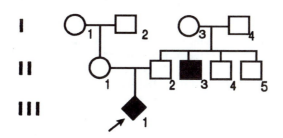

423. Tay-Sachs disease (272800) causes cherry red spots in the eye, "startle" responses in infancy, neurodegeneration, and death. Heterozygotes with an abnormal Tay-Sachs allele are termed carriers. What is the risk that the grandmother of an affected child is a carrier?

a. 100%
b. 67%
c. 50%
d. 25%
e. Virtually 0

424. Isolated cleft lip and palate is a multifactorial trait. The recurrence risk of isolated cleft lip and palate is

a. The same in all families
b. Not dependent upon the number of affected family members
c. The same in all ethnic groups
d. The same in males and females
e. Affected by the severity of the cleft

425. Individuals with achondroplastic dwarfism have about 80% fewer viable offspring than do normal persons, but the incidence of achondroplasia seems to have remained constant for generations. These observations imply

a. Decreased fitness, negative selection, and relatively high mutation rates
b. Increased fitness, negative selection, and relatively high mutation rates
c. Decreased fitness, positive selection, and relatively low mutation rates
d. Increased fitness, positive selection, and relatively low mutation rates
e. Decreased fitness, positive selection, and relatively high mutation rates

426. Many disorders that present in adult life, such as coronary artery disease and hypertension, are multifactorial traits. A multifactorial trait results from

a. The interaction between the environment and a single gene
b. The interaction between the environment and multiple genes
c. Multiple postnatal environmental factors
d. Multiple pre- and postnatal environmental factors
e. Multiple genes independent of environmental factors

427. Which of the following genetic disorders has a similar incidence in different ethnic groups?

a. Cystic fibrosis
b. Thalassemias
c. Tay-Sachs disease
d. Down's syndrome
e. Sickle cell anemia

428. The ship *Hopewell* arrived on a small island several hundred years ago, carrying numerous pilgrims with diabetes insipidus. This disease is now known to be caused by mutant allele A, and residents of the island have 10 times the frequency of this allele as do those on the mainland. Which of the following terms describes this phenomenon?

a. Selection for allele A
b. Linkage disequilibrium with allele A
c. Linkage to allele A
d. Founder effect for allele A
e. Assortative mating for allele A

429. Increased resistance to malaria is seen in persons with hemoglobin AS, where A is the normal allele and S is the allele for sickle hemoglobin. Which of the following terms applies to this situation?

a. Founder effect
b. Heterozygote advantage
c. Genetic lethal
d. Fitness
e. Natural selection

430. Assume that frequencies for the different blood group alleles are as follows: A = 0.3; B = 0.1; O = 0.6. What is the expected percentage of individuals with blood type B?

a. 7%
b. 13%
c. 27%
d. 36%
e. 45%

431. What proportion of genes do a brother and half-sister have in common?

a. One
b. One-half
c. One-fourth
d. One-eighth
e. One-sixteenth

432. A man whose brother has cystic fibrosis wants to know his risk of having an affected child. The prevalence of cystic fibrosis is 1 in 1600 individuals. The risk in this case is

a. 1/8
b. 1/16
c. 1/60
d. 1/120
e. 1/256

433. An African American couple with a normal family history wants to know their chance of having a child with sickle cell anemia. The incidence of sickle cell trait is 1 in 8 for African Americans. The risk in this case is

a. 1/8
b. 1/16
c. 1/60
d. 1/120
e. 1/256

434. A woman who married her first cousin wants to know the risk of having a child with cystic fibrosis because her grandmother, who is also her husband's grandmother, died of cystic fibrosis. Her risk is

a. 1/8
b. 1/16
c. 1/60
d. 1/120
e. 1/256

Inheritance Mechanisms/Risk Calculations

Answers

381. The answer is e. (*Murray, pp 812–828. Scriver, pp 3–45. Sack, pp 1–40. Wilson, pp 1–20.*) The term *familial* indicates that a trait or disorder tends to cluster in families. A genetic disorder is one in which there is evidence that a gene or chromosome is involved in the susceptibility to the disease. Evidence for vertical transmission (e.g., father to daughter) is necessary for a disorder to be labeled inherited. *Sporadic* indicates that evidence for vertical transmission or familial clustering is lacking. *Congenital* simply means present at birth. Note that many congenital diseases (e.g., congenital AIDS) are not genetic, that adult-onset diseases may be genetic without being congenital, and that diseases may be familial (e.g., chickenpox) without being inherited or genetic. The eugenics movement was based on a fallacy about genetics, as it proposed breeding restrictions based on the assumption that all genetic traits (e.g., Down's syndrome) have a high risk of transmission.

382. The answer is b. (*Murray, pp 812–828. Scriver, pp 3–45. Sack, pp 1–40. Wilson, pp 1–20.*) Many common diseases are caused by a combination of environmental and genetic factors, and are described as multifactorial diseases. Examples include diabetes mellitus, schizophrenia, alcoholism, and many common birth defects such as cleft palate or congenital dislocation of the hip. The proportion of genetically identical monozygous twins who share a trait such as diabetes mellitus provides a measure of the genetic contribution to etiology (heritability). Mendelian disorders are completely determined by the genotype of an individual, and exhibit 100% concordance in identical twins. Sporadic disorders have no genetic predisposition and do not cluster in families except by chance or through similar environmental exposure. Congenital disorders are present at birth, in contrast to juvenile diabetes mellitus, which usually presents during childhood. Sex-limited disorders occur predominantly in males or females, in contrast to the approximately equal sex distribution of juvenile diabetes mellitus.

383. The answer is c. (*Murray, pp 812–828. Scriver, pp 3–45. Sack, pp 205–222. Wilson, pp 45–57.*) Genetic disorders may be classified into several major categories. Multifactorial disorders, the most common type of human genetic disease, represent the composite effects of multiple genes, each of which contributes a component to the disorder. Environmental factors also play a role in multifactorial disorders. Many common diseases, such as coronary artery disease or diabetes mellitus, are multifactorial disorders. Chromosomal disorders are caused by the deletion or duplication of either pieces of chromosomes or entire chromosomes and are a common cause of miscarriage. Single-gene disorders, also known as Mendelian disorders, are due to defects in single genes. Since mitochondria are cytoplasmic organelles inherited via the cytoplasm of the ovum, Mitochondrial disorders may be maternally inherited.

384. The answer is e. (*Murray, pp 812–828. Scriver, pp 3–45. Sack, pp 1–40. Wilson, pp 1–20.*) During meiotic segregation, each parental gamete receives one allele from every genetic locus. The probability of a parental allele being transmitted to offspring is thus 1/2, and the probability of a given genotype appearing in offspring is thus a joint probability. For a maternal Aa versus paternal aa mating, the probability of maternal alleles A or a being transmitted is 1/2, and the probability of transmission of the paternal allele a is 1. The joint probability for an Aa genotype in offspring is thus 1/2 × 1 = 1/2, the same as for an aa genotype. For a maternal Aa versus paternal Aa mating, the probabilities for AA, Aa, or aa genotypes in offspring are all 1/2 × 1/2 = 1/4, but the Aa genotype can occur in two ways (A from mother, a from father, or vice versa).

385. The answer is f. (*Murray, pp 812–828. Scriver, pp 3–45. Sack, pp 1–40. Wilson, pp 23–98.*) It is important that the pedigree be an accurate reflection of the family history and that information not be recorded unless specifically mentioned. Pedigree B in the figure omits the double line needed to indicate consanguinity, and pedigree C assumes that the father's affected cousin is the offspring of his uncle rather than being unspecified. Pedigree F correctly illustrates the birth order (third) of the affected female (indicated by arrow) and the consanguinity (double line) represented by the first-cousin marriage.

386. The answer is c. (*Murray, pp 812–828. Scriver, pp 3–45. Sack, pp 57–84. Wilson, pp 123–148.*) The standard karyotype is an arrangement of chromosomes from one cell that is undergoing division at metaphase. At other mitotic stages, the chromosomes are not sufficiently condensed or are too dispersed to allow counting and comparison of pairs under the microscope. After growth, metaphase arrest, separation, hypotonic treatment, and fixing of white blood cells, smearing on a slide yields only about 3% cells that can be analyzed (metaphase spreads). In high-resolution chromosome analysis, less condensed chromosomes in late prophase may be analyzed (prometaphase analysis); however, this process is extremely time-consuming and usually requires focus on a particular chromosome region (e.g., chromosome 15 in a patient suspected of Prader-Willi syndrome, a condition marked by obesity and mental retardation).

387. The answer is d. (*Murray, pp 812–828. Scriver, pp 3–45. Sack, pp 57–84. Wilson, pp 123–148.*) The case described represents one of the more common chromosomal causes of reproductive failure, Turner mosaicism. Turner's syndrome represents a pattern of anomalies including short stature, heart defects, and infertility. Turner's syndrome is often associated with a 45,X karyotype (monosomy X) in females, but mosaicism (i.e., two or more cell lines with different karyotypes in the same individual) is common. However, chimerism (i.e., two cell lines in an individual arising from different zygotes, such as fraternal twins who do not separate) is extremely rare. Trisomy refers to three copies of one chromosome, euploidy to a normal chromosome number, and monoploidy to one set of chromosomes (haploidy in humans).

388. The answer is e. (*Murray, pp 812–828. Scriver, pp 3–45. Sack, pp 57–84. Wilson, pp 123–148.*) Chromosomal abnormalities may involve changes in number (i.e., polyploidy and aneuploidy) or changes in structure (i.e., rearrangements such as translocations, rings, and inversions). Extra material (i.e., extra chromatin) seen on chromosome 5 implies recombination of chromosome 5 DNA with that of another chromosome to produce a rearranged chromosome. Since this rearranged chromosome 5 takes the place of a normal chromosome 5, there is no change in number of the autosomes (nonsex chromosomes) or sex chromosomes (X and Y chromosomes). The question implies that all cells karyotyped from the patient (usually 11 to 25 cells) have the same chromosomal constitution, ruling out mosaicism. The patient's clinical findings are similar to those occurring in trisomy 13, suggesting that the extra material on chromosome 5 is derived from chromosome 13, producing an unbalanced karyotype called dup(13) or partial trisomy 13.

389. The answer is d. *(Murray, pp 812–828. Scriver, pp 3–45. Sack, pp 57–84. Wilson, pp 123–148.)* The hallmarks of children with chromosomal anomalies are mental retardation and multiple congenital anomalies. In this case, the individual has learning problems that have not yet been recognized as mental retardation, and he has minor anomalies rather than major birth defects that cause cosmetic or surgical problems. The physician was astute to suspect a chromosomal anomaly even when the developmental disability and alterations in physical appearance were subtle. Other indications for a karyotype include a couple with multiple miscarriages, an individual at risk for inheriting or transmitting a chromosomal rearrangement, a child with ambiguous external genitalia, or an individual with characteristics of a chromosomal syndrome such as Down's, Turner's, or Klinefelter's syndrome. Chromosome translocations are characteristic of many types of cancer, but these occur in somatic cancer cells rather than in the patient's germ line.

390. The answer is c. *(Murray, pp 812–828. Scriver, pp 3–45. Sack, pp 57–84. Wilson, pp 123–148.)* The 47,XYY karyotype is an example of sex chromosome aneuploidy, as are Klinefelter's syndrome (47,XXY), Turner's syndrome (45,X), and triple X syndrome (47,XXX). Sex chromosome mixoploidy implies mosaicism, such as 45,X/46,XX with two cell lines in one individual. Autosomal trisomies include Down's syndrome [47,XX+21 (trisomy 21)], Patau's syndrome [47,XX+13 (trisomy 13)], and Edwards' syndrome [47,XY+18 (trisomy 18)].

391. The answer is c. *(Murray, pp 812–828. Scriver, pp 3–45. Sack, pp 57–84. Wilson, pp 123–148.)* The sex chromosomes with differently named homologues allow easy visualization of chromosome sorting during meiosis. Female meiosis only involves X chromosomes; thus, Y chromosomal abnormalities must arise during paternal meiosis or occur spontaneously in offspring. Nondisjunction at paternal meiosis I produces XY secondary spermatocytes and a 24,XY gamete. Fertilization with a 23,X ovum yields a 47,XXY individual (Klinefelter's syndrome). Only nondisjunction at paternal meiosis II produces a 24,YY gamete that yields a 47,XYY individual after fertilization.

392. The answer is b. (*Murray, pp 812–828. Scriver, pp 3–45. Sack, pp 57–84. Wilson, pp 123–148.*) The recurrence risk for aneuploidies caused by meiotic nondisjunction is about 1% in addition to the maternal age-related risk. It is not known why the risk for aneuploidy increases slightly after an affected child is born, but parental karyotypes are almost always normal. Surveys of penal institutions have revealed an increased incidence of 47,XYY individuals, but other conditions with mental disability are increased as well. As with other chromosomal syndromes, the phenotype of 47,XYY is variable and can be found coincidentally in normal males. It would therefore be inappropriate to label a child as abnormal in school unless there have been previous concerns about a medical disorder. Males with Klinefelter's syndrome (47,XXY), rather than those with 47,XYY syndrome, are often sterile and may require supplementation with male hormones.

393. The answer is e. (*Murray, pp 812–828. Scriver, pp 3–45. Sack, pp 57–84. Wilson, pp 123–148.*) Aneuploidy involves extra or missing chromosomes that do not arise as increments of the haploid chromosome number *n*. Polyploidy involves multiples of *n*, such as triploidy (3*n* = 69,XXX) or tetraploidy (4*n* = 92,XXXX). Diploidy (46,XX) and haploidy (23,X) are normal karyotypes in gametes and somatic cells, respectively. A 90,XX karyotype represents tetraploidy with two missing X chromosomes, which has been seen in one patient who had features that resembled those of Turner's syndrome.

394. The answer is d. (*Murray, pp 812–828. Scriver, pp 3–45. Sack, pp 57–84. Wilson, pp 123–148.*) Mosaicism occurs when a chromosomal anomaly affects one of several precursor cells of an embryo or tissue. The two or more karyotypes that characterize the mosaic cells are separated by a slash in cytogenetic notation. The notation 47,XX,+21 denotes a cell line typical of a female with trisomy 21 (Down's syndrome), while 46,XX is the karyotype expected for a normal female.

395. The answer is b. (*Murray, pp 812–828. Scriver, pp 3–45. Sack, pp 57–84. Wilson, pp 123–148.*) Cytogenetic notation provides the chromosome number (e.g., 46), the sex chromosomes, and a shorthand description of anomalies. Examples include the following: 45,X indicates a female with monosomy X or Turner's syndrome; 47,XX+21 indicates a female with trisomy 21 or Down's syndrome; 46,XX,t(14;21) indicates a female with translocation Down's syndrome; 45,XX–21 indicates a female with monosomy 21. Note the absence of spaces between symbols, and the use of 47,XXX for sex chromosomal aneuploidy ("triple X" syndrome) rather than the more awkward 47,XX+X. (Note also that 45,X is sufficient for X chromosome monosomy, since absence of an X is indicated by the convention of listing sex chromosomes). Translocations that join two chromosomes with minuscule short arms (acrocentric chromosomes—13, 14, 15, 21, and 22) are called Robertsonian translocations. The joined acrocentric chromosomes in a Robertsonian translocation have a single centromere between them and are counted as one chromosome. A normal person who "carries" a Robertsonian translocation therefore has a chromosome number of 45, as in 45,XX,t(14;21). This female has a 5 to 20% risk of transmitting the Robertsonian 14:21 translocation to her offspring and having a child with Down's syndrome—e.g., 46,XX,t(14;21).

396. The answer is a. (*Murray, pp 812–828. Scriver, pp 3–45. Sack, pp 57–84. Wilson, pp 123–148.*) Reciprocal translocations (diagram A) involve the exchange of segments between two chromosomes. Robertsonian translocations (diagram B) involve the joining of two acrocentric chromosomes by breakage and reunion of their short arms. Translocations that produce no duplication or deficiency are called balanced. Individuals who have balanced translocations are called "carriers"; they have normal phenotypes unless the translocation alters the expression of an important gene at the breakpoint region. Isochromosomes involve duplication of short (diagram C) or long (diagram E) arms, which produces perfectly metacentric chromosomes deficient in long- or short-arm material, respectively. Paracentric inversions (diagram D) alter the banding pattern but not the shape of the chromosome because they do not involve the centromere.

397. The answer is e. (*Murray, pp 812–828. Scriver, pp 3–45. Sack, pp 57–84. Wilson, pp 123–148.*) The abbreviations i and t describe isochromosomes and translocation chromosomes, respectively. Isochromosomes create chromosomes with mirror-image duplications of the long arm (diagram E) or short arm (diagram C). Reciprocal translocations (diagram A) involve exchange of segments between two chromosomes. A semicolon (;) indicates this exchange and is placed between the breakpoints, as in 46,XX,t(2;6)(q23;p14). Robertsonian translocations join together two acrocentric chromosomes to form a metacentric chromosome (diagram B). Carriers of balanced reciprocal translocations have a normal chromosome number, while carriers of balanced Robertsonian translocations have only 45 chromosomes.

398. The answer is a. *(Murray, pp 812–828. Scriver, pp 3–45. Sack, pp 57–84. Wilson, pp 123–148.)* A chromosome study or karyotype delineates the number and kinds of chromosomes in one cell karyon (nucleus). Blood is conveniently sampled, so most chromosomal studies or karyotypes are performed on peripheral leukocytes in blood. A number of leukocytes are karyotyped under the microscope (10 to 25, depending on the laboratory), and a representative photograph is taken. The chromosome images are then arranged (cut out by hand or moved by computer) in order of size from the #1 pair to the #22 pair, and this ordered array is also called a karyotype. Except in cases of mosaicism (different karyotypes in different tissues), the peripheral blood karyotype is indicative of the germ-line karyotype that is characteristic for an individual. In most cases of Turner's syndrome there is a lack of one X chromosome, as in panel A, which shows one X (arrow) and no Y chromosome. Other cases involve mosaicism (45,X/46,XX or 45,X/46,XY) or isochromosomes (e.g., 46,X,isoXq). Correlation of karyotypes and phenotypic features of girls with Turner's syndrome has demonstrated that haploinsufficiency (partial monosomy) of the short arm (Xp) is what generates the characteristic manifestations (web neck, shield chest, puffy feet, coarctation). Women with Turner's syndrome also have short stature and infertility due to maldevelopment of the ovaries (streak gonads).

399. The answer is c. *(Murray, pp 812–828. Scriver, pp 3–45. Sack, pp 57–84. Wilson, pp 123–148.)* Panel c in question 398 demonstrates normal X and Y sex chromosomes, but one pair of autosomes is not homologous (arrow). Given the family history of Down's syndrome, the appearance of extra material on the short arm of chromosome 14 (arrow) can be interpreted as material from chromosome 21. Together with the two normal chromosomes 21, this extra 21 material would give three doses of chromosome 21 and result in Down's syndrome. The abnormal chromosome 14 can thus be interpreted as a Robertsonian 14;21 translocation that was inherited by this child and by the previous child with Down's syndrome [i.e., karyotypes of 46,XY,t(14;21) causing Down's syndrome]. Karyotyping the parents would then be important to determine which was the carrier of the 14;21 translocation—45,XX,t(14;21) or 45,XY,t(14;21). Genetic counseling using the appropriate recurrence risk (5 to 10% for male carriers, 10 to 20% for female carriers) could include the option of prenatal diagnosis (fetal karyotyping) for future pregnancies.

400. The answer is e. (*Murray, pp 812–828. Scriver, pp 3–45. Sack, pp 57–84. Wilson, pp 123–148.*) Children with chromosome abnormalities often exhibit poor growth (failure to thrive) and developmental delay with an abnormal facial appearance. This baby is too young for developmental assessment, but the catlike cry should provoke suspicion of cri-du-chat syndrome. Cri-du-chat syndrome is caused by deletion of the terminal short arm of chromosome 5 [46,XX,del(5p), also abbreviated as 5p–] as depicted in panel e. When a partial deletion or duplication like this one is found, the parents must be karyotyped to determine if one carries a balanced reciprocal translocation. The other karyotypes show (a) deletion of the short arm of chromosome 4 [46,XY,del(4p) or 4p–]; (b) XYY syndrome (47,XYY); (c) deletion of the long arm of chromosome 13 [46,XX,del(13q) or 13q–]; (d) Klinefelter's syndrome (47,XXY). Most disorders involving excess or deficient chromosome material produce a characteristic and recognizable phenotype (e.g., Down's, cri-du-chat, or Turner's syndrome). The deletion of 4p– (panel A) produces a pattern of abnormalities (syndrome) known as Wolf-Hirschhorn syndrome; deletion of 13q– produces a 13q– syndrome (no eponym). The mechanism(s) by which imbalanced chromosome material produces a distinctive phenotype is completely unknown.

401. The answer is a. (*Murray, pp 812–828. Scriver, pp 3–45. Sack, pp 97–158. Wilson, pp 23–39.*) Autosomal recessive conditions tend to have a horizontal pattern in the pedigree. Men and women are affected with equal frequency and severity. It is the pattern of inheritance most often seen in cases of deficient enzyme activity (inborn errors of metabolism). Autosomal recessive conditions tend to be more severe than dominant conditions and are less variable than dominant phenotypes. Both alleles are defective but do not necessarily contain the exact same mutation. All individuals carry 6 to 12 mutant recessive alleles. Fortunately, most matings involve persons who have mutations at different loci. Since related persons are more likely to inherit the same mutant gene, consanguinity increases the possibility of homozygous affected offspring.

402. The answer is e. (*Murray, pp 812–828. Scriver, pp 521–524. Sack, pp 85–96. Wilson, pp 23–39.*) The father is affected with Gardner's syndrome

(175100), an autosomal dominant disease. Therefore, each of his four children has a 1/2 chance of receiving the allele that causes Gardner's syndrome and a 1/2 chance of receiving the normal allele. The probability that none of his four children received the allele for Gardner's syndrome is thus the joint probability of four independent events, computed by the product $1/2 \times 1/2 \times 1/2 \times 1/2 = 1/16$. The probability that at least one child has received the abnormal Gardner's syndrome allele is thus $1 - 1/16 = 15/16$. Gardner's syndrome is one of many genetic disorders that may not be obvious in early childhood. Intestinal cancer in particular has a later onset, with 50% of patients being affected by age 30 to 35. More extensive evaluation of the children for internal signs of disease (e.g., the bony tumors) is required before the father can conclude that he has not transmitted the gene. Late-onset disorders are an important category of adult genetic disease, and presymptomatic testing for these diseases is a novel application of DNA diagnosis.

403. The answer is a. (*Murray, pp 812–828. Scriver, pp 3–45. Sack, pp 97–158. Wilson, pp 23–39.*) Incomplete penetrance applies to a normal individual who is known from the pedigree to have an allele responsible for an autosomal dominant trait. Variable expressivity refers to family members who exhibit signs of the autosomal dominant disorder that vary in severity. When this severity seems to worsen with progressive generations, it is called anticipation. A new mutation in the grandson would be extremely unlikely given the affected grandfather. The father could be an example of somatic mosaicism if a back-mutation occurred to allow normal limb development, but there is no reason to suspect mosaicism of his germ cells (germinal mosaicism).

404. The answer is d. (*Murray, pp 812–828. Scriver, pp 3–45. Sack, pp 97–158. Wilson, pp 23–39.*) The fact that the mother of the affected child has an affected brother and an affected nephew through her sister suggests X-linked recessive inheritance. This is made more likely because the symptoms suggest a mucopolysaccharidosis (storage of glycosaminoglycans) and because one type exhibits X-linked recessive inheritance [Hunter's syndrome or MPS type II (309900)]. When evaluating the possibility of an X-linked disorder, it is important to remember the pattern of inheritance of the X chromosome. Females have two X chromosomes, which are passed along in a random fashion. They pass any given X chromosome to 50% of their sons and 50% of their daughters. For an X-linked recessive condition, those daughters who inherit the affected allele are heterozygous carriers of the disorder but are not affected. Since males have only one X chromosome, those who inherit the affected allele are affected with the disorder. Given X-linked recessive inheritance, the mother must have the abnormal allele on one of her X chromosomes (she is an obligate carrier) in order for her son and brother to be affected. The fetus thus has a 1/2 chance of being a boy and a 1/2 chance of being affected given male sex, resulting in a 1/4 (25%) overall risk of being affected.

405. The answer is d. (Murray, pp 812–828. Scriver, pp 3–45. Sack, pp 97–158. Wilson, pp 23–39.) The family history and the likelihood that the boys have a metabolic disease suggest autosomal recessive inheritance. Autosomal recessive conditions tend to have a horizontal pattern in the pedigree. Although there may be multiple affected individuals within a sibship, parents, offspring, and other relatives are generally not affected. Most autosomal recessive conditions are rare; however, consanguinity greatly increases the likelihood that two individuals will inherit the same mutant allele and pass it along to their offspring. The recurrence risk for the fetus will be that for an autosomal recessive condition with carrier parents—1/4 or 25%. This risk is not affected by the sex of the fetus. The disease caused by cystathionine-β-synthase (CS) deficiency is homocystinuria (236300). S-adenosylmethionine accepts methyl groups and is converted to S-adenosylhomocysteine, which yields homocysteine; homocysteine is converted to cystathionine by CS. Methionine and homocysteine (dimerized to homocystine) accumulate, and homocystine is excreted in urine. Pyridoxine is a cofactor for CS and is beneficial in some forms of homocystinuria. Other causes of homocystinuria include defective cobalamin (vitamin B_{12}) metabolism.

406. The answer is c. (Murray, pp 812–828. Scriver, pp 3–45. Sack, pp 97–158. Wilson, pp 23–39.) In an autosomal dominant pedigree, there is a vertical pattern of inheritance. Assuming the disorder is not the result of a new mutation, every affected person has an affected parent. The same is true of X-linked dominant pedigrees. However, male-to-male transmission, as seen in this family, excludes the possibility of an X-linked disorder. A person with an autosomal dominant phenotype has one mutant allele and one normal allele. These people randomly pass one or the other of these alleles to their offspring, giving a child a 50% chance of inheriting the mutant allele and therefore being affected with the disorder. This risk is unaffected by the genotypes of the previous offspring.

407. The answer is c. *(Murray, pp 812–828. Scriver, pp 3–45. Sack, pp 97–158. Wilson, pp 23–39.)* Males always transmit their single X chromosome to their daughters. Therefore, a daughter of a male affected with an X-linked disorder is an obligate carrier for that disorder. When the condition is X-linked recessive, as with most forms of color-blindness, the daughter is unlikely to show any phenotypic evidence that she is carrying this abnormal gene. Offspring of female carriers are of four types: (1) female carrier with one normal and one mutant allele, (2) normal female with two normal alleles, (3) affected male with a single mutant allele, and (4) normal male with a single normal allele. The chance of having an affected child is thus 1/4 or 25%. If the obligate carrier female gives birth to a son, the chance of the son being color-blind is 50%.

408. The answer is b. *(Murray, pp 812–828. Scriver, pp 3–45. Sack, pp 97–158. Wilson, pp 23–39.)* The genotype of each dwarf can be represented as Aa, with the uppercase A representing the achondroplasia allele. The Punnett square below demonstrates that 3/4 possible gamete combinations yield individuals with at least one A allele. Homozygous AA achondroplasia is a severe disease that is usually lethal in the newborn period. The increased likelihood of individuals with achondroplasia marrying each other because of their similar phenotypes is an example of assortative mating.

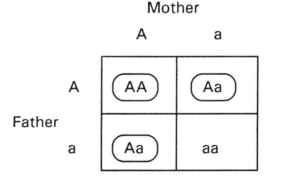

409. The answer is c. (*Murray, pp 812–828. Scriver, pp 3–45. Sack, pp 97–158. Wilson, pp 23–39.*) The McKusick number for cystic fibrosis (219700) begins with 2, indicating an autosomal recessive disorder. The genotype of the affected woman with cystic fibrosis is therefore best represented as the two lowercase letters cc. Her parents are obligate carriers for the disorder (genotypes Cc), and one of her grandparents must also be a carrier (barring new mutations). Her first cousin then has a 1/4 chance of being a carrier, since one of their common grandparents is a carrier, one of his parents has a 1/2 chance of being a carrier, and he has a 1/2 chance of inheriting the c allele from his parent. The affected woman can only transmit c alleles to her fetus, while her cousin has 1/2 chance of transmitting his c allele if it is present. Thus, the probability that the first child will have cystic fibrosis is 1/4 (cousin is carrier) × 1/2 (cousin transmits c allele) = 1/8 (fetus has cc genotype).

410. The answer is e. (*Murray, pp 812–828. Scriver, pp 3–45. Sack, pp 97–158. Wilson, pp 23–39.*) The common forms of color blindness are X-linked recessive, as indicated by the initial 3 of the McKusick number (304000). The couple's daughters will be obligate carriers—that is, carriers implied by the pedigree. Using a lowercase c to represent the recessive color blindness allele, the woman is $X^C X^c$, while her husband is $X^c Y$. The Punnett square below indicates that all daughters will be carriers ($X^C X^c$), while sons will be normal ($X^C Y$). Note again that loci on the X chromosome cannot be transmitted from father to son, since the son receives the father's Y chromosome.

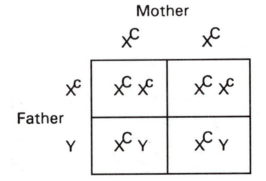

411. The answer is c. (*Murray, pp 812–828. Scriver, pp 3–45. Sack, pp 97–158. Wilson, pp 23–39.*) Autosomal dominant inheritance is suggested by the pedigree because of the vertical pattern of affected individuals and the affliction of both sexes. Autosomal recessive inheritance is ruled out by transmission through three generations, and X-linked recessive inheritance is made unlikely by the presence of affected females. Maternal inheritance should demonstrate transmission to all or most offspring of affected mothers. Polygenic or multifactorial inheritance is not associated with such a high frequency of transmission. Note that X-linked dominant inheritance would also be an explanation for the pedigree. Because the most likely mechanism responsible for the pedigree is autosomal or X-linked dominant inheritance, individual III-3 is affected with the disorder, and she has a 50% risk of transmitting the disease. Discrimination between autosomal and X-linked dominant inheritance could be made by noting the offspring of affected males, such as individual III-4. If X-linked dominant inheritance were operative, affected males would have normal sons and affected daughters. The likely diagnosis is an autosomal dominant form of Charcot-Marie-Tooth disease (118200). Charcot-Marie-Tooth disease exhibits genetic heterogeneity and can exhibit autosomal dominant, autosomal recessive (214380), and X-linked inheritance (302800). Note that the physician could provide counseling based on knowledge of genetics even though the disease is unfamiliar.

412. The answer is e. (*Murray, pp 812–828. Scriver, pp 3–45. Sack, pp 97–158. Wilson, pp 23–39.*) The presence of consanguinity (double line in the figure) is a red flag for autosomal recessive inheritance because, although disease-causing alleles are rare, the probability of a homozygous individual escalates dramatically when the same rare allele descends through two branches of a family. Using a lowercase r to denote the retinitis pigmentosa allele, the affected male (individual II-2 in the pedigree) has a genotype of rr. His prospective mate has a very low risk to be a carrier for this rare disease, making her genotype RR. Their children will all have genotypes Rr, making them carriers but not affected. Retinitis pigmentosa is another disease manifesting genetic heterogeneity, with autosomal dominant (180100), autosomal recessive (268000), and X-linked recessive (312650) forms. Carriers of autosomal recessive diseases are heterozygotes with one normal and one abnormal allele. Many autosomal recessive diseases involve enzyme deficiencies, indicating that 50% levels of enzymes found in heterozygotes are sufficient for normal function. The probability that an affected individual will encounter a mate who is a carrier is approximately twice the square root of the disease incidence. This figure derives from the Hardy-Weinberg law. Since most recessive diseases have incidences lower than 1/10,000, the risk for unrelated mates to be carriers is less than 1/50, and the chance of having an affected child is less than $1/50 \times 1/4 = $ less than 1/200. Disorders that are fairly common in certain ethnic groups, such as cystic fibrosis, are exceptions to this very low risk.

413. The answer is d. (*Murray, pp 812–828. Scriver, pp 3–45. Sack, pp 97–158. Wilson, pp 23–39.*) X-linked recessive inheritance is characterized by a predominance of affected males and an oblique pattern. Transmission must be through females with no evidence of male-to-male transmission. The lack of affected females would make autosomal dominant inheritance less likely, and the sex ratio plus transmission through three generations would eliminate autosomal recessive inheritance. Polygenic inheritance usually exhibits less frequent transmission, although it is certainly not ruled out in this pedigree. The many normal offspring of affected females rule out maternal inheritance. Individual II-4 in the pedigree that accompanies the question is an obligate carrier because she has an affected brother and affected son. This means that her daughter (III-3) has a 1/2 chance of inheriting the X chromosome with an abnormal allele and 1/2 chance of inheriting the X chromosome with the normal allele. If individual III-3 is a carrier, she has a 1/2 chance of transmitting her abnormal allele to her son. The risk that her son will be affected is thus $1/2 \times 1/2 = 1/4$, or 25%. Since the daughters of individual III-3 might be carriers (1/2 chance) but will not be affected, individual III-3 has a 1/8 chance of having an affected child.

414. The answer is e. (*Murray, pp 812–828. Scriver, pp 3–45. Sack, pp 97–158. Wilson, pp 23–39.*) If two individuals in a sibship are affected with an autosomal dominant disease, then the usual implication is that one of the parents has the abnormal allele. Parents with one normal and one abnormal allele have a 50% chance of transmitting the abnormal allele with each pregnancy. Complicating the recognition of autosomal dominant inheritance are incomplete penetrance, where there are no signs of the disease phenotype after all relevant medical evaluations, and variable expressivity, where a parent may have more subtle disease than the offspring.

Incomplete penetrance applies to this family because the parents have no signs or symptoms of disease. If a mutation occurs in the primordial germ cells, then these cells may have abnormal alleles despite the lack of these alleles in the rest of the body tissues (germinal mosaicism). Germinal mosaicism was thought to be very rare until testing for type I collagen gene mutations in osteogenesis imperfecta allowed verification of germinal mosaicism in this condition. Germinal mosaicism explained why autosomal recessive inheritance had been incorrectly postulated for families with normal parents and multiple affected children. Once a child has received the abnormal allele through the gamete of the mosaic parent, the child has the abnormal allele in all cells, with the usual 50% risk of transmission.

415. The answer is a. (*Murray, pp 812–828. Scriver, pp 3–45. Sack, pp 97–158. Wilson, pp 23–39.*) Females have two alleles for each locus on the X chromosome because of their 46,XX karyotype. One normal allele is by definition sufficient for normal function in X-linked recessive disorders, so that females with one abnormal allele are carriers instead of affected individuals. Only when the companion normal allele is disrupted or missing does the abnormal allele cause disease. The Lyon hypothesis predicts that X inactivation is early, irreversible, and random, but some females inactivate only the X chromosome carrying the normal allele. X autosome translocations may disrupt an X chromosome locus and cause disease because the translocated autosome must remain active to avert embryonic death; nonrandom inactivation of the normal X chromosome thus ablates expression of its normal allele. Females with Turner's syndrome, like males with 46,XY karyotypes, have only one X chromosome and can be affected with X-linked recessive diseases. Conversely, females with triple X or trisomy X syndrome have three alleles at each X chromosome locus and are not affected with X-linked recessive disorders. Since choices c, d, and e each require two genetic changes, they are less common than choice a.

416. The answer is e. (*Murray, pp 812–828. Scriver, pp 3–45. Sack, pp 97–158. Wilson, pp 23–39.*) The fact that a disorder is lethal in utero in males does not alter the normal sex ratios for conception. Women who are affected with such conditions still conceive 50% males and 50% females. One-half of the males inherit the affected X chromosome and present as spontaneous abortions. Since the disorder does not affect the in utero viability of females, twice as many females as males are born. The high percentage of new mutations means that many isolated cases will occur. In disorders such as this one, where affected individuals may have mild manifestations, careful examination of the mother is required before assuming that an affected daughter is a new mutation.

417. The answer is e. (*Murray, pp 812–828. Scriver, pp 3–45. Sack, pp 97–158. Wilson, pp 23–39.*) An increasing recurrence risk according to the number of relatives affected is characteristic of polygenic inheritance. The more affected relatives there are, the more evidence there is that an individual's genetic background is shifted toward the threshold for a particular trait; for example, the expectation for tall parents with tall grandparents is to have tall children. Inheritance risks for Mendelian disorders are unaffected by outcomes in prior offspring.

418. The answer is b. (*Murray, pp 812–828. Scriver, pp 3–45. Sack, pp 97–158. Wilson, pp 23–39.*) Albinism is one of many genetic diseases that exhibit locus heterogeneity, which means that mutations at several different loci can produce identical phenotypes. The two McKusick numbers provide a clue that there is more than one locus for albinism, both causing autosomal recessive disease. Each parent must be homozygous for a mutant allele from one albinism locus but heterozygous or homozygous normal at the other locus. Their child would then be an obligate carrier for each type of albinism. A new mutation in the child is also possible, converting one of the parental mutant alleles to normal, but this would be very rare. Autosomal dominant disorders often vary in severity within families (variable expressivity) but occasionally are clinically silent in a person known to carry the abnormal allele (incomplete penetrance).

419. The answer is c. (*Murray, pp 812–828. Scriver, pp 3–45. Sack, pp 97–158. Wilson, pp 23–39.*) For each pregnancy, the probability that the child will be affected is 1/2. Therefore, the probability that all three children will be affected is the product of the three independent events—that is, $1/2 \times 1/2 \times 1/2 = 1/8$. The probability that all three children will be unaffected is the same. When evaluating the probability that one of the three children will be affected, it must be noted that there are three of eight possible birth orders that have one affected child (Www, wWw, wwW). For two of three children to be affected, there are also three of eight possible birth orders (WWw, WwW, wWW).

420. The answer is d. (*Murray, pp 812–828. Scriver, pp 3–45. Sack, pp 97–158. Wilson, pp 23–39.*) Diploid persons have two alleles per autosomal locus, with one being transmitted to each gamete (Mendel's law of segregation). The key to blood group problems is to recognize that a blood type is ambiguous regarding possible alleles—type A persons may have AA or AO genotypes. Once the possible genotypes are deduced from the blood types, potential offspring will represent all combinations of parental alleles. Parents with AB and OO genotypes can only have offspring with genotypes AO (type A) or BO (type B).

421. The answer is b. (*Murray, pp 812–828. Scriver, pp 3–45. Sack, pp 97–158. Wilson, pp 23–39.*) If the abnormal allele is represented as p and the normal as P, an infant affected with phenylketonuria (PKU) has the genotype pp. Parents must be heterozygotes or carriers (Pp) for the child to inherit the p allele from both the mother and father (assuming correct paternity and the absence of unusual chromosomal segregation). Subsequent children have a 1/2 chance of inheriting allele p from the mother and a 1/2 chance of inheriting allele p from the father; the chance that both events will occur to give genotype pp is thus $1/2 \times 1/2 = 1/4$, or 25%. A normal sibling may be genotype PP (1/4 probability) or Pp (1/2 probability since two different combinations of parental alleles give this genotype). The ratio of these probabilities results in a 2/3 chance (67%) of genotype Pp. Note that genotype pp is excluded because a normal sibling (the first child) is specified.

422. The answer is d. (*Murray, pp 812–828. Scriver, pp 3–45. Sack, pp 97–158. Wilson, pp 23–39.*) The figure shows the correctly drawn pedigree with generations indicated by Roman numerals and individuals by Arabic numbers. As the McKusick numbers indicate, achondroplasia is autosomal dominant, cystic fibrosis autosomal recessive. Since neither parent is affected with achondroplasia, the risk for their next child to be affected is virtually zero (rare chances for germ-line mosaicism or incomplete penetrance are ignored). The person who prompted genetic concern is the proband (III-1). George has a brother with cystic fibrosis, making his parents (I-3, I-4) obligate carriers. He has a 1/4 chance of being normal, a 2/4 chance of being a carrier, and a 1/4 chance of being affected with cystic fibrosis. Since George's possibility of being affected is eliminated by circumstance (he is normal), his odds of being a carrier are 2/3. George's wife is definitely a carrier, giving their next child a 1/6 chance to have cystic fibrosis

(2/3 chance George is a carrier × 1/4 chance the child is affected if both are carriers). Although the ΔF_{508} (three–base pair deletion of phenylalanine codon at position 508 in the cystic fibrosis transmembrane regulator gene) accounts for 70% of cystic fibrosis mutations in whites, George's family may have a different mutation than was detected by DNA analysis in his wife. Their child may therefore have a risk of being a compound heterozygote (two different abnormal cystic fibrosis alleles) but will still be affected.

423. The answer is c. (*Murray, pp 812–828. Scriver, pp 3–45. Sack, pp 97–158. Wilson, pp 23–39.*) Parents of children with autosomal recessive disorders are obligate carriers if nonpaternity and rare examples of uniparental disomy (inheritance of chromosomal homologues from the same parent) are excluded. Normal siblings have a 2/3 chance of being carriers because they cannot be homozygous for the abnormal allele. Grandparents have a 1/2 chance of being carriers because one or the other must have transmitted the abnormal allele to the obligate carrier parent. First cousins share a set of grandparents of whom one must be a carrier. There is a 1/2 chance for the aunt or uncle to be a carrier and a 1/4 chance for the first cousin. Half-siblings share an obligate carrier parent and have a 1/2 chance of being carriers. These calculations assume a lack of mutations (Tay-Sachs is rare) and a lack of coincidental alleles (no consanguinity).

424. The answer is e. (*Murray, pp 812–828. Scriver, pp 3–45. Sack, pp 205–222. Wilson, pp 45–57.*) Cleft lip with or without cleft palate [CL(P)] is one of the most common congenital malformations. Because of the genetic component of this trait, it tends to be more common in certain families. The more family members affected and the more severe the cleft, the higher the recurrence risk. In addition, CL(P) is more common in males and in certain ethnic groups (i.e., Asians > whites > African Americans).

425. The answer is a. (*Murray, pp 812–828. Scriver, pp 3–45. Sack, pp 97–158. Wilson, pp 59–79.*) If an abnormal allele is as likely to be transmitted to the next generation as its corresponding normal allele, it is said to have a fitness of 1. Loss of fitness (decrease in allele frequency after one generation) is also referred to as negative selection. The decreased fitness of achondroplast alleles that are eliminated by negative selection must be balanced by new mutations if the disorder has not disappeared or declined in incidence. Thus, the mutation rate of achondroplasia would be expected to be high relative to those of more benign dominant diseases.

426. The answer is b. (*Murray, pp 812–828. Scriver, pp 3–45. Sack, pp 205–222. Wilson, pp 45–58.*) Many common disorders tend to run in families but are not single-gene or chromosomal disorders. These disorders are multifactorial traits, which are caused by multiple genetic and environmental factors. For quantitative traits like height or blood pressure, it is easy to visualize how the alleles at multiple loci plus environmental factors might make additive contributions toward a final phenotype such as a height of 6 ft. For qualitative traits such as cleft lip/palate and other congenital anomalies, a threshold is envisioned that divides normal from abnormal phenotypes. Individuals with more clefting alleles, in combination with an unfavorable intrauterine environment, can cross the threshold and manifest the anomaly. The likelihood of inheriting clefting alleles is increased if there are relatives in the family with cleft lip/palate. Recurrence risks for cleft lip/palate and other multifactorial disorders are thus modified according to the family history.

427. The answer is d. (*Murray, pp 812–828. Scriver, pp 3–45. Sack, pp 97–158. Wilson, pp 59–78.*) Allele frequencies may differ among populations when there has been geographic isolation, founder effect, or selection for certain alleles based on different environments. Although African Americans have intermixed with whites in the United States for over 400 years, they retain a higher frequency of sickle cell alleles, which are thought to protect individuals from malarial infection. Each ethnic group has frequencies of polymorphic alleles that reflect its origin; for example, Ashkenazi Jews have a higher frequency of Tay-Sachs alleles; Greeks and other Mediterranean peoples of thalassemia alleles; and whites of cystic fibrosis alleles. Down's syndrome, a chromosomal disorder, has virtually the same frequency of 1 in 600 births in all ethnic groups. The preservation of genetic differences after migration allows the use of highly polymorphic mitochondrial genes to trace relationships among ancient and modern human populations.

428. The answer is d. (*Murray, pp 812–828. Scriver, pp 3–45. Sack, pp 97–158. Wilson, pp 59–78.*) Linkage disequilibrium describes an association between a particular polymorphic allele and a trait. Many autoimmune diseases exhibit association with particular human leukocyte antigen (HLA) alleles (i.e., HLA-B27 and ankylosing spondylitis). The association is not necessarily cause and effect (e.g., when viral infections that trigger a disease preferentially infect certain HLA genotypes). Founder effects represent a special case of genetic drift in which rare alleles are introduced into a small population by the migration of ancestors. Genetic linkage implies physical proximity of the allele locus to the gene causing the disease. Linkage differs from allele association in that either allele A or a may be linked in a given family, depending on which allele is present together with the offending gene. Neither assortative mating (preferential mating by genotype) or selection (advantageous alleles) applies to the examples in the questions.

429. The answer is b. (*Murray, pp 812–828. Scriver, pp 3–45. Sack, pp 97–158. Wilson, pp 59–78.*) Sickle cell anemia is the classic example of a disorder with a high frequency in a specific population because of heterozygote advantage. Persons who are heterozygous for this mutant allele (hemoglobin AS) have increased resistance to malaria and are therefore at an advantage in areas where malaria is endemic. Founder effect is a special type of genetic drift. In these cases, the founder or original ancestor of a population has a certain mutant allele. Because of genetic isolation and inbreeding in populations such as the Pennsylvania Amish, certain disorders such as maple syrup urine disease (248600) are maintained at a relatively high frequency. Fitness is a measure of the ability to reproduce. A genetic lethal implies that affected individuals cannot reproduce and, therefore, cannot pass on their mutant alleles. Natural selection is a theory introduced by Charles Darwin, which postulates that the fittest individuals have a selective advantage for survival.

430. The answer is b. (*Murray, pp 812–828. Scriver, pp 3–45. Sack, pp 97–158. Wilson, pp 59–78.*) It is important to remember that individuals with blood type A can have either genotype AA or AO, and individuals with blood type B can have either genotype BB or BO. Therefore, the frequency of blood type A is the frequency of homozygotes—that is, 0.3×0.3—plus the frequency of heterozygotes—that is, $2(0.3) \times 0.6$—for a total of 0.45. The frequency of blood type B is $0.1 \times 0.1 + 2(0.1) \times 0.6$ for a total of 0.13. The frequency of individuals with blood type O is simply the frequency of homozygotes—that is, $0.6 \times 0.6 = 0.36$.

431. The answer is c. (*Murray, pp 812–828. Scriver, pp 3–45. Sack, pp 97–158. Wilson, pp 59–78.*) Although all individuals, other than identical twins, are genetically unique, we all share some genes in common with our relatives. The more closely we are related, the more genes we have in common. First-degree relatives, such as siblings, parents, and children, share one-half of their genes. Second-degree relatives share one-fourth, and third-degree relatives share one-eighth.

432. The answer is d. *(Murray, pp 812–828. Scriver, pp 3–45. Sack, pp 97–158. Wilson, pp 59–787.)* According to the Hardy-Weinberg equilibrium, the frequency of heterozygotes (2pq) is twice the square root of the rare homozygote frequency (q^2). The man in the question has a 2/3 chance of being a carrier and a 1/20 chance that his wife is a carrier. His risk for an affected child is 2/3 × 1/20 × 1/4 = 1/120.

433. The answer is e. *(Murray, pp 812–828. Scriver, pp 3–45. Sack, pp 97–158. Wilson, pp 59–78.)* The African American man and woman each have a 1/8 chance of having sickle trait. They have a 1/64 × 1/4 = 1/256 chance of having a child with sickle cell anemia. There is also a 1/64 × 1/2 = 1/128 chance that their child will have sickle trait.

434. The answer is b. *(Murray, pp 812–828. Scriver, pp 3–45. Sack, pp 97–158. Wilson, pp 59–78.)* The grandmother has cystic fibrosis, so her children are obligate carriers. Each cousin therefore has a 1/2 chance of being a carrier. The woman's risk is 1/2 × 1/2 × 1/4 = 1/16 chance of having an affected child. This illustrates the effects of consanguinity.

Genetic and Biochemical Diagnosis

Questions

DIRECTIONS: Each item below contains a question or incomplete statement followed by suggested responses. Select the **one best** response to each question.

435. A 48-year-old woman is diagnosed with Parkinson's disease and requests a DNA test to confirm the diagnosis. Her physician explains that 1% of people over 50 may contract the disease, that monozygotic twins have a 3% concordance rate, that there is little variation among ethnic groups, that siblings of affected individuals have a 2 to 3% incidence of parkinsonism, and that low levels of dopamine have been found in the substantia nigra of the brains of people with Parkinson's. A definitive DNA test is not possible because

a. Parkinson's disease exhibits polygenic inheritance
b. Parkinson's disease is a metabolic disorder
c. Parkinson's disease has no genetic basis
d. Parkinson's disease is a Mendelian disorder
e. Parkinson's disease has not been attributed to or associated with a specific gene mutation

436. The strategy for therapy for dopamine deficiency in the substantia nigra of individuals with Parkinson's disease is indicated by which of the following?

a. Feedback inhibition of dopamine oxidation
b. Competitive inhibition of biosynthesis from histidine
c. Provision of metabolites in the tyrosine pathway
d. Stimulation of monoamine oxidase
e. Provision of metabolites in the alanine pathway

437. A three-year-old girl is scheduled for a tonsillectomy. As she is prepared for the operating room, her father becomes agitated and insists on accompanying her. He says that 2 of his 6 siblings have died during operations, one having a "reaction" to the anesthetic, the other never waking up. Which of the following options is the best response to the father's anxiety?

a. Postpone the operation until the psychiatric state of the father can be evaluated
b. Proceed after explaining that problems in the father's siblings are unlikely to be transmitted to his daughter
c. Proceed after reassuring the father that drug reactions are environmental and unlikely to have a genetic basis
d. Postpone the operation until a more detailed family history is obtained
e. Proceed after explaining that modern anesthetic procedures are much safer than in the past

438. In the operating room, a child receives succinylcholine as a muscle relaxant to facilitate intubation and anesthesia. The operation proceeds until it is time for recovery, when the child does not begin breathing. A hurried discussion with the father discloses no additional problems in the family, but he does say that he and his wife are first cousins. The most likely possibility is

a. An autosomal dominant disorder that interferes with succinylcholine metabolism
b. An autosomal recessive disorder that interferes with succinylcholine metabolism
c. An X-linked disorder that interferes with succinylcholine metabolism
d. A lethal gene transmitted through consanguinity that affects the respiratory system
e. Mismanagement of halothane anesthesia during the operation

439. Succinylcholine relaxes muscles during anesthesia by competing with the molecule normally responsible for neuromuscular transmission. Which of the following phrases describes the appropriate treatment for a disease involving this neurotransmitter?

a. L-dopa treatment of parkinsonism
b. Haldol treatment of schizophrenia
c. Neostigmine treatment of myasthenia gravis
d. Prozac treatment of schizophrenia
e. Diisopropylfluorophosphate (DFP) treatment of myasthenia gravis

440. A man with early-onset emphysema undergoes protein electrophoresis for analysis of α_1 antitrypsin (AAT) deficiency (107400). The result shows two electrophoretic bands that react with AAT, one at the normal position and one at an abnormal position. Which of the following best describes this result?

a. The man is homozygous and has normal AAT activity
b. The man is heterozygous and has normal AAT activity
c. The man is homozygous and has deficient AAT activity
d. The man is homozygous and has an altered AAT protein
e. The man is heterozygous and has an altered AAT protein

441. A girl seems normal at birth but begins flinching at loud noises (enhanced startle response) at age 6 months. Ophthalmologic examination reveals a central red area of the retina surrounded by white tissue (cherry red spot). The child initially can sit up, but then regresses so that she cannot roll over or recognize her parents. Her physician suspects a lipid storage disease (neurolipidosis). If the diagnosis is correct, what is the risk that the next child of these parents will be affected with the same disease?

a. 1/2
b. 1/4
c. 3/4
d. 1/12
e. 1/24

442. The cause of Tay-Sachs disease (272800) is best described by which of the following?

a. Excess of a lysosomal enzyme in blood due to defective uptake
b. Deficiency of a lysosomal enzyme that digests proteoglycans
c. Deficiency of a membrane receptor that takes up proteoglycans
d. Deficiency of a mitochondrial enzyme that degrades glycogen
e. Deficiency of a mitochondrial triglyceride lipase

443. The frequency of Tay-Sachs carriers among Ashkenazi Jews is 1/30. The frequency of Tay-Sachs carriers among whites of Western European descent is approximately 1/300. If a mother is an Ashkenazi Jew and a father is a white from Western Europe, what is the chance that a child of this union will have Tay-Sachs disease?

a. 1/120
b. 1/240
c. 1/3,600
d. 1/9,000
e. 1/36,000

444. The parents of a girl with Tay-Sachs disease decide to pursue bone marrow transplantation in an attempt to provide a source for the missing lysosomal enzyme. Preliminary testing of the girl's normal siblings is performed to assess their carrier status and their human leukocyte antigen (HLA) locus compatibility with their affected sister. What is the chance that one of the three siblings is homozygous normal (i.e., has a good supply of enzyme) and HLA-compatible?

a. 1/2
b. 1/3
c. 1/4
d. 1/6
e. 1/12

445. A sibling donor is found for a patient with Tay-Sachs disease, and the physician writes to the patient's insurance company explaining the diagnosis of Tay-Sachs disease and the reasons for the bone marrow transplant. Not only does the insurance company refuse payment for transplantation, it also discontinues coverage for the family based on anticipated medical expenses. From the ethical perspective, these events fall under which of the following categories?

a. Patient confidentiality
b. Nondisclosure
c. Informed consent
d. Failure to provide ongoing care
e. Discrimination

446. A couple decide to have prenatal diagnosis because their previous child has Tay-Sachs disease. Which prenatal diagnostic technique is optimal for fetal diagnosis?

a. Chorionic villi sampling (CVS)
b. Percutaneous umbilical blood sampling
c. Amniotic fluid α-fetoprotein levels
d. Maternal serum α-fetoprotein (MSAFP)
e. Fetal x-rays

447. A patient with the Marfan's syndrome is evaluated at a clinic. He is noted to have a tall, thin body habitus, loose joints, and arachnodactyly (spider fingers). Ophthalmologic examination reveals lens dislocation. Echocardiogram reveals dilation of the aortic root. A family history reveals that the patient's parents are medically normal, but that his paternal grandfather and great-grandfather died in their forties with lens dislocation and dissecting aortic aneurysms. A sister is found to have a similar body habitus, dilation of the aortic root, and normal lenses. The different findings in these different family members with the same disease are best described by which of the following terms?

a. Pleiotropy
b. Founder effect
c. Variable expressivity
d. Incomplete penetrance
e. Genetic heterogeneity

448. Marfan's syndrome is caused by which of the following mechanisms?

a. Mutation that prevents addition of carbohydrate residues to the fibrillin glycoprotein
b. Mutation in a carbohydrate portion of fibrillin that interferes with targeting
c. Mutation that disrupts the secondary structure of fibrillin and blocks its assembly into microfibrils
d. Mutation in a lysosomal enzyme that degrades fibrillin
e. Mutation in a membrane receptor that targets fibrillin to lysosomes

449. The diagnosis of osteogenesis imperfecta (166200) is most accurately performed by

a. PCR amplification and DNA sequencing of type I collagen gene segments to look for point mutations
b. Gel electrophoresis of labeled type I collagen chains synthesized in fibroblasts
c. PCR amplification and ASO hybridization to detect particular mutant alleles
d. Northern blotting to evaluate type I collagen mRNAs
e. Purification and trypsin digestion of type I collagen chains to visualize altered peptides after two-dimensional gel electrophoresis

450. Studies of the eye tumor retinoblastoma have revealed an Rb locus on the long arm of chromosome 13 that influences retinoblastoma occurrence. Patients with 13q– deletions often develop bilateral tumors (both sides), in contrast to more common forms of retinoblastoma that occur at one site. Which of the following phrases best explains this phenomenon?

a. Rb is an oncogene
b. Rb is a tumor suppressor gene
c. Rb mutations ablate a promoter sequence
d. Rb mutations ablate an enhancer sequence
e. Rb mutations must always involve chromosome abnormalities

451. In Burkitt's lymphoma, there is increased expression of a hybrid protein with an amino-terminus similar to immunoglobulin (Ig) heavy chain and an unknown carboxyterminus. Which of the following best explains this phenomenon?

a. Chromosome translocation that brings together an Ig heavy chain with an oncogene
b. Chromosome duplication involving a segment with an oncogene
c. Chromosome translocation involving a segment with Ig heavy chains
d. Chromosome deletion removing an oncogene
e. Chromosome deletion removing a tumor suppressor gene

452. A couple request genetic counseling because the wife has contracted early-onset breast cancer at age 23. The husband has a benign family history, but the wife has several relatives who developed cancers at relatively early ages. Affected relatives include a sister (colon cancer, age 42), a brother (colon cancer, age 46), mother (breast cancer, age 56), maternal aunt (leukemia, age 45), maternal uncle (muscle sarcoma, age 49), and a nephew through the brother with colon cancer (leukemia, age 8). The most likely conclusion from the family history is

a. No genetic predisposition to cancer since most individuals have different types of cancer
b. Possible autosomal dominant inheritance or multifactorial inheritance of cancer predisposition
c. Germ-line mutations in an oncogene, with somatic mutations that suppress the oncogene
d. Germ-line mutations in a tumor suppressor gene, with neoplasia from chemical exposure
e. Mitochondrial inheritance of tumor predisposition evidenced by the affected maternal relatives

453. A normal 6-year-old girl has a strong family history of cancer, including several relatives with Li-Fraumeni syndrome, an autosomal dominant condition that predisposes to breast and colon cancer. Her parents request that she have genetic testing for a possible cancer gene. The major ethical concern about such testing is

a. Nonmaleficence
b. Beneficence
c. Autonomy
d. Informed consent
e. Confidentiality

454. A 45-year-old male is hospitalized for treatment of myocardial infarction. His father and a paternal uncle also had heart attacks at an early age. His cholesterol is elevated, and lipoprotein electrophoresis demonstrates an abnormally high ratio of low- to high-density lipoproteins (LDL to HDL). Which of the following is the most likely explanation for this problem?

a. Mutant HDL is not responding to high cholesterol levels
b. Mutant LDL is not responding to high cholesterol levels
c. Mutant caveolae proteins are not responding to high cholesterol levels
d. Mutant LDL receptors are deficient in cholesterol uptake
e. Intracellular cholesterol is increasing the number of LDL receptors

455. A patient with myocardial infarction is treated with nitroglycerin to dilate his coronary arteries. Which of the following best describes the action of nitroglycerin?

a. Methylation occurs to produce S-adenosylmethionine
b. GTP hydrolysis accomplishes oxidation of LDL proteins
c. Arginine is converted to a neurotransmitter that activates guanyl cyclase
d. Acetyl CoA and choline are condensed to form a neurotransmitter
e. Tyrosine is converted to serotonin

456. A woman presents with fatigue, pallor, and pale conjunctival blood vessels. She gives a recent history of metrorrhagia (heavy menstrual periods). Which of the following laboratory findings is most likely?

a. High serum haptoglobin
b. High serum iron
c. High numbers of transferrin receptors
d. High saturation of transferrin
e. High serum ferritin

457. A man is evaluated for mild liver disease, arthritis, fatigue, and grayish skin pigmentation. A liver biopsy shows marked increase in iron. Which of the following laboratory values is most likely?

a. Low serum iron
b. High serum copper
c. Low saturation of transferrin
d. High serum ferritin
e. Low serum haptoglobin

458. The regulation of transferrin receptors is studied in tissue culture. There is increased synthesis of transferrin receptor protein with no changes in transferrin mRNA transcription. The most plausible explanation is

a. Change in amounts or types of transcription factors
b. Allosteric regulation of transferrin receptor function
c. Activation of transferrin receptor function by a protein kinase
d. Stabilization of transferrin mRNA
e. Increased GTP levels to accelerate protein elongation

459. A 2-year-old child is hospitalized for evaluation of poor growth and low muscle tone. The most striking physical finding is unruly, "kinky" hair, but the child also has increased joint laxity and thin skin. Which of the following laboratory findings is most likely?

a. High ceruloplasmin
b. High serum copper
c. Low serum iron
d. Low saturation of transferrin
e. Low serum haptoglobin

460. Deletions of 11p13 may result in Wilms tumor, aniridia, genitourinary malformations, and mental retardation (WAGR syndrome). In some patients, however, not all features are seen. Additionally, individual features of this syndrome may be inherited separately in a Mendelian fashion. Limited features may also be seen in patients without visible chromosomal deletions. The most likely mechanism for this finding is

a. Mitochondrial inheritance
b. Imprinting
c. Germ-line mosaicism
d. Uniparental disomy
e. Contiguous gene syndrome

461. Polycystic kidney disease is a significant cause of renal failure that presents from early infancy to adulthood. Early-onset cases tend to affect one family member or siblings, while adult-onset cases often show a vertical pattern in the pedigree. Which of the following offers the best explanation of these facts?

a. Pleiotropy
b. Allelic heterogeneity
c. Locus heterogeneity
d. Multifactorial inheritance
e. Variable expressivity

462. A male child presents with delayed development and scarring of his lips and hands. His parents have restrained him because he obsessively chews on his lips and fingers. Which of the following is likely to occur in this child?

a. Increased levels of 5-phosphoribosyl-1-pyrophosphate (PRPP)
b. Decreased purine synthesisis
c. Decreased levels of uric acid
d. Increased levels of hypoxanthine-guanosine phosphoribosyl transferase (HGPRT)
e. Glycogen storage

463. A couple request prenatal diagnosis because a maternal uncle and male cousin on the wife's side were diagnosed with Lesch-Nyhan syndrome (308000). DNA analysis of the family is performed using Southern blotting with VNTR probes near the HGPRT gene. What is the chance that the fetus will have Lesch-Nyhan syndrome?

a. 100%
b. 50%
c. 33%
d. 25%
e. Virtually 0%

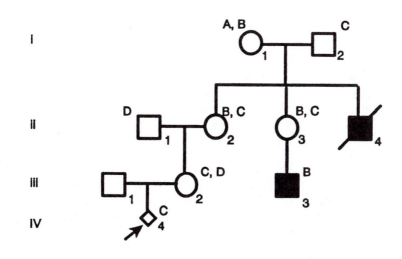

464. A 6-year-old girl is referred to a physician for evaluation. She is known to have mild mental retardation and a ventricular septal defect (VSD). On physical examination, the patient is noted to have some facial dysmorphism, including a long face, a prominent nose, and flattening in the malar region. In addition, the patient's speech has an unusual quality. Which description best explains the patient's condition?

a. Sequence
b. Syndrome
c. Disruption
d. Deformation
e. Single birth defect

465. A standard karyotypic analysis is ordered for a girl with heart defects, developmental delay, and an unusual appearance. The results are normal, but a colleague recommends performing fluorescent in situ hybridization (FISH) analysis on the patient's chromosomes, using probes for chromosome 22. Only one signal is seen for each chromosomal spread. Which of the following statements regarding these analyses is true?

a. The initial karyotype results are inconsistent with the FISH results
b. This is a normal result
c. A small deletion is present on one of the patient's number 22 chromosomes
d. FISH is only helpful when the initial karyotype results are abnormal
e. The chromosome with the positive signal is paternal in origin

466. As exemplified by HLA-DQβ haplotypes in type I diabetes mellitus, an individual's HLA status may be relevant to genetic counseling for certain multifactorial diseases. The relation of HLA haplotypes to disease and the use of this information in genetic counseling are referred to as

a. Genetic linkage and the frequency of recombination
b. Allele association and risk modification
c. Positional cloning and gene isolation
d. Gene mapping and gene segregation
e. Genotyping and phenotypic correlation

467. Screening of an African American population in Minnesota yields allele frequencies of 7/8 for the A globin allele and 1/8 for the sickle globin allele. A companion survey of 6400 of these people's ancestors in central Africa reveals 4600 individuals with genotype AA, 1600 with genotype AS (sickle trait), and 200 with genotype SS (sickle cell disease). Compared to their descendants in Minnesota, the African population has

a. A lower frequency of AS genotypes consistent with inbreeding
b. A lower frequency of AS genotypes consistent with malarial exposure
c. A higher frequency of AS genotypes consistent with heterozygote advantage
d. A higher frequency of AS genotypes consistent with selection against the S allele
e. Identical A and S allele frequencies as predicted by the Hardy-Weinberg law

468. If all SS individuals in the Minnesota population were sterilized, the SS genotype frequency in the next generation would be

a. Reduced by 2/3
b. Reduced by 1/2
c. Reduced by 1/3
d. Reduced to 0
e. Approximately the same

469. A newborn infant presents with poor feeding, vomiting, jaundice, and an enlarged liver. The urine tests positive for reducing substances, indicating the presence of sugars with aldehyde groups. Which of the following processes is most likely to be abnormal?

a. Conversion of glucose to galactose
b. Conversion of lactose to galactose
c. Conversion of activated galactose to activated glucose
d. Excretion of glucose by the kidney
e. Excretion of galactose by the kidney

470. The frequency of galactosemia is approximately 1 in 40,000 live births. The frequency of the carrier state can be calculated as

a. 1 in 50 live births
b. 1 in 100 live births
c. 1 in 200 live births
d. 1 in 500 live births
e. 1 in 1000 live births

471. A woman who has two brothers with hemophilia A (306700) and two normal sons is again pregnant. She requests counseling for the risk of her fetus to have hemophilia. What is the risk that her next child will have hemophilia?

a. 1
b. 1/2
c. 1/4
d. 1/8
e. 1/16

472. Which of the following statements about hemophilia A (306700) is true?

a. The extrinsic clotting pathway is impaired
b. The cleavage of fibrinogen is impaired
c. Tissue factor activation is impaired
d. Activation of factor XII is impaired
e. Activation of factor X is impaired

473. A woman who is at risk to be a carrier of hemophilia A desires prenatal diagnosis. She does not want her extended family to know about her pregnancy if the fetus is affected. Which of the following prenatal diagnostic techniques should be advised?

a. Amniocentesis with western blot analysis of factor VIII
b. Chorionic villus sampling with DNA analysis for factor VIII mutations
c. Percutaneous umbilical blood sampling with testing of factor VIII levels
d. Amniocentesis with DNA analysis for factor VIII mutations
e. Chorionic villus sampling with assay of factor VIII activity

474. The figure below shows a pedigree that includes individuals with Charcot-Marie-Tooth disease (CMT), a neurologic disorder that produces dysfunction of the distal extremities with characteristic footdrop. If individual III-4 becomes pregnant, what is her risk of having a child with CMT?

a. 1/2
b. 1/4
c. 1/8
d. 1/16
e. Virtually 0

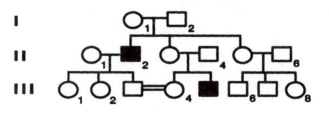

475. In another family with Charcot-Marie-Tooth disease (CMT), restriction analysis using sites flanking the CMT gene on 17 yields one large abnormal fragment and one smaller fragment that is seen in controls. What is the probable inheritance mechanism in this family?

a. X-linked recessive
b. Autosomal dominant
c. Autosomal recessive
d. Multifactorial
e. X-linked dominant

476. Prader-Willi syndrome involves a voracious appetite, obesity, short stature, hypogonadism, and mental disability. At least 50% of Prader-Willi patients have a small deletion on the proximal long arm of chromosome 15. In detecting the Prader-Willi deletion, which of the following techniques would be most accurate?

a. Standard karyotyping of peripheral blood leukocytes
b. Northern blotting of mRNAs transcribed from the deletion region
c. Restriction analysis to detect DNA fragments from the deletion region
d. Rapid karyotyping of bone marrow
e. Fluorescent in situ hybridization (FISH) analysis of peripheral blood lymphocytes using fluorescent DNA probes from the deleted region

477. A child is referred for evaluation because of low muscle tone and developmental delay. Shortly after delivery the child was a poor feeder and had to be fed by tube. In the second year, the child began to eat voraciously and became obese. He has a slightly unusual face with almond-shaped eyes and downturned corners of the mouth. The hands, feet, and penis are small, and the scrotum is poorly formed. The diagnostic category and laboratory test to be considered for this child are

a. Sequence, serum testosterone
b. Single birth defect, serum testosterone
c. Deformation, karyotype
d. Syndrome, karyotype
e. Disruption, karyotype

478. A karyotype is performed on an obese child and is entirely normal. Because the physician suspects Prader-Willi syndrome, Southern blotting is performed to determine the origin of the patient's number 15 chromosomes. In the figure below, a hypothetical Southern blot with DNA probe D15S8 defines which of four restriction fragment length polymorphisms (RFLPs) are present in DNA from mother (M), child (C), and father (F). Based on the D15S8 locus, what is the origin of the child's two number 15 chromosomes?

a. One from the mother, one from the father
b. Both from the father
c. Both from the mother
d. From neither parent
e. Cannot tell because the locus is deleted in the child

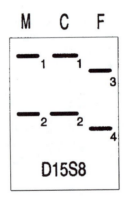

479. Because the figure in question 478 demonstrates that the child is missing both paternal chromosome 15 alleles, nonpaternity is a more plausible explanation than uniparental disomy. The hypothetical Southern blot shown below illustrates a DNA "fingerprinting" analysis to examine paternity, where maternal (M), child (C), and paternal (F) DNA samples have been restricted, blotted, and hybridized simultaneously to the probes D7Z5 and D20Z1. The distributions of restriction fragment alleles suggest

a. The child is adopted
b. False maternity (i.e., baby switched in the nursery)
c. False paternity
d. Correct maternity and paternity
e. None of the above

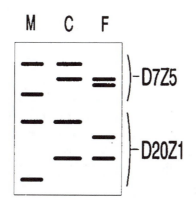

480. Many family studies employing DNA have the potential to demonstrate nonpaternity. If the physician ordering these analyses does not discuss this possibility with the couples involved, he or she is in violation of

a. Patient confidentiality
b. Patient rights
c. Informed consent
d. Standards of care
e. Malpractice guidelines

481. The genesis of Prader-Willi syndrome by inheritance of two normal chromosomes from a single parent is an example of

a. Germinal mosaicism
b. Genomic imprinting
c. Chromosome deletion
d. Chromosome rearrangement
e. Anticipation

482. A child with severe epilepsy, autistic behavior, and developmental delay has characteristics of a condition known as Angelman's syndrome. Because of the syndromic nature of the disorder and the developmental delay, a karyotype is performed that shows a missing band on one chromosome 15. Which of the following best describes this abnormality?

a. Interstitial deletion of 15
b. Terminal deletion of 15
c. Pericentric inversion of 15
d. Paracentric inversion of 15
e. 15q−

483. An infant with severe muscle weakness is born to a mother with mild muscle weakness and myotonia (sustained muscle contractions manifested clinically by the inability to release a handshake). The mother's father is even less affected, with some frontal baldness and cataracts. Worsening symptoms in affected individuals of successive generations suggest which of the following inheritance mechanisms?

a. Genomic imprinting
b. Heteroplasmy
c. Unstable trinucleotide repeats
d. Multifactorial inheritance
e. Mitochondrial inheritance

484. A child is born with spina bifida, a defect in the lower spinal cord and meninges that may cause bladder and lower limb dysfunction. The family history reveals that the father had a small spina bifida that was repaired by surgery. The most critical aspect of the medical evaluation as it pertains to genetic counseling is

a. A search for additional anomalies to determine if the child has a syndrome
b. A karyotype on the child
c. A serum folic acid level on the child
d. A spinal x-ray on the mother
e. A spinal x-ray on the father

485. Most isolated congenital anomalies exhibit

a. Mendelian inheritance
b. Chromosomal inheritance
c. Multifactorial inheritance
d. Maternal inheritance
e. Atypical inheritance

486. Spina bifida exhibits female predilection and recurrence risks of 3% for first-degree relatives and 0.5% for second-degree relatives. A father and child have spina bifida, but the mother is normal. The risk that the couple's next child will have spina bifida is

a. >1%
b. <1%
c. >6%
d. <6%
e. 10%

487. Neural tube defects, such as spina bifida and anencephaly, are best diagnosed by

a. Chorionic villus biopsy and karyotype at 10 weeks after the last menstrual period (LMP)
b. Maternal serum α-fetoprotein (MSAFP) levels and ultrasound at 16 weeks after conception
c. Amniotic fluid α-fetoprotein (AFP) levels and ultrasound at 16 weeks after the LMP
d. Amniotic fluid acetylcholinesterase levels at 16 weeks after conception
e. Amniotic fluid karyotype and ultrasound at 16 weeks after the LMP

488. Every prenatal evaluation should include which of the following diagnostic procedures?

a. Level I ultrasound
b. Chorionic villus sampling (CVS)
c. Doppler analysis
d. Amniocentesis
e. Genetic counseling

489. A couple has a child who has been diagnosed with medium-chain acyl coenzyme A (CoA) dehydrogenase deficiency (MCAD), a condition that affects the body's ability to metabolize medium-chain fatty acids. This couple is now expecting another child. What is the risk that this child will have MCAD?

a. 2/3
b. 1/2
c. 1/3
d. 1/4
e. 1/5

490. A 1-year-old child develops fever and vomiting and is unable to keep food down for 2 days. The physical examination discloses no congenital anomalies, and the baby resembles his parents. Which of the following laboratory findings are most likely if the child has a disorder of fatty acid oxidation?

a. Hypoglycemia, acidosis, and elevated urine dicarboxylic acids
b. Alkalosis and elevated serum ammonia
c. Acidosis and elevated urine reducing substances
d. Hypoglycemia, acidosis, and elevated serum leucine, isoleucine, and valine
e. Hepatomegaly, elevated serum liver enzymes, and elevated tyrosine

491. Laboratory tests on a sick child reveal a low white blood cell count, metabolic acidosis, increased anion gap, and mild hyperammonemia. Measurement of plasma amino acids reveals elevated levels of glycine, and measurement of urinary organic acids reveals increased amounts of propionic acid and methyl citrate. Which of the following processes is most likely?

a. Diabetes mellitus
b. A fatty acid oxidation disorder
c. Vitamin B_{12} deficiency
d. Propionic acidemia
e. A disorder in glycine catabolism

492. In the treatment of propionic acidemia, which of the following is contraindicated?

a. Antibiotics
b. A diet high in fatty acids
c. Caloric supplementation
d. Aggressive fluid and electrolyte management
e. Hemodialysis

493. DNA analysis is performed on a family because the first child has propionic acidemia. The parents desire prenatal diagnosis, and the fetal DNA is also analyzed. The results are shown below. Which of the following risk figures reflect the risk of the fetus being affected before and after testing?

a.   1/2, virtually 0
b.   1/4, 2/3
c.   1/4, 1/2
d.   1/4, 2/3
e.   1/4, virtually 0

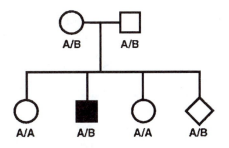

494. The screening test for phenylketonuria (PKU) is called the Guthrie test. Based on this screening method, which of the following is the most likely explanation of a false-negative screen in a newborn?

a.   Bacteria placed on the agar plate
b.   Excess infant blood on the agar plate
c.   Sampling of infant blood before adequate dietary intake due to early discharge requirements
d.   Sampling of infant blood after the newborn period
e.   Adding an inhibitor of bacterial growth to the plate

495. The aspect of PKU that provides the most important reason for newborn screening is

a.   The severity of the disorder
b.   The high frequency of carriers
c.   The availability of effective treatment
d.   The value of genetic counseling
e.   The availability of prenatal diagnosis for the disorder

496. Which of the following is most likely in an untreated child with PKU?

a. Elevated tyrosine
b. Increased skin pigmentation
c. Decreased skin pigmentation
d. Normal phenylalanine hydroxylase levels
e. Elevated alanine

497. A newborn presents with ambiguous genitalia, having an enlarged clitoris or small phallus and labial fusion or hypoplastic scrotum. The newborn's sex can most reliably be established by

a. Buccal smear to determine if there are one or two Barr bodies
b. Buccal smear to determine if there is one Barr body or none
c. Peripheral blood karyotype
d. Bone marrow karyotype
e. Polymerase chain reaction (PCR) using primers specific for the long arm of the Y chromosome

498. The dot-blot shown below examines DNA from a child with ambiguous genitalia after polymerase chain reaction (PCR) amplification and hybridization with DNA probes from the X and Y chromosome. In this case, the Y chromosome probe is from the SRY region of Yp that has recently been characterized as the male-determining region. DNA from control male and female patients is also applied to the dot-blot. Based on the dot-blot results, which is the most likely conclusion?

a. The proband is a genetic male
b. The proband is a genetic female
c. The proband is male
d. The proband is female
e. The proband is mosaic 46,XX/46,XY

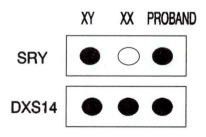

499. A child has ambiguous genitalia including an apparent small phallus and scrotum. The child's DNA hybridizes to probes from the sex-determining region of the Y (SRY). Based on the clinical findings and dot-blot analysis, which of the following terms applies?

a. Female pseudohermaphroditism
b. Male pseudohermaphroditism
c. True hermaphroditism
d. XY female
e. XX male

500. A newborn with ambiguous genitalia and a 46,XY karyotype develops vomiting, low serum sodium concentration, and high serum potassium. Which of the following proteins is most likely to be abnormal?

a. 21-hydroxylase
b. An ovarian enzyme
c. 5α-reductase
d. An androgen receptor
e. A testicular enzyme

Genetic and Biochemical Diagnosis

Answers

435. The answer is e. (*Murray, pp 812–828. Scriver, pp 3–45. Sack, pp 97–158. Wilson, pp 361–391.*) Specific gene mutations must be characterized for a disease before DNA testing to reveal those mutations that can be employed for diagnosis. Some diseases, such as diabetes mellitus with autoimmune pathogenesis, can exhibit associations with particular HLA alleles that would allow DNA testing. However, such testing merely increases or decreases the likelihood of diagnosis rather than being definitive. Parkinson's disease gives little evidence of genetic predisposition because twin concordance rates (the fraction of pairs of twins that are both affected) are low and the incidence in siblings of affected individuals is minimally elevated. Monozygotic twin concordance rates should be 100% for Mendelian disorders and 20 to 40% for multifactorial disorders such as cleft palate. Slight elevations in twin concordance or sibling rates may reflect cohabitation and exposure to similar environmental factors rather than genetic predisposition. However, a genetic basis cannot be excluded for Parkinson's disease since novel gene mutations can occur in somatic cells (i.e., substantia nigra), particularly in older individuals. Metabolic alterations in dopamine would support some type of somatic gene mutation, since most metabolic diseases are genetic.

436. The answer is c. (*Murray, pp 347–358. Scriver, pp 3–45. Sack, pp 97–158. Wilson, pp 361–391.*) Dopamine is produced from L-dopa, which in turn is made from tyrosine. Therapy with the L-dopa precursor increases dopamine concentrations and improves the rigidity and immobility that occur in Parkinson's disease. Dopamine is degraded in the synaptic cleft by monoamine oxidases A and B (MAO-A and MAO-B), producing 3,4-dihydroxyphenylacetaldehyde (DOPAC). DOPAC is in turn broken down to homovanillic acid, which can be measured in spinal fluid to assess dopamine metabolism. Inhibitors of MAO-A and MAO-B have some use in treating Parkinson's disease. The metabolism of histidine or alanine is not related to that of dopamine, but phenylalanine is a precursor of tyrosine and L-dopa.

437. The answer is d. (*Murray, pp 812–828. Scriver, pp 3–45. Sack, pp 97–158. Wilson, pp 1–22.*) A family history is an important precedent for anesthesia, and awareness of individual differences is important when administering any drug. Pharmacogenetics is the area of study that examines genetic influences on drug metabolism. The extensive human genetic variation revealed by DNA analysis has important implications for pharmacology, since drug effects often vary according to each patient's unique genome.

438. The answer is b. (*Murray, pp 812–828. Scriver, pp 3–45. Sack, pp 97–158. Wilson, pp 361–391.*) Succinylcholine is metabolized by a plasma enzyme formerly called pseudocholinesterase [now called butyryl-cholinesterase (BChE) to designate its favored substrate]. Approximately 1 in 100 individuals are homozygous for a variant of BChE that has 60% activity, while 1 in 150,000 individuals are homozygous for a variant with 33% activity. The latter group exhibits prolonged recovery from succinylcholine-induced anesthesia, a phenotype known as succinylcholine apnea. As with most enzyme defects, succinylcholine apnea exhibits autosomal recessive inheritance. The father is presumably homozygous for a BChE variant, like his two deceased siblings, but has not undergone anesthesia to display the phenotype. His daughter is also likely to be homozygous, implying that her mother is a heterozygote. (Note that the BChE variant with 60% activity has a heterozygote frequency of 1/5 by application of the Hardy-Weinberg law.)

439. The answer is c. (*Murray, pp 812–828. Scriver, pp 3–45. Sack, pp 97–158. Wilson, pp 81–97.*) Succinylcholine competes with acetylcholine, the molecule that is released by motor nerve endings to activate muscle end plates. Antibodies to acetylcholine arise in myasthenia gravis (weak muscles), prompting therapies to elevate acetylcholine levels. Acetylcholine is synthesized from acetyl coenzyme A and choline and incorporated into synaptic vesicles. Depolarization of the nerve causes calcium uptake and acetylcholine release by exocytosis. The released acetylcholine binds to acetylcholine receptors on the motor end plate, causing sodium uptake, depolarization of the muscle membrane, and contraction. Acetylcholine is degraded by acetylcholinesterase, and the choline is recycled by active transport back into the nerve ending. Inhibitors of acetylcholinesterase are of three types—irreversible poisons like DFP, transient inhibitors like Tensilon that are used as diagnostic tests for myasthenia gravis, and longer-acting agents like neostigmine that are used as therapy. Treatments of schizophrenia and Parkinson's disease involve manipulation of other neu-rotransmitter pathways.

440. The answer is e. (*Murray, pp 48–62. Scriver, pp 5559–5586. Sack, pp 97–158. Wilson, pp 361–391.*) Serum protein electrophoresis separates pro-teins according to their structure and charge. Two bands for AAT in this man imply that two types of AAT protein with different structures or charges are present. The electrophoresis does not reveal whether the abnormal AAT protein has normal or abnormal activity. The McKusick number indicates that AAT deficiency is autosomal dominant, implying that two homologous loci encode AAT proteins. The man is thus heterozygous, one locus encod-ing a normal and one an abnormal protein. The AAT locus is located on chromosome 14 within a family of protease inhibitors called serpins. Altered AAT proteins termed M, S, or Z variants have normal inhibitory activity but are defective in their rates of secretion across the liver membrane into the blood. Lower levels of AAT protein apparently expose lung proteins to damage, causing emphysema. Heterozygotes are usually not affected, so the man may have emphysema because of cigarette smoking or other fac-tors. Homozygous ZZ individuals may have liver disease in addition to lung disease because the abnormally secreted AAT accumulates in liver cells.

441. The answer is b. (*Murray, pp 259–267. Scriver, pp 3827–3876. Sack, pp 97–158. Wilson, pp 287–320.*) Metabolic diseases usually exhibit autoso-mal or X-linked recessive inheritance. Autosomal recessive inheritance is most likely because the affected patient is female. In this case, the parents are obligate carriers and there is a 1/4 chance (25% recurrence risk) that their next child will be affected. The symptoms suggest Tay-Sachs disease (272800), an autosomal recessive disorder involving severe neurodegener-ation and early death.

442. The answer is b. (*Murray, pp 259–267. Scriver, pp 3827–3876. Sack, pp 97–158. Wilson, pp 287–320.*) The lysosomal enzyme hexosaminidase A is deficient in Tay-Sachs disease. The enzyme cleaves aminohexose groups from gangliosides, complex lipids formed from ceramide (a derivative of sphingosine). Ceramide is synthesized in the endoplasmic reticulum from palmitoyl coenzyme A (16-carbon acyl CoA) and serine in a reaction cat-alyzed by pyridoxal phosphate. Uridine diphosphoglucose (UDP-glucose) or UDP-galactose moeities and sialic acid groups are then added in the Golgi apparatus and the gangliosides contribute to myelin in nerve cells.

Neurolipidoses like Tay-Sachs disease lack certain lysosomal enzymes necessary to degrade the gangliosides, causing severe effects on nerve cells (neurodegeneration). A parallel group of disorders called mucopolysaccharidoses result from the absence of lysosomal enzymes that degrade complex carbohydrate chains and their associated proteins (called proteoglycans). Proteoglycans are more widely distributed than gangliosides, occurring in the ground substance of many tissues. Accumulation of the glycosaminoglycans from these proteoglycans thus causes a wide spectrum of symptoms including coarsening of the face and hair, cardiopulmonary problems, and bony deformities such as kyphosis (beaked spine). There is a specific lysosomal receptor that recognizes mannose-6-phosphate on certain lysosomal enzymes and targets them to lysosomes. Mutations in this receptor can cause increased blood levels and lysosomal deficiencies of several enzymes that are normally targeted to lysosomes. One such disease is I (inclusion) cell disease (252500). The slow accumulation of abnormal gangliosides in lipidoses and of abnormal proteoglycans in mucopolysaccharidoses causes a characteristic clinical course of normal early development that plateaus and then regresses. The age of regression and lifespan vary widely among the lysosomal storage diseases, with Tay-Sachs being one of the most severe.

443. The answer is e. (*Murray, pp 259–267. Scriver, pp 3827–3876. Sack, pp 97–158. Wilson, pp 287–320.*) To determine the joint probability of two or more independent events, the product of their separate probabilities must be determined. If the parents were both Ashkenazi Jews, they would have a 1/30 chance of carrying an abnormal gene for Tay-Sachs disease; for each pregnancy, they would have a 1/2 chance of passing that gene along should they carry it. The probability that all of these four independent events would occur is $1/30 \times 1/2 \times 1/30 \times 1/2$ or 1/3600. The joint probability for a mother who is an Ashkenazi Jew and a father who is not is $1/30 \times 1/2 \times 1/300 \times 1/2$ or 1/36,000.

444. The answer is c. (*Murray, pp 259–267. Scriver, pp 3827–3876. Sack, pp 97–158. Wilson, pp 287–320.*) The probability that any one sibling is homozygous normal is 1/3. The human leukocyte antigen (HLA) cluster on chromosome 6 consists of several loci that are each highly polymorphic. Because the loci are clustered together, their polymorphic products form haplotypes (i.e., A1-B8-DR2 on one chromosome and A9-B5-DR3 on another chromosome). Since recombination among HLA loci is unlikely, the chances of two siblings being HLA-identical are essentially those of inheriting the same parental chromosomes, that is, 1/4. The chance for a sibling to be both homozygous normal for Tay-Sachs disease and HLA-compatible is $1/3 \times 1/4$ = 1/12. Since there are three siblings, the total chance is $1/12 \times 3$, or 1/4.

445. The answer is e. *(Murray, pp 259–267. Scriver, pp 3827–3876. Sack, pp 97–158. Wilson, pp 287–320.)* The physician is obligated to describe a patient's disease accurately in the medical record and to share such records with legally entitled entities, such as health insurance companies. Although care should be exercised that records containing confidential information are not shared inappropriately, there was no such breach of confidentiality in this case. If the physician had declined further care without appropriate notice, then this would be a breach of ongoing care. However, insurance companies and managed care plans have excluded patients because of prior conditions or excessive expenses (i.e., capitation limits). This does constitute discrimination, but application of the Americans with Disabilities Act to patients with genetic diseases is not yet routine. These dilemmas will grow dramatically with the increasing ability to test for genetic diseases and predispositions. Although the administration of exogenous normal enzyme (enzyme therapy) or transplantation to provide a cellular source of normal enzyme has been successful in correcting lysosomal deficiencies, the enzymes fail to cross the blood-brain barrier in sufficient amounts to remit neurological symptoms in patients with lipidoses. This form of enzyme therapy has the advantage of targeting the defective organelle via the mannose-6-phosphate residues on the enzyme. It is very expensive but effective in lipidoses that have few neurological symptoms, such as Gaucher's disease (230800).

446. The answer is a. *(Murray, pp 259–267. Scriver, pp 3827–3876. Sack, pp 97–158. Wilson, pp 287–320.)* Most enzymes are expressed in chorionic villi or amniocytes and allow prenatal diagnosis of metabolic disorders through cell culture and enzyme assay. Percutaneous umbilical blood sampling (PUBS), or cordocentesis, offers another strategy if the enzyme is normally present in leukocytes. However, transabdominal aspiration of the umbilical cord is difficult and must be performed later in pregnancy (18+ weeks) than CVS (8 to 10 weeks). α-fetoprotein (AFP) is not known to be involved in any metabolic disorders, but it is used as an index of fetal tissue differentiation and integrity. Amniotic or maternal serum α-fetoprotein (MSAFP) is most often used to detect, respectively, neural tube defects or chromosomal disorders and would not be useful in a case of normal fetal development with hexosaminidase A deficiency.

447. The answer is c. (*Murray, pp 812–828. Scriver, pp 5287–5312. Sack, pp 97–158. Wilson, pp 287–320.*) Although a mutation at a single locus generally alters a single gene, the result being the abnormal synthesis or lack of production of a single RNA molecule or polypeptide chain, the results of this mutation may be far-reaching. When there are multiple phenotypic effects involving multiple systems, the result is referred to as pleiotropy. Penetrance is the all-or-none expression of an abnormal genotype, whereas expressivity is the degree of expression of that genotype. Incomplete or reduced penetrance implies that some individuals have a mutant allele with absolutely no phenotypic expression of that allele. Variable expressivity implies that all individuals with a mutant allele have some phenotypic effects, although the severity and range of effects differ in different people. Marfan's syndrome (154700) exhibits pleiotropy of its single-gene mutation by causing lens dislocation, loose connective tissue (joint laxity, tall stature, sternal and vertebral deformities), and fragile aortic tissue that can lead to aortic valve insufficiency or aortic dissection. Individuals with the disease exhibit variable combinations and severity of these symptoms due to variable expressivity of this single gene.

448. The answer is c. (*Murray, pp 812–828. Scriver, pp 5287–5312. Sack, pp 97–158. Wilson, pp 287–320.*) Mutations in structural proteins often exhibit autosomal dominant inheritance, while mutations in enzymes often exhibit autosomal recessive inheritance. Structural proteins such as collagen or fibrillin must interact to form scaffolds in the extracellular matrix of connective tissue. Mutation at one of the homologous autosomal loci can introduce an abnormal polypeptide throughout the scaffold much like a misshapen brick in a wall—the distorted polypeptide from the abnormal locus subverts that from the normal locus and weakens the connective tissue matrix, causing autosomal dominant disease. Sometimes the abnormal polypeptide complexes with normal polypeptides and causes them to be degraded, a mechanism called protein suicide. The suicidal effects of mutations at some loci are referred to generally as "dominant negative" mutations. Fibrillin is a glycoprotein used to form a scaffold in the connective tissue filaments called microfibrils. It is distributed in the suspensory ligament for the lens of the eye, the aorta, and the bones and joints, accounting for the symptoms of Marfan's syndrome (154700). Similar pathogenetic mechanisms occur in the osteogenesis imperfectas (e.g., 166200) with multiple fractures and in the Ehlers-Danlos syndromes (e.g., 130060) with skin fragility (scarring) and vascular disease due to mutations in various collagens. The mutations disrupt the α helix secondary structure of collagens, which is dependent on the glycine-X-Y triplet amino acid repeats; the distorted collagen polypeptides then disrupt the collagen fibrils with symptoms dependent on its tissue distribution (2 types of fibrillin and more than 15 types of collagen are known).

449. The answer is b. (*Murray, pp 812–828. Scriver, pp 5241–5286. Sack, pp 97–158. Wilson, pp 287–320.*) The spectrum of mutations in collagen (and fibrillin) disorders is very broad, making it more efficient to evaluate electrophoretic mobility of their polypeptide chains as a clue to structural abnormality. Almost every patient with osteogenesis imperfecta (and other collagen disorders) has a different type of mutation. PCR amplification followed by allele-specific oligonucleotide (ASO) hybridation to detect specific alleles is thus impractical—hundreds of PCR/ASO reactions would be required to screen for all of the possible mutant alleles. Similarly, DNA sequencing would be extraordinarily time-consuming and give many false positives due to nucleotide polymorphisms or silent mutations that do not cause structural abnormalities in the polypeptide. Northern blotting would detect mutations that affect RNA processing and generate RNAs of altered size, but these are a small fraction of possible collagen mutations.

As DNA chip technology becomes practical, screening for thousands of mutations at a locus may be possible. DNA chips contain thousands of different oligonucleotides embedded on a solid matrix. Hybridization of colored or labeled gene fragments with randomized sequences from that gene on a chip gives signals corresponding to the gene sequences that are present. The chip can then be washed and used again. Hybridization of the chip with suitably digested DNAs from patients and controls can thus detect any variant gene fragment (complementary oligonucleotide). Use of numerous control DNAs would separate true mutant alleles (sequence variants associated with disease) from polymorphisms or silent mutations.

450. The answer is b. (*Murray, pp 787–811. Scriver, pp 521–524. Sack, pp 85–96. Wilson, pp 187–224.*) The two-hit hypothesis was developed by Knudsen to explain why patients with hereditary retinoblastoma [germline mutations (180200)] have multiple, bilateral tumors while those with sporadic tumors (no family history) have single tumors. A germ-line mutation (first hit) alters one Rb allele and confers enhanced susceptibility to retinoblastoma. A somatic mutation (second hit) inactivating the other homologous Rb allele can then occur in any tissue. If it occurs in the retina, a tumor is born. The multiple tumors thus represent the sites at which somatic mutations have occurred in the retina. In sporadic cases, two somatic mutational events must take place. Since these somatic mutations are relatively rare events, it is extremely uncommon for more than one tumor to develop. It is curious that, although retinoblastoma susceptibility is inherited in a dominant fashion, tumor development is a recessive event, requiring the inactivation of both alleles. Genes such as Rb are called tumor suppressor genes, in contrast to oncogenes, in which only one of the two homologous alleles must be altered to initiate malignant transformation. Alteration of an enhancer or promoter site on one Rb allele would thus not be sufficient to cause cancer, since the other Rb allele would not be affected. Obvious chromosome changes such as 13q− are rare compared to other mutations that alter Rb function.

451. The answer is a. (*Murray, pp 787–811. Scriver, pp 521–552. Sack, pp 85–96. Wilson, pp 187–224.*) Chromosome translocations may often promote tumors in somatic cells by placing regulatory genes next to promoters that aberrantly increase their expression. Burkitt's lymphoma, a B cell lymphoma that usually occurs in childhood, often involves reciprocal translocation of chromosomes 8 and 14. The result of this is to place the *c-myc* protooncogene from 8q24 into the immunoglobulin heavy chain locus at 14q32. Since immunoglobulin genes are actively transcribed, this move alters the normal regulatory control of *c-myc*. Another example is the Philadelphia chromosome, a shortened chromosome 22 caused by translocation t(9:22)(q34:q11). This translocation is seen in almost all patients with chronic myelogenous leukemia (CML) and in a percentage of patients with acute lymphoblastic leukemia (ALL). The Philadelphia chromosome is seen with increased frequency in individuals with Down's syndrome.

452. The answer is b. (*Murray, pp 787–811. Scriver, pp 521–552. Sack, pp 85–96. Wilson, pp 187–224.*) Genetic predisposition to cancer is best understood by the Knudsen hypothesis, where two independent mutations or "hits" are required to produce neoplasia of a somatic tissue. In many hereditary cancers, the "first hit" is a germ-line mutation that is transmitted in families. Individuals who inherit this mutation are much more likely to develop cancer through a "second hit" in their somatic cells. The second hit can be any mutation that removes the homologous allele (loss of heterozygosity); mechanisms include missense mutation, chromosome deletion, and chromosome nondisjunction. For tumor suppressor genes like those responsible for neurofibromatosis 1 (162200) or the Li-Fraumeni syndrome (114480), the first hit removes one suppressor allele and the second hit removes the homologous suppressor allele. The family in the question is an example of a "cancer family" that exhibits the bone, breast, colon, and blood cancers that are typical of Li-Fraumeni syndrome. The mechanism involves mutations in the *src* tumor suppressor gene.

453. The answer is d. (*Murray, pp 787–811. Scriver, pp 521–552. Sack, pp 85–96. Wilson, pp 187–224.*) Presymptomatic DNA testing of individuals in cancer families is increasingly available. However, testing of minors is controversial because they may not be old or mature enough to understand the personal, medical, and financial implications. They therefore cannot give truly informed consent. Beneficence is the ethical imperative to do good for patients, while nonmaleficence is the imperative to do no harm. Autonomy refers to a patient's right to make decisions regarding his or her health care, and confidentiality to the privilege of doctor-patient communication.

454. The answer is d. (*Murray, pp 258–284. Scriver, pp 2863–2914. Sack, pp 205–222. Wilson, pp 361–391.*) This man has familial hypercholesterolemia (143890), an autosomal dominant phenotype defined by studying men who experienced heart attacks at young ages. Mutations in the LDL receptor lead to decreased cellular cholesterol uptake and increased serum cholesterol. Since LDL has a high cholesterol content, the LDL fraction is elevated compared to the HDL fraction on lipoprotein electrophoresis. In normal individuals, the LDL is taken up by its specific receptor and imported via caveolae to the cell interior. Cholesterol then produces feedback inhibition on the rate-limiting enzyme of cholesterol synthesis (hydroxymethylglutaryl CoA reductase) and also leads to a decrease in the number of LDL receptors. In rare cases, two individuals with familial hypercholesterolemia marry and produce a child with homozygous familial hypercholesterolemia. These children develop severe atherosclerosis and xanthomas (fatty tumors) at an early age.

455. The answer is c. (*Murray, pp 258–284. Scriver, pp 2863–2914. Sack, pp 205–222. Wilson, pp 361–391.*) Nitroglycerin causes release of nitric oxide (NO), which activates guanyl cyclase, produces cyclic GMP, and causes vasodilation. NO is formed from one of the guanidino nitrogens of the arginine side chain by the enzyme nitric oxide synthase. NO has a short half-life, reacting with oxygen to form nitrite, then nitrates that are excreted in urine. Coronary vasodilation caused by nitroglycerin is thus short-lived, making other measures necessary for long-term relief of coronary occlusion. The neurotransmitter formed by condensation of acetyl CoA and choline is acetylcholine.

456. The answer is c. *(Murray, pp 763–779. Scriver, pp 2961–3062. Sack, pp 205–222. Wilson, pp 361–391.)* The symptoms are typical of iron-deficiency anemia, in this case caused by increased blood loss through menstruation. Transferrin is a glycoprotein that transports iron among tissues. Its amounts in serum can be measured as the total iron-binding capacity. Under conditions of iron deficiency, the percentage of transferrin saturated with iron (normally about 33%) is decreased. A specific transferrin receptor brings the iron-ferritin complex into cells, and it is regulated in response to iron stores. When iron is deficient, the number of transferrin receptors is increased. Ferritin is a protein that stores iron in tissues and is minimally present in serum unless there is iron excess. About 10% of the hemoglobin released by normal red cell destruction is bound by haptoglobin. The remainder is salvaged from damaged red cells that are degraded in the reticuloendothelial system. Haptoglobins are decreased in hemolytic anemias in which there is increased release of hemoglobin.

457. The answer is d. *(Murray, pp 763–779. Scriver, pp 3127–3162. Sack, pp 121–138. Wilson, pp 361–391.)* The man has symptoms of hemochromatosis (235200), an autosomal recessive disorder with increased iron absorption from the small intestine. There is increased serum iron, higher saturation of transferrin, and increased amounts of ferritin-iron complex so that it appears in serum. The red cell lifetime is normal in hemochromatosis, resulting in normal release of hemoglobin and normal serum haptoglobin. Hemochromatosis is caused by mutations at a locus in the histocompatibility region of chromosome 6; the protein product is localized to the small intestine and influences iron absorption by an unknown mechanism.

458. The answer is d. *(Murray, pp 763–779. Scriver, pp 3127–3162. Sack, pp 121–138. Wilson, pp 361–391.)* The regulation of mammalian gene expression is selective: specific genes are up- or downregulated by controls at the gene dosage, mRNA transcription, mRNA splicing, mRNA stability, or protein function levels. Under conditions of iron deficiency, transferrin receptor mRNA is stabilized so that more protein is synthesized. Regulation thus occurs at the protein translation level, without changes in transferrin mRNA transcription through transcription factors or transferrin receptor activity through interaction with small molecules (allostery) or through phosphorylation by protein kinases. Overall increases in rates of RNA transcription or protein elongation are not employed for gene regulation by mammalian cells.

459. The answer is b. (*Murray, pp 763–779. Scriver, pp 3105–3126. Sack, pp 121–138. Wilson, pp 287–326.*) This child's kinky hair is a symptom of Menke's disease, an alteration in a copper-binding ATPase. Dysfunction of the ATPase imprisons copper in cells and prevents its normal absorption from the intestine. Enzymes that use copper as cofactor have diverse roles in metabolism, including some that modify and degrade amino acids in collagen. This accounts for the connective tissue symptoms (lax joints, thin skin) in Menke's disease. Wilson's disease (277900) is also caused by mutations in a copper-binding ATPase that lead to copper storage in liver (causing hepatitis and cirrhosis) and the brain (sometimes causing psychosis). Ceruloplasmin, the major copper transporter in serum, is decreased in both diseases.

460. The answer is e. (*Murray, pp 787–811. Scriver, pp 521–524. Sack, pp 85–96. Wilson, pp 187–224.*) Contiguous gene syndromes, also known as microdeletion syndromes, occur when deletions result in the loss of several different closely linked loci. Depending on the size of the deletion, different phenotypes may result. Mutations in the individual genes may result in isolated features that may be inherited in a Mendelian fashion.

461. The answer is c. (*Murray, pp 812–828. Scriver, pp 5467–5492. Sack, pp 97–158. Wilson, pp 287–320.*) Polycystic kidney disease occurs in two distinctive genetic forms—adult-onset and infantile. Infantile disease is autosomal recessive, while adult-onset disease is autosomal dominant. Confusion between these types can occur due to variable expressivity in the adult, dominant form. Occasional onset in young children may occur in adult-type disease. Consistency of early onset, the presence of consanguinity, and the lack of vertical transmission distinguish the infantile, recessive form. Polycystic kidney disease is an example of genetic heterogeneity, in which different mutations may cause similar phenotypes. This may be further divided into allelic and nonallelic (locus) heterogeneity. Allelic heterogeneity implies that there are different mutations at the same locus that both result in similar disease [i.e., the many fibrillin mutations in Marfan's syndrome (154700)]. In locus heterogeneity, mutations occur at different loci, yet the phenotype is similar. Locus heterogeneity also explains why certain disorders, such as polycystic kidney disease, Charcot-Marie-Tooth disease, sensorineural hearing loss, and retinitis pigmentosa may be inherited in several different fashions. A general rule predicts that the autosomal recessive forms of these diseases will be more severe, the autosomal dominant forms less so. It is especially important to recognize the possibility of genetic heterogeneity when counseling patients in regard to recurrence risks.

462. The answer is a. (*Murray, pp 812–828. Scriver, pp 2537–2570. Sack, pp 97–158. Wilson, pp 287–320.*) The child has Lesch-Nyhan syndrome (308000), an X-linked recessive disorder that is caused by HGPRT enzyme deficiency. HGPRT is responsible for the salvage of purines from nucleotide degradation, and its deficiency elevates levels of PRPP, purine synthesis, and uric acid. PRPP is also elevated in glycogen storage diseases due to increased amounts of carbohydrate precursors.

463. The answer is e. (*Murray, pp 812–828. Scriver, pp 2537–2570. Sack, pp 97–158. Wilson, pp 287–320.*) Polymorphic DNA regions with variable numbers of tandem repeats (VNTRs) yield an assortment of DNA fragment sizes after restriction endonuclease digestion. The visualization of variable fragments (alleles) from a particular VNTR region can be performed by hybridization with a DNA probe after electrophoresis and transfer (Southern blotting). If the VNTR region is near (linked to) a disease locus, the VNTR alleles can be used to determine which accompanying allele at the disease locus is present. Transmission of VNTR allele B to the affected individual III-3 in the figure that accompanies the question establishes phase and indicates that the abnormal Lesch-Nyhan (L-N) allele is cosegregating with VNTR allele B in this family. Individual I-1 is an obligate carrier because both II-4 and III-3 received abnormal L-N alleles (the rare chance of two L-N mutations in one family is discounted). Individuals II-2 and II-3 are thus carriers by virtue of inheriting the B allele from their mother. Individual III-2 is not a carrier because she did not inherit the B allele, and her fetus is not at risk for L-N. These conclusions do not reflect the possibility of recombination between the VNTR allele and the abnormal L-N allele. If one of the affected individuals had a common mutant allele that could be detected by direct analysis of the HGPRT gene, then fetal DNA analysis could be performed without concern about recombination.

464. The answer is b. (*Murray, pp 812–828. Scriver, pp 3–45. Sack, pp 57–76. Wilson, pp 123–149.*) The child described in the question has multiple independent anomalies that are characteristic of a syndrome. Although they are likely to be causally related, they do not appear to be sequential. These problems do not appear to be caused by the breakdown of an originally normal developmental process as in a disruption, nor do they appear to be related to a nondisruptive mechanical force as in a deformation.

465. The answer is c. (*Murray, pp 812–828. Scriver, pp 3–45. Sack, pp 57–76. Wilson, pp 123–149.*) Fluorescent in situ hybridization (FISH) analysis is a technique in which molecular probes that are specific for individual chromosomes or chromosomal regions are used to identify these regions. FISH probes frequently identify chromosomal regions that are submicroscopic and therefore may be useful when standard karyotypic analysis is normal. In this case, the fact that only one signal is present, despite the fact that there are two number 22 chromosomes, indicates that a submicroscopic deletion has occurred. The parental chromosome of origin cannot be determined using this technique unless that parent also carries a similar deletion and his or her chromosomes are evaluated.

466. The answer is b. (*Murray, pp 812–828. Scriver, pp 3–45. Sack, pp 191–204. Wilson, pp 81–97.*) Individuals affected with autoimmune disorders such as juvenile diabetes mellitus, ankylosing spondylitis, or rheumatoid arthritis often have increased frequencies of particular HLA alleles, termed allele associations. Genetic linkage differs from allele association in that the linking of allele and phenotype depends on the family context; one family may exhibit segregation of the nail-patella phenotype with allele A of the ABO blood group while another family exhibits segregation with allele O. Allele association or linkage disequilibrium implies that the same allele is always seen at higher frequency in affected individuals from different families (e.g., HLA-B27 in ankylosing spondylitis). Allele association implies neither a genotype-phenotype relation between allele and disease nor a common chromosomal location for allele and disease. It may indicate a role for the allele in facilitating disease pathogenesis. In contrast, genetic linkage places a disease gene on the chromosome map, facilitating its isolation by positional cloning. Gene mutations in various individuals can then be characterized, allowing genotype-phenotype correlations. HLA testing for autoimmune disorders, like cholesterol testing for heart disease, exemplifies the use of risk factors to modify risks for multifactorial diseases.

467. The answer is c. *(Murray, pp 812–828. Scriver, pp 3–45. Sack, pp 121–144. Wilson, pp 59–79.)* Under certain conditions, the Hardy-Weinberg law allows one to interconvert genotype and allele frequencies in a population by using the formula $(p + q)_2 = p_2 + 2pq + q_2$. For a locus with two alleles, p represents the frequency of the more common allele, q of the less common allele, and $p + q = 1$. The Minnesota population therefore has $p^2 = 7/8 \times 7/8 = 49/64$ (4900 individuals) with the AA genotype, $2pq = 2 \times 7/8 \times 1/8 = 14/64$ (1400 individuals) with sickle trait (AS genotype), and $q_2 = 1/8 \times 1/8 = 1/64$ (100 individuals) with sickle cell disease (SS genotype). The African population has a higher frequency of AS and SS genotypes caused by heterozygote advantage for the AS genotype that confers resistance to malaria.

468. The answer is e. *(Murray, pp 812–828. Scriver, pp 3–45. Sack, pp 121–144. Wilson, pp 59–79.)* Even if SS individuals were prevented from contributing to the next generation by sterilization, breeding between AS individuals would replenish SS genotype frequencies. This stability of populations in accord with the Hardy-Weinberg law is often referred to as the Hardy-Weinberg equilibrium. During the decades of 1900 to 1920 in America, the eugenics movement succeeded in passing laws obligating sterilization of those with mental disabilities. These laws were based on two false premises—the idea that mental retardation is always due to Mendelian transmission (ignoring chromosomal and multifactorial disease) and the idea that elimination of affected people will always change gene frequencies.

469. The answer is c. *(Murray, pp 812–828. Scriver, pp 1553–1588. Sack, pp 121–144. Wilson, pp 59–79.)* This infant may have galactosemia (230400), a deficiency of galactose-1-phosphate uridyl transferase (GALT). Galactose from lactose in breast milk or infant formula is phosphorylated by galactokinase, activated to uridine diphosphogalactose (UDP-galactose) by GALT, and converted to UDP-glucose by UDP-galactose epimerase. The elevation of galactose metabolites is thought to cause liver toxicity, and their urinary excretion produces reducing substances. Infants with the signs and symptoms listed are placed on lactose-free formulas until enzyme testing is complete. Deficiencies of epimerase or kinase can cause mild forms of galactosemia.

470. The answer is b. (*Murray, pp 812–828. Scriver, pp 1553–1588. Sack, pp 121–144. Wilson, pp 59–79.*) The Hardy-Weinberg expansion, $p^2 + 2pq + q^2$, describes the frequency of genotypes for allele frequencies p and q. In the case of rare disorders ($q^2 < \frac{1}{10,000}$), p approaches 1. The heterozygote frequency $2pq$ is thus approximately $2q$. In this case, $q^2 = \frac{1}{40,000}$, $q = \frac{1}{200}$, and $2q = \frac{1}{100}$. Since carriers are still quite rare compared with normal individuals, the matching of rare recessive alleles is greatly enhanced when there is common descent through consanguinity.

471. The answer is d. (*Murray, pp 812–828. Scriver, pp 3–45. Sack, pp 121–144. Wilson, pp 23–98.*) The mother of the pregnant woman (consultand) is an obligate carrier since she has two affected sons with hemophilia. The consultand thus has a 1/2 chance of receiving the X that carries the abnormal gene and being a carrier. The risk for her fetus to have hemophilia A is thus $1/2 \times 1/4 = 1/8$. In practice, this risk could be modified by recognizing that the woman has already had two normal boys. Among carriers with two boys, the boys would be normal only 1/4 of the time. The a priori 1/2 chance the woman is a carrier could then be modified to $1/2 \times 1/4 = 1/8$. The a priori 1/2 chance that she is not a carrier could also be modified by the 100% chance that women who are not carriers will have two normal boys ($1/2 \times 1 = 1/2$). The modified risk that the woman is a carrier now becomes the modified chance she is a carrier (1/8) divided by all the possibilities (1/8 + 1/2 or 4/8), giving a modified risk of 1/5. The risk of her fetus having hemophilia would then be lower at 1/20. This process for weighting probabilities according to conditional facts is derived from Bayes theorem, named after an English statistician.

472. The answer is e. (*Murray, pp 812–828. Scriver, pp 3–45. Sack, pp 121–144. Wilson, pp 23–98.*) Hemophilia A is caused by deficiency of factor VIII and hemophilia B by deficiency of factor IX. Both factors are involved in the intrinsic blood coagulation pathway that results in activation of factor X. Alternatively, factor X can be activated by tissue factors through the extrinsic blood coagulation pathway. Activated factors X and V produce thrombin from prothrombin, which in turn cleaves fibrinogen to produce fibrin monomers. The fibrin monomers are polymerized and cross-linked to produce a fibrin polymer, which interacts with platelets and other factors to produce a blood clot. The genes for factor VIII and factor IX are on the X chromosome, making hemophilia A and B X-linked recessive diseases.

473. The answer is b. *(Murray, pp 812–828. Scriver, pp 3–45. Sack, pp 121–144. Wilson, pp 23–98.)* Chorionic villus sampling (CVS) is performed at 8 to 10 weeks gestation, before a woman is obviously pregnant. This technique preserves the confidentiality of prenatal decisions since diagnostic results are available by 11 to 12 weeks gestation rather than the 18 to 20 weeks for standard amniocentesis. DNA analysis must be employed because factor VIII is not expressed in chorion or amniotic cells. Percutaneous umbilical blood sampling (PUBS) must be performed later in gestation (18+ weeks). Since some factor VIII gene mutations may give normal amounts of structurally abnormal factor VIII, activity rather than amounts of factor VIII protein must be measured for diagnosis.

474. The answer is c. *(Murray, pp 812–828. Scriver, pp 3–45. Sack, pp 121–144. Wilson, pp 23–98.)* The predominance of affected males with transmission through females makes this pedigree diagnostic of X-linked recessive inheritance. Individual I-1 is an obligate carrier, as demonstrated by her affected son and grandson. Individual II-2 cannot transmit an X-linked disorder, although his daughters are obligate carriers. Individual II-3 must be a carrier because of her affected son, which results in a 1/4 probability of recurrence of CMT in her offspring. Individual II-5 has a 1/2 probability of being a carrier with a 1/8 probability for affected offspring. Individual III-4 also has a 1/2 probability of being a carrier; her risk for affected offspring is also 1/8 despite the consanguineous marriage. Individual III-8 has a 1/4 chance of being a carrier and a 1/16 chance of having affected offspring. CMT is one of the disorders exhibiting genetic heterogeneity, with autosomal dominant (118200), autosomal recessive (214380), and X-linked recessive (302800) forms.

475. The answer is b. *(Murray, pp 812–828. Scriver, pp 3–45. Sack, pp 121–144. Wilson, pp 23–98.)* The large fragment could derive from a mutation ablating one flanking restriction site or from extra DNA inserted between the restriction sites. The fact that there are two DNA fragment sizes in the affected individual but one in controls suggests alteration of only one of the two homologous CMT regions on chromosome 17. The production of disease by alteration of one homologous locus (one abnormal allele) causes autosomal dominant inheritance. This form of CMT is caused by a duplication of the PMP22 gene, a gene encoding a peripheral myelin protein. The extra copy of PMP22 increases protein abundance and interferes with nerve conduction. DNA duplication is one form of atypical inheritance discovered through DNA analysis.

476. The answer is e. *(Murray, pp 812–828. Scriver, pp 3–45. Sack, pp 57–76. Wilson, pp 227–246.)* The Prader-Willi deletion is quite small and is not usually detected by standard metaphase karyotyping. Fluorescent in situ hybridization (FISH) is the most efficient and accurate method for detecting the deletion in Prader-Willi syndrome. Fluorescent DNA probes from the deletion region (chromosome band 15q11) give two signals in normal subjects and one signal in patients with a deletion. Detection of RNA or DNA fragments from this region would require quantitation to reveal one-half normal amounts, since genes on the homologous 15 chromosome would be normal. It is much easier to visualize one versus two fluorescent signals. Standard karyotypes typically display about 300 bands over the 23 chromosomes or about 10 bands on chromosome 10. This is adequate for detecting aneuploidy but inadequate for small deletions seen in conditions like Prader-Willi syndrome. Rapid karyotyping of bone marrow samples is possible because marrow contains actively dividing cells. Results are available in 2 to 3 h rather than the 2 to 3 days for standard karyotyping because peripheral blood T leukocytes must be stimulated to divide using lectins like phytohemagglutinin. Resolution of bone marrow karyotypes is usually even less than for standard karyotypes from blood, necessitating the use of FISH probes for accurate diagnosis. Newborns suspected of one of the common trisomies can have bone marrow karyotypes with FISH using probes from chromosomes 13, 18, and 21. Diagnosis is thus available in several hours, allowing guidance of management decisions.

477. The answer is d. *(Murray, pp 812–828. Scriver, pp 3–45. Sack, pp 57–76. Wilson, pp 227–246.)* This child has several minor anomalies, a major anomaly that affects the genitalia, and developmental delay. These multiply affected and embryologically unrelated body regions suggest a syndrome rather than a sequence. Because of the multiple anomalies and developmental delay, the first diagnostic test to be considered is a karyotype rather than a test for specific organ function, such as serum testosterone.

478. The answer is c. (*Murray, pp 812–828. Scriver, pp 3–45. Sack, pp 57–76. Wilson, pp 227–246.*) The hypothetical probe D15S8 implies a unique DNA segment that recognizes a single locus on chromosome 15— the eighth such anonymous DNA probe to be isolated. Since normal individuals have two number 15 chromosomes, they should have two alleles visualized after DNA restriction and hybridization with probe D15S8. Since both parents are heterozygous for the D15S8 locus, as shown in the question, the child's result suggests that he has only received the maternal alleles (alleles 1 and 2) for locus D15S8. This implies that he has received both number 15 chromosomes from his mother. This is known as uniparental disomy and may occur due to correction of trisomy 15 conceptions through loss of the paternal number 15 chromosome.

479. The answer is d. (*Murray, pp 812–828. Scriver, pp 3–45. Sack, pp 57–76. Wilson, pp 227–246.*) DNA fingerprinting is used in both paternity and forensic analyses and relies on highly variable DNA polymorphisms called variable numbers of tandem repeats (VNTRs). The multicopy repeats include $(CA)_n$ and minisatellite sequences that are present throughout the genome. The usual VNTR probe is directed against single-copy DNA that flanks these repeats and yields multiple restriction fragment sizes that reflect the number of intervening repeats. The hypothetical probes D7Z5 and D20Z1 shown in the question recognize VNTR loci on chromosomes 7 and 20 that yield at least three alleles. Since the child's two alleles for D7Z5 (and D20Z1) match those of the mother and father, correct maternity and paternity are established with a degree of error equal to the chance that these allele combinations would occur in an unrelated individual. In practice, at least five VNTR probes are employed so that the odds for paternity (or nonpaternity) are very high indeed.

480. The answer is c. (*Murray, pp 812–828. Scriver, pp 3–45. Sack, pp 57–76. Wilson, pp 227–246.*) Informed consent requires that the patient be informed of all adverse effects that might result from a procedure. Evidence for nonpaternity may result from various types of DNA analysis and should be discussed with the concerned parties at the time of blood collection. Some physicians speak to the mother and father separately about this issue to maximize the opportunity for independent decision making.

481. The answer is b. (*Murray, pp 812–828. Scriver, pp 3–45. Sack, pp 57–76. Wilson, pp 227–246.*) In humans and other mammals, the source of genetic material may be as important as its content. Mice manipulated to receive two male pronuclei develop as abortive placentas, while those receiving two female pronuclei develop as abortive fetuses. The different impact of the same genetic material according to whether it is transmitted from mother or father is due to genomic imprinting. The term *imprinting* is borrowed from animal behavior and refers to parental marking during gametogenesis—the physical basis may be DNA methylation or chromatin phasing. Both maternally derived and paternally derived haploid chromosome sets are thus necessary for normal fetal development. This is why parthenogenesis does not occur in mammals. The imprint is erased in the fetal gonads and reestablished based on fetal sex. Certain cases of Prader-Willi syndrome are disorders of imprinting with the absence of the paternally imprinted chromosome 15.

482. The answer is a. (*Murray, pp 812–828. Scriver, pp 3–45. Sack, pp 57–76. Wilson, pp 227–246.*) A missing band suggests an interstitial (internal) deletion rather than removal of the distal short or long arm (known as a terminal deletion). The shorthand notation 15q– implies a terminal deletion of the long arm of chromosome 15. Pericentric (surrounding the centromere) or paracentric (not including the centromere) inversions result from crossover of a chromosome with itself, then breakage and reunion to produce an internal inverted segment. Interstitial deletion 15q11q13 is seen in approximately 50% of patients with Prader-Willi and Angelman's syndromes. Other patients with these syndromes inherit both chromosomes 15 from their mother (Prader-Willi) or both from their father (Angelman's), a situation known as uniparental disomy. Genomic imprinting of the 15q11q13 region is different on the chromosome inherited from the mother than on the chromosome inherited from the father. The normal balance of maternal and paternal imprints is thus disrupted by deletion or uniparental disomy, leading to reciprocal differences in gene expression that present as Angelman's or Prader-Willi syndromes.

483. The answer is c. (*Murray, pp 812–828. Scriver, pp 3–45. Sack, pp 57–76. Wilson, pp 227–246.*) Anticipation refers to the worsening of the symptoms of disease in succeeding generations. The famous geneticist L.S. Penrose dismissed anticipation as an artifact, but the phenomenon has been validated by the discovery of expanding trinucleotide repeats. Steinert myotonic dystrophy is caused by unstable trinucleotide repeats near a muscle protein kinase gene on chromosome 19; the repeats are particularly unstable during female meiosis and may cause a severe syndrome of fetal muscle weakness and joint contractures. Variable expressivity could also be used to describe the family in the question, but the concept implies random variation in severity rather than progression with succeeding generations. Diseases that involve triplet repeat instability exhibit a bias for exaggerated repeat amplification during meiosis (e.g., women with the fragile X syndrome or myotonic dystrophy and men with Huntington's chorea). The explanation for this bias is unknown.

484. The answer is a. *(Murray, pp 812–828. Scriver, pp 3–45. Sack, pp 167–180. Wilson, pp 287–324.)* Spina bifida is a defect of neural tube development that can be partially prevented by encouraging preconceptional folic acid supplementation in women desiring to become pregnant. Examination for subtle evidence of dysmorphology in children with major birth defects is necessary to rule out a syndrome. Syndromes often exhibit Mendelian or chromosomal inheritance.

485. The answer is a. *(Murray, pp 812–828. Scriver, pp 3–45. Sack, pp 167–180. Wilson, pp 287–324.)* When present as an isolated anomaly, spina bifida (meningomyelocele) exhibits multifactorial inheritance. Chromosomal inheritance usually causes a syndrome rather than isolated anomalies. Atypical inheritance (genomic imprinting, trinucleotide repeat instability, mitochondrial inheritance) has not been implicated in neural tube defects.

486. The answer is c. *(Murray, pp 812–828. Scriver, pp 3–45. Sack, pp 167–180. Wilson, pp 287–324.)* The father and child are affected with spina bifida. The next child will be related to them as a primary (first-degree) relative. The existence of two affected primary relatives predicts a recurrence risk of >6%. Had the child had a Mendelian syndrome, the risk could have been as high as 25% from autosomal recessive inheritance.

487. The answer is c. *(Murray, pp 812–828. Scriver, pp 3–45. Sack, pp 167–180. Wilson, pp 395–421.)* Any defect of the fetal skin may elevate the amniotic α-fetoprotein (AFP) level, causing a parallel rise of this substance in the maternal blood. Neural tube defects such as anencephaly or spina bifida elevate the AFP in amniotic fluid or maternal serum; other causes of increased AFP include fetal kidney disease with leakage of fetal proteins into amniotic fluid. Mild forms of spina bifida or meningomyelocele may be covered by the skin, so that the AFP is not elevated, and maternal serum AFP is less sensitive than amniotic fluid AFP for such cases. Ultrasound is required to detect covered neural tube defects that do not leak fetal AFP into the amniotic fluid and maternal blood. Acetylcholinesterase is an enzyme produced at high levels in neural tissue that is somewhat more specific than AFP for neural tube defects; it is used for confirmation rather than as a primary prenatal test. Chorionic villus biopsy is performed at about 10 weeks after the last menstrual period (LMP) and amniocentesis at 14 to 16 postmenstrual weeks. Since conception often occurs 2 weeks prior to the LMP, distinction between postconceptional and postmenstrual timing is important for early stages of pregnancy. Neural tube defects are usually localized, multifactorial anomalies rather than part of a malformation syndrome that can result from chromosomal aberrations. For this reason, documentation of the fetal karyotype by chorionic villus biopsy or amniocentesis does not influence the risk for neural tube defects.

488. The answer is e. *(Murray, pp 812–828. Scriver, pp 3–45. Sack, pp 167–180. Wilson, pp 395–421.)* Genetic counseling is an essential component of every prenatal diagnostic test. Couples must understand their risks and options before selecting a prenatal diagnostic procedure. There must also be adequate provisions for explaining the results. Since additional obstetric procedures, such as pregnancy termination, may follow prenatal diagnosis, obstetricians need to be comprehensive and thorough with the genetic counseling process.

489. The answer is d. *(Murray, pp 238–249. Scriver, pp 2297–2326. Sack, pp 121–144. Wilson, pp 287–324.)* Assuming that nonpaternity or an unusual method of inheritance is not operative, the parents of a child with an autosomal recessive condition are obligate heterozygotes. Therefore, their risk of having a child with medium-chain acyl-coenzyme A (CoA) dehydrogenase deficiency (MCAD) is 1/4 or 25% for each future pregnancy.

490. The answer is a. *(Murray, pp 238–249. Scriver, pp 2297–2326. Sack, pp 121–144. Wilson, pp 287–324.)* Catastrophic metabolic disease often begins after the first few feedings, when the baby is exposed to nutrients that cannot be metabolized and are toxic. Often there are misguided attempts to encourage feeding, which further poisons the child. Inborn errors of carbohydrate, amino acid, or organic/fatty acid metabolism can present in the newborn period. They are characterized by a similar pattern of symptoms that include spitting up, vomiting, exaggeration of the usual physiologic jaundice, lethargy progressing to coma, hypoglycemia, acidosis, hyperammonemia, and, in the case of maple syrup urine disease or isovaleric acidemia, unusual odors. Disorders of fatty acid oxidation worsen during fasting to cause carnitine depletion, failure of fatty acid oxidation, and excretion of dicarboxylic acid intermediates. Deficiencies in medium-chain fatty acid oxidation are milder, and may present after a period of illness with calorie deprivation in children aged 2 to 6 years. Urea cycle disorders worsen during fasting (catabolic breakdown) or protein feeding, producing excess ammonia, rapid breathing, and respiratory alkalosis. Galactosemia worsens on exposure to lactose-containing formula, producing hypoglycemia, liver failure, and excretion of urinary sugars (reducing substances). Tyrosinemia and maple syrup urine disease are amino acid disorders that worsen after protein feeding and produce elevated levels of tyrosine or branch chain amino acids (leucine, isoleucine, valine). Tyrosinemia is associated with severe liver failure and maple syrup urine disease with severe acidosis due to conversion of excess amino acids to ketoacids.

491. The answer is d. (*Murray, pp 238–249. Scriver, pp 2165–2194. Sack, pp 121–144. Wilson, pp 287–324.*) Propionic acidemia (232000) results from a block in propionyl CoA carboxylase (PCC), which converts propionic to methylmalonic acid. Excess propionic acid in the blood produces metabolic acidosis with a decreased bicarbonate and increased anion gap (the serum cations sodium plus potassium minus the serum anions chloride plus bicarbonate). The usual values of sodium (~140 meq/L) plus potassium (~4 meq/L) minus those for chloride (~105 meq/L) plus bicarbonate (~20 meq/L) thus yield a normal anion gap of ~20 meq/L. A low bicarbonate of 6 to 8 meq/L yields an elevated gap of 32 to 34 meq/L, a "gap" of negative charge that is supplied by the hidden anion (propionate in propionic acidemia). Biotin is a cofactor for PCC and its deficiency causes some types of propionic acidemia. Vitamin B_{12} deficiency can cause methylmalonic aciduria because vitamin B_{12} is a cofactor for methylmalonyl coenzyme A mutase. Glycine is secondarily elevated in propionic acidemia, but no defect of glycine catabolism is present.

492. The answer is b. (*Murray, pp 238–249. Scriver, pp 2165–2194. Sack, pp 121–144. Wilson, pp 287–324.*) In treating inborn errors of metabolism that present acutely in the newborn period, aggressive fluid and electrolyte therapy and caloric supplementation are important to correct the imbalances caused by the disorder. Calories spare tissue breakdown that can increase toxic metabolites. Since many of the metabolites that build up in inborn errors of metabolism are toxic to the central nervous system, hemodialysis is recommended for any patient in stage II coma (poor muscle tone, few spontaneous movements, responsive to painful stimuli) or worse. Dietary therapy should minimize substances that cannot be metabolized—in this case fatty acids, since the oxidation of branched-chain fatty acids results in propionate. Antibiotics are frequently useful because metabolically compromised children are more susceptible to infection.

493. The answer is c. (*Murray, pp 238–249. Scriver, pp 2165–2194. Sack, pp 121–144. Wilson, pp 287–324.*) The proband in this case has inherited the A allele from one parent and the B allele from the other. However, it is impossible to determine which allele came from which parent. The fetus has the same genotype as his affected brother. However, it cannot be determined if he inherited these alleles from the same parents as the affected boy and is thus affected, or from the opposite parents and is thus an unaffected noncarrier. It can be said that he is definitely not an unaffected carrier. Assuming no recombination has occurred, the risk for the fetus to be affected is 1/2, or 50%.

494. The answer is c. (*Murray, pp 323–346. Scriver, pp 1667–1724. Sack, pp 121–144. Wilson, pp 287–324.*) For the Guthrie test, infant blood from a heel or finger stick is placed on filter paper discs and mailed to the central screening laboratory. Discs are arrayed on agar plates containing a competitive inhibitor of bacterial growth (thienylalanine), which must be overcome by sufficient amounts of phenylalanine for bacterial colonies to be visible. Rapid scanning of agar plates with hundreds of filter discs is thus possible by eye, and discs surrounded by bacterial growth constitute a positive result.

495. The answer is c. (*Murray, pp 323–346. Scriver, pp 1667–1724. Sack, pp 121–144. Wilson, pp 287–324.*) The prime justification for newborn screening is that early diagnosis results in benefits through prevention or treatment. Although early identification of PKU carriers through diagnosis of their affected newborns is a benefit of newborn screening, its chief rationale is the prevention of mental retardation by early diagnosis and lowering of dietary protein intake. False-positive screens are the most frequent problem with screening, and repeat screens are sometimes needed for borderline results.

496. The answer is c. *(Murray, pp 323–346. Scriver, pp 1667–1724. Sack, pp 121–144. Wilson, pp 287–324.)* Decreased melanin can occur in PKU because melanin is produced from phenylalanine and tyrosine. The defect in most children with PKU is deficiency of phenylalanine hydroxylase. Rare children have deficiency of biopterin cofactor due to a defect in its synthetic enzyme that is also autosomal recessive. Phenylalanine is converted to tyrosine by phenylalanine hydroxylase, so deficient tyrosine can occur in children on restrictive diets.

497. The answer is c. *(Murray, pp 575–587. Scriver, pp 4077–5016. Sack, pp 121–144. Wilson, pp 287–324.)* A peripheral blood karyotype provides the most reliable examination of the sex chromosomes. A bone marrow karyotype is more rapid (it uses rapidly dividing bone marrow cells) but usually has less resolution for defining subtle X and Y chromosome rearrangements. A buccal smear would theoretically show one Barr body in females (representing inactivation of one X chromosome) and none in males. In practice, this test is not very reliable and is rarely used. Detection of material of the Y long arm by polymerase chain reaction (PCR) would be useful but does not examine the Y short arm that contains the sex-determining region.

498. The answer is a. *(Murray, pp 575–587. Scriver, pp 4077–5016. Sack, pp 121–144. Wilson, pp 287–324.)* The dot-blot demonstrates hybridization of the proband's DNA with the DXS14 and SRY DNA probes and suggests the diagnosis of a genetic male. The presence of a Y rules out the possibility of the proband being a genetic female but not the rare occurrence of 46,XX/46,XY mosaicism. Gender assignment is not based solely on genetic testing but must include surgical and reproductive prognoses for male versus female adult function. For these reasons, the patient with ambiguous genitalia is a medical emergency that requires delicate management until gender assignment is agreed upon. In the past, individuals judged not to have adequate phallic tissue for reconstruction of normal male genitalia underwent appropriate surgery for female gender assignment. However, recent follow-up studies suggest that at least some XY individuals who had feminizing surgery including orchiectomy have developed a male sexual identity. These findings make management more complex in that sexual identity may be at least partly determined during fetal life.

499. The answer is b. *(Murray, pp 575–587. Scriver, pp 4077–5016. Sack, pp 121–144. Wilson, pp 287–324.)* True hermaphroditism implies the presence of both male and female genitalia in the same patient and is extremely rare. Male pseudohermaphroditism implies a genetic male with incomplete development of his genitalia, as in the proband. Causes can range from abnormalities of the pituitary-adrenal-gonadal hormone axis to local defects in tissue responsiveness to testosterone. The XY female and XX male refer to phenotypically normal individuals whose genetic sex does not match their phenotypic sex. Examples include testicular feminization and pure gonadal dysgenesis (XY females) and offspring of fathers with Y translocations that inherit a cryptic SRY region without a visible Y chromosome (XX males).

500. The answer is a. *(Murray, pp 575–587. Scriver, pp 4077–5016. Sack, pp 121–144. Wilson, pp 287–324.)* Sex steroids are synthesized from cholesterol by side chain cleavage (employing a P450 enzyme) to produce pregnenolone. Pregnenolone is then converted to testosterone in the testis, to estrogen in the ovary, and to corticosterone and aldosterone in the adrenal gland. The enzymes 3β-hydroxysteroid dehydrogenase, 21-hydroxylase, 11β-hydroxylase, and 18-hydroxylase modify pregnenolone to produce other sex and adrenal steroids. Deficiencies in adrenal 21-hydoxylase can thus lead to inadequate testosterone production in males and produce ambiguous external genitalia. Such children can also exhibit low sodium and high potassium due to deficiency of the more distal steroids, cortisol and aldosterone. 5α-reductase converts testosterone to dihydrotestosterone, and its deficiency produces milder degrees of hypogenitalism without salt wasting. Deficiency of the androgen receptor is called testicular feminization, producing normal-looking females who may not seek medical attention until they present with infertility.

Appendix I

Summary of Questions as Related to Items in the USMLE Content Outline

USMLE#	Subject	Question Numbers
1.1	Biochemistry and molecular biology	
1.1.1	Gene expression: DNA structure, replication, and exchange	
	DNA structure, single- and double-stranded DNA, stabilizing forces, supercoiling	2, 3, 7, 19, 21, 28
	Analysis of DNA: sequencing, restriction analysis, PCR amplification, hybridization	5, 8, 23, 24
	DNA replication: mutation, repair, degradation, and inactivation	6, 9, 11–16, 18, 20, 22, 25, 26, 36
	Gene structure and organization, chromosomes, centromere, telomere	10, 32, 92, 386–400
	Recombination, insertion sequences, transposons, mechanisms of genetic exchange (transformation, transduction, conjugation), plasmids and bacteriophages, di- and tri-nucleotide repeats	17, 27, 483
1.1.2	Gene expression: transcription	
	Transcription of DNA into RNA, enzymatic reactions, RNA, RNA degradation	30, 35, 38–40, 43–45, 46, 48, 50–52, 57, 58

(continued)

USMLE#	Subject	Question Numbers
	Regulation: *cis*-regulatory elements, transcription factors, enhancers, promoters, silencers, repressants, splicing	41–42, 71, 72, 74, 84–87, 91, 139
	Defects in transcription and RNA processing	36, 37, 53, 76, 80, 89
1.1.3	Gene expression: translation	
	The genetic code	33, 35, 37, 38, 49, 77, 78, 79, 81, 83
	Structure and function of tRNA, ribosomes	47, 61, 63, 66, 67
	Protein synthesis, regulation of translation	54, 56, 58, 59, 62–64, 65, 68, 69
	Posttranslational modifications, protein degradation, defects in translation and protein structure	34, 55, 60, 64, 70, 82, 88
1.1.4	Structure and function of proteins	
	Principles of protein structure and folding	4, 21, 109, 110, 113, 117, 118, 122,128, 129, 139
	Enzymes: kinetics, reaction mechanisms	151, 152–163
	Structural and regulatory proteins, ligand binding, self-assembly, regulatory properties	90, 108, 111, 119, 123, 125, 127, 130–132, 134, 137, 138, 141–146, 150
	Mutations that alter proteins	73–77, 116, 117, 121, 147–149, 440, 447–449, 471–473 487, 488
1.1.5	Energy metabolism: metabolic sequences and regulation	
	Generation of energy from carbohydrates, fatty acids, and essential amino acids	106, 164–183, 188–200, 469, 470

USMLE#	Subject	Question Numbers
	Storage of energy thermodynamics: free energy, chemical equilibria and group transfer potential, acid-base balance, disorders of energy metabolism, e.g., mitochondrial myopathies, diabetic ketoacidosis	107–108, 230–268, 318, 412
1.1.6	Metabolic pathways of small molecules and associated diseases	
	Biosynthesis and degradation of amino acids, e.g., PKU	107, 112, 114, 126, 133, 135, 242, 243, 245–255, 435, 436, 454, 455, 494–496
	Biosynthesis and degradation of purines and pyrimidine nucleotides, gout, Lesch-Nyhan syndrome	290–292, 482, 483
	Biosynthesis and degradation of fatty acids, phospholipids and cholesterol, dyslipidemias, carnitine deficiency	258, 259, 263–289, 439, 454, 455, 489–493
	Biosynthesis and degradation of steroid hormones, bile acids (e.g., adrenogenital syndromes)	256, 338, 340–342, 353–355, 497–500
	Prostaglandins and leukotrienes, biosynthesis and degradation of porphyrins	256, 257, 348, 352, 356–360
1.1.7	Biosynthesis and degradation of other macromolecules and associated abnormalities	184–187, 201–206, 260, 273, 404, 423, 441–446

(continued)

USMLE#	Subject	Question Numbers
1.3	Human development and genetics	
1.3.1	Embryogenesis, homeotic	389, 403, 406, 419, 424, 464,
1.3.2	genes: congenital	465, 484–487, 497–500
	abnormalities	
1.3.3	Gene analysis: pedigree analysis, genetic markers, linkage analysis, gene mapping	384, 385, 401–433
1.3.4	Population genetics: Hardy-Weinberg law, founder effects, mutation-selection equilibrium	412, 427, 429–433
1.3.5	Disease-producing mutations	
	Chromosomal abnormalities (aneuploidy): translocations, deletions, duplications (including nucleotide repeats and inversions), missense, nonsense mutations	92, 386–400, 460, 464, 465
	Imprinting and mosaicism, e.g., Prader-Willi syndromes	394, 476–482
	Single-gene defects: homozygosity, heterozygosity, autosomal dominant, autosomal recessive, X-linked, phenotypic variation, pleiotropy, variable expression, delayed onset, anticipation	1, 384, 385, 401–434, 437–440, 447–449, 454, 455, 461

USMLE#	Subject	Question Numbers
1.3.6	Multifactorial diseases	381–383, 426, 435, 436, 466
1.3.7	Principles of therapy	
	Application of diagnostic methods, predictive testing-screening, counseling (recurrence risk assessment), prenatal diagnosis	24, 73, 385, 435, 436, 441–446, 464, 465, 473–475, 488–493, 497–500
	Potentials for gene therapy, antisense oligonucleotides, genes, viral vectors, ex vivo therapy, ethical issues	71, 72, 76
1.3.8	Pharmacogenetics	75, 189, 437–439
1.4.4	Neoplasia: karyotypic abnormalities, predisposing Mendelian conditions	13, 31, 92, 401, 450–453, 480
1.6	Multisystem processes	
1.6.1	Nutrition: generation, expenditure, and storage of energy at the whole-body level, functions of essential nutrients, protein-calorie malnutrition	304, 339, 343–355, 349, 350, 362–380
	Vitamin deficiencies and toxicities (e.g., A, B, C, D, E, K), mineral deficiencies and toxicities	303, 305–337, 456–459

Appendix 2

Medical Disorders and Processes Used as Examples

Disease or Process	Question Numbers
Acetyl CoA carboxylase deficiency	229
Achondroplasia	408, 422
Acidosis	93, 94
Adenosine deaminase deficiency	71
AIDS	25
Albinism	16, 418
Alkaptonuria	114
Alcoholism	168
α_1 antitrypsin deficiency	70, 440
Ambiguous genitalia	497–500
Anemia	110, 111, 121, 377
Anesthesia	438, 439
Angelman's syndrome	482
Aspirin effects	357
Bee sting	359
Beriberi	313
Blood types	420, 430
Burkitt's lymphoma	92, 451
Carnitine acyltransferase deficiency	228
Carnitine deficiency	379
Charcot-Marie-Tooth disease	411, 474, 475
Cleft lip/palate	424
Cholera	237

(continued)

Disease or Process	Question Numbers
Cockayne's syndrome	12
Color blindness	407, 410
Congenital adrenal hyperplasia	497–500
Congestive heart failure	355
Chromosome disorders	386–400
Chromosome mosaicism	394
Chromosome translocation	396, 397, 420, 430
Copper excess	459
Cri-du-chat syndrome	400
Crouzon's syndrome	406
Cushing's syndrome	340
Cyanide poisoning	195
Cystic fibrosis	385, 409, 432, 434
Diabetes insipidus	428
Diabetes mellitus	95, 96, 106, 378, 382, 466
Dinitrophenol poisoning	201
Diphtheria	64, 379
Down's syndrome	399
Duchenne's muscular dystrophy	415
Emphysema	141, 169
Ethics	392, 468, 480
Ethylene glycol poisoning	259
Fructokinase deficiency	175
Galactosemia	176, 469, 470
Gardner's polyposis syndrome	401
Glucose-6-phosphate dehydrogenase deficiency	75, 189
Glycogen storage diseases	201
Gyrate atrophy of the retina	74
Hartnup disease	253
Heart attack	135, 147, 426, 454, 455

(continued)

Disease or Process	Question Numbers
Mushroom poisoning	43
Myasthenia gravis	343
Myotonic dystrophy of Steinert	483
Neonatal jaundice	256
Neural tube defects (spina bifida, anencephaly)	336, 484–486
Neurolipidoses	263, 273, 423, 441–444
Orotic aciduria	294
Osteogenesis imperfecta	116, 242, 414, 449
Parkinson's disease	435 436
Paternity analysis, DNA fingerprinting	479
Pernicious anemia	305
Phenylketonuria (PKU)	421, 494–496
Polycystic kidney disease	461
Prader-Willi syndrome	476–479, 481
Prenatal diagnosis	473, 487, 488
Propionic acidemia	491, 492
Recurrent abortion	387
Renal failure	376
Retinitis pigmentosa	412
Retinoblastoma	450
Rickets	337
Scheie's mucopolysaccharidosis syndrome	272
Shprintzen's velocardiofacial syndrome	464, 465
Sickle cell anemia	4, 34, 149, 429, 433, 487, 488
Starvation	380
Statin therapy	282
Stickler skeletal dysplasia syndrome	73
Succinyl choline apnea	438, 439
Tay-Sachs disease	423, 441–444

Disease or Process	Question Numbers
Tetany	377
Thalassemia	80, 89, 91, 148
Triploidy	393
Turner's syndrome	395, 398
Urea cycle disorders	247
Waardenburg syndrome	419
Wilms tumor	460
Wilson's disease	459
Xeroderma pigmentosum	20

Bibliography

McKusick VA: *Mendelian Inheritance in Man,* 13/e. Baltimore, Johns Hopkins University Press, 1996. Internet address (updated monthly): www3.ncbi.nlm.nih.gov/omim

Murray RK, Granner DK, Mayes PA, Rodwell, VW: *Harper's Biochemistry,* 25/e. New York, McGraw-Hill, 2000.

Sack GH Jr: *Medical Genetics.* New York, McGraw-Hill, 1999.

Scriver CR, Beaudet AL, Sly WS, Valle D: *The Metabolic and Molecular Bases of Inherited Disease,* 7/e. New York, McGraw-Hill, 1995.

Wilson GN: *Clinical Genetics: A Short Course.* New York, Wiley-Liss, 2000.

The primary references cited in the answers include the Murray and Scriver textbooks, which are more directed toward biochemistry, and the Sack and Wilson textbooks, which are more directed toward medical genetics. The appropriate texts should thus be consulted for questions 1 to 380, which emphasize biochemistry, and for questions 381 to 435, which emphasize genetics. All four texts are useful for the integrated biochemistry and genetics questions (436 to 500).

Many genetic diseases cited in this book include a six-digit McKusick number that allows reference to the compendium of genetic diseases that is available in hard copy or online. This compendium is now maintained by the National Institutes of Health and lists more than 4000 genetic diseases and genetic loci. For all but the most recently entered disorders, the McKusick number provides the inheritance mechanism. Those numbers beginning with 1 designate autosomal dominant diseases, those beginning with 2 autosomal recessive diseases, those beginning with 3 X-linked recessive diseases, those beginning with 4 Y-linked diseases (so far only gene loci), and those beginning with 5 mitochondrial DNA–encoded diseases.

Index